D1264604

THE HARVEY LECTURES

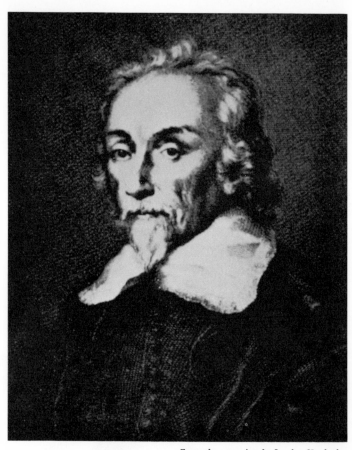

From the engraving by Jacobus Houbraken

WILLIAM HARVEY

BORN APRIL 1, 1578 - DIED JUNE 3, 1657

THE HARVEY LECTURES

DELIVERED UNDER THE AUSPICES OF

The HARVEY SOCIETY of NEW YORK

1975–1976

UNDER THE PATRONAGE OF THE NEW YORK
ACADEMY OF MEDICINE

BY

EDWARD A. BOYSE   ROGER GUILLEMIN
EUGENE BRAUNWALD   SEYMOUR S. KETY
JOSEPH G. GALL   BEATRICE MINTZ
DONALD R. GRIFFIN   LLOYD J. OLD
WALLACE P. ROWE

SERIES 71

1978

ACADEMIC PRESS   New York   San Francisco   London
A Subsidiary of Harcourt Brace Jovanovich, Publishers

ACADEMIC PRESS, INC.
111 Fifth Avenue, New York, New York 10003

United Kingdom Edition published by
ACADEMIC PRESS, INC. (LONDON) LTD.
24/28 Oval Road, London NW1 7DX

LIBRARY OF CONGRESS CATALOG CARD NUMBER: 7–2726

ISBN 0–12–312071–3

PRINTED IN THE UNITED STATES OF AMERICA

CONTENTS

HARVEY LECTURES 1975–1976

THE HARVEY SOCIETY*

A SOCIETY FOR THE DIFFUSION OF KNOWLEDGE
OF THE MEDICAL SCIENCES

CONSTITUTION

I

This Society shall be named the Harvey Society.

II

The object of this Society shall be the diffusion of scientific knowledge in selected chapters in anatomy, physiology, pathology, bacteriology, pharmacology, and physiological and pathological chemistry, through the medium of public lectures by men who are workers in the subjects presented.

III

The members of the Society shall constitute two classes: Active and Honorary members. Active members shall be workers in the medical or biological sciences, residing in the metropolitan New York area, who have personally contributed to the advancement of these sciences. Active members who leave New York to reside elsewhere may retain their membership. Honorary members shall be those who have delivered lectures before the Society and who are not Active members. Honorary members shall not be eligible to office, nor shall they be entitled to a vote.

Active members shall be elected by ballot. They shall be nominated to the Executive Committee and the names of the nominees shall accompany the notice of the meeting at which the vote for their election will be taken.

IV

The management of the Society shall be vested in an Executive Committee to consist of a President, a Vice-President, a Secretary, a Treasurer, and

*The Constitution is reprinted here for historical interest only; its essential features have been included in the Articles of Incorporation and By-Laws.

three other members, these officers to be elected by ballot at each annual meeting of the Society to serve one year.

V

The Annual Meeting of the Society shall be held at a stated date in January of each year at a time and place to be determined by the Executive Committee. Special meetings may be held at such times and places as the Executive Committee may determine. At all meetings ten members shall constitute a quorum.

VI

Changes in the Constitution may be made at any meeting of the Society by a majority vote of those present after previous notification to the members in writing.

THE HARVEY SOCIETY, INC.

A SOCIETY FOR THE DIFFUSION OF KNOWLEDGE
OF THE MEDICAL SCIENCES

BY-LAWS

ARTICLE I

Name and Purposes of the Society

SECTION 1. The name of the Society as recorded in the Constitution at the time of its founding in 1905 was the Harvey Society. In 1955, it was incorporated in the State of New York as The Harvey Society, Inc.

SECTION 2. The purposes for which this Society is formed are those set forth in its original Constitution and modified in its Certificate of Incorporation as from time to time amended. The purposes of the Society shall be to foster the diffusion of scientific knowledge in selected chapters of the biological sciences and related areas of knowledge through the medium of public delivery and printed publication of lectures by men and women who are workers in the subjects presented, and to promote the development of these sciences.

It is not organized for pecuniary profit, and no part of the net earnings, contributions, or other corporate funds of the Society shall inure to the benefit of any private member or individual, and no substantial part of its activities shall be carrying on propaganda, or otherwise attempting, to influence legislation.

ARTICLE II

Offices of the Society

SECTION 1. The main office and place of business of the Society shall be in the City and County of New York. The Board of Directors may designate additional offices.

ARTICLE III

Members

SECTION 1. The members of the Society shall consist of the incorporators, members of the hitherto unincorporated Harvey Society, and persons elected from time to time. The members of the Society shall constitute two classes: Active and Honorary Members. Active members shall be individuals with either the Ph.D. or the M.D. degree or its equivalent, residing or carrying on a major part of their work in the New York metropolitan area at the time of their election, who are personally making original contributions to the literature of the medical or biological sciences. Honorary members shall be those who have delivered a lecture before the Society and who are not Active members. Honorary members shall be exempted from the payment of dues. Active members who have remained in good standing for 35 years or who have reached the age of 65 and have remained in good standing for 25 years shall be designated Life members. They shall retain all the privileges of their class of membership without further payment of dues. Honorary members shall not be eligible to office, nor shall they be entitled to participate by voting in the affairs of the Society. Volumes of The Harvey Lectures will be circulated only to Active and Life members. Honorary members will receive only the volume containing their lecture. New Active members shall be nominated in writing to the Board of Directors by an Active member and seconded by another Active member. They shall be elected at the Annual Meeting of the Society by a vote of the majority of the Active members present at the meeting. Members who leave New York to reside elsewhere may retain their membership. Active members who have given a Harvey Lecture and who have moved out of the New York metropolitan area may, if they wish, become Honorary members. Membership in the Society shall terminate on the death, resignation, or removal of the member.

SECTION 2. Members may be suspended or expelled from the Society by the vote of a majority of the members present at any meeting of members at which a quorum is present, for refusing or failing to comply with the By-Laws, or for other good and sufficient cause.

SECTION 3. Members may resign from the Society by written declaration, which shall take effect upon the filing thereof with the Secretary.

ARTICLE IV

Meetings of the Members of the Society

SECTION 1. The Society shall hold its annual meeting of Active members for the election of officers and directors, and for the transaction of such other business as may come before the meeting in the month of January or

February in each year, at a place within the City of New York, and on a date and at an hour to be specified in the notice of such meeting.

SECTION 2. Special meetings of members shall be called by the Secretary upon the request of the President or Vice-President or of the Board of Directors, or on written request of twenty-five of the Active members.

SECTION 3. Notice of all meetings of Active members shall be mailed or delivered personally to each member not less than ten nor more than sixty days before the meeting. Like notice shall be given with respect to lectures.

SECTION 4. At all meetings of Active members of the Society ten Active members, present in person, shall constitute a quorum, but less than a quorum shall have power to adjourn from time to time until a quorum be present.

ARTICLE V

Board of Directors

SECTION 1. The number of directors constituting The Board of Directors shall be seven: the President, the Vice-President, the Secretary, and the Treasurer of the Society, and the three members of the Council. The number of directors may be increased or reduced by amendments of the By-Laws as hereinafter provided, within the maximum and minimum numbers fixed in the Certificate of Incorporation or any amendment thereto.

SECTION 2. The Board of Directors shall hold an annual meeting shortly before the annual meeting of the Society.

Special meetings of the Board of Directors shall be called at any time by the Secretary upon the request of the President or Vice-President or of one-fourth of the directors then in office.

SECTION 3. Notice of all regular annual meetings of the Board shall be given to each director at least seven days before the meeting and notice of special meetings, at least one day before. Meetings may be held at any place within the City of New York designated in the notice of the meeting.

SECTION 4. The Board of Directors shall have the immediate charge, management, and control of the activities and affairs of the Society, and it shall have full power, in the intervals between the annual meetings of the Active members, to do any and all things in relation to the affairs of the Society.

SECTION 5. Council members shall be elected by the members of the Society at the Annual Meeting. One Council member is elected each year to serve for three years, there being three Council members at all times. Vacancies occurring on the Council for any cause may be filled for the unexpired term by the majority vote of the directors present at any meeting at which a quorum is present. Only Active members of the Society shall be eligible for membership on the Council.

SECTION 6. A majority of the Board as from time to time constituted shall be necessary to constitute a quorum, but less than a quorum shall have power to adjourn from time to time until a quorum be present.

SECTION 7. The Board shall have power to appoint individual or corporate trustees and their successors of any or all of the property of the Society, and to confer upon them such of the powers, duties, or obligations of the directors in relation to the care, custody, or management of such property as may be deemed advisable.

SECTION 8. The directors shall present at the Annual Meeting a report, verified by the President and Treasurer, or by a majority of the directors, showing the whole amount of real and personal property owned by the Society, where located, and where and how invested, the amount and nature of the property acquired during the year immediately preceding the date of the report and the manner of the acquisition; the amount applied, appropriated, or expended during the year immediately preceding such date, and the purposes, objects, or persons to or for which such applications, appropriations, or expenditures have been made; and the names of the persons who have been admitted to membership in the Society during such year, which report shall be filed with the records of the Society and an abstract thereof entered in the minutes of the proceedings of the Annual Meeting.

ARTICLE VI

Committees

SECTION 1. The Board of Directors may appoint from time to time such committees as it deems advisable, and each such committee shall exercise such powers and perform such duties as may be conferred upon it by the Board of Directors subject to its continuing direction and control.

ARTICLE VII

Officers

SECTION 1. The officers of the Society shall consist of a President, a Vice-President, a Secretary, and a Treasurer, and such other officers as the Board of Directors may from time to time determine. All of the officers of the Society shall be members of the Board of Directors.

SECTION 2. The President shall be the chief executive officer of the Society and shall be in charge of the direction of its affairs, acting with the advice of the Board of Directors. The other officers of the Society shall have the powers and perform the duties that usually pertain to their respective offices, or as may from time to time be prescribed by the Board of Directors.

SECTION 3. The officers and the directors shall not receive, directly or indirectly, any salary or other compensation from the Society, unless authorized by the concurring vote of two-thirds of all the directors.

SECTION 4. The officers shall be elected at the Annual Meeting of the Active members. All officers shall hold office until the next Annual Meeting and until their successors are elected or until removed by vote of a majority vote of the directors. Vacancies occurring among the officers for any cause may be filled for the unexpired term by the majority vote of the directors present at any meeting at which a quorum is present. Officers must be Active members of the Society.

ARTICLE VIII

Fiscal Year—Seal

SECTION 1. The fiscal year of the Society shall be the calendar year.

SECTION 2. The seal of the Society shall be circular in form and shall bear the words "The Harvey Society, Inc., New York, New York, Corporate Seal."

ARTICLE IX

Amendments

SECTION 1. These By-Laws may be added to, amended, or repealed, in whole or in part, by the Active members or by the Board of Directors, in each case by a majority vote at any meeting at which a quorum is present, provided that notice of the proposed addition, amendment, or repeal has been given to each member or director, as the case may be, in the notice of such meeting.

THE BIOLOGICAL ROOTS OF MENTAL ILLNESS: THEIR RAMIFICATIONS THROUGH CEREBRAL METABOLISM, SYNAPTIC ACTIVITY, GENETICS, AND THE ENVIRONMENT*

SEYMOUR S. KETY

*Department of Psychiatry, Harvard Medical School,
Mailman Research Center, McLean Hospital, Belmont, Massachusetts*

THE inference that the major mental illnesses have important biological bases is not easily validated. The unique feature of the brain, especially that of higher animals is its ability to process, encode, and store experiential information and to utilize that store adaptively in later behavior. To a considerable extent normal human behavior is determined by experience, which, though mediated by biological mechanisma, cannot be reduced to them (Kety, 1961). The language we speak, the principles we value, the decisions that motivate our daily actions, are to a greater extent a reflection of what we have learned than the resultant of how we were constituted, and the differences among us in regard to these qualities lie largely in the scope of the psychological and social sciences.

But what of the severe disturbances of thought, behavior, and feeling that are seen in schizophrenia or in the affective extremes of manic-depressive illness? Are these merely the result of unusual rearing and interpersonal relationships, or an adaptation to extremes of social stress, as some would have us believe? Or do they come about as the result of alterations in the biological mechanisms through which experience must operate? If that is the case, our understanding of these disorders will depend upon increased knowledge in the biological disciplines and their interfaces with the brain and behavior. Over the past several decades, knowledge in the fundamental neurobiological disciplines has increased at a gratifying rate. Their relevance to the major mental disorders, such

*Lecture delivered September 18, 1975.

as schizophrenia and affective illness, is becoming clearer, and, in some places, links between that body of knowledge and the clinical problems are being forged. The following account, which does not pretend to be exhaustive, describes some of these developments in physiology, biochemistry, pharmacology, and anatomy from the vantage point of one observer.

Modern neurochemistry began with an examination and characterization of the components of the brain (Thudichum, 1884) and, when studies on metabolism became possible, focused on energy-yielding oxidative processes (Quastel, 1939), in slices and homogenates of brain *in vitro,* using the paradigms of general biochemistry. This produced a wealth of information under conditions that could be rigorously controlled, but faltered at the crucial link between metabolism and function. The activity of any part of the brain is uniquely dependent upon its connection with many other regions, and there was need for information regarding the metabolism of the intact, normally functioning brain. Dumke and Schmidt (1943) had succeeded in making accurate measurements of the cerebral blood flow in lightly anesthetized monkeys under reasonably physiological conditions, and this permitted the measurement of cerebral oxygen consumption in the same state and during deeper anesthesia as well as convulsive activity (Schmidt *et al.,* 1945).

Just as the brain is unique among organs for its complexity, so is the human brain unique for its plasticity and capacity, its ability to symbolize in concept and speech, to experience and express ecstasy and grief. It is also the human brain that falls prey to serious disorders of these functions for which no comparable animal model exists. There was need to examine the nutrition and energy metabolism of the human brain in health and in disease.

Cournand (1945) had demonstrated the feasibility of making accurate measuurements of cardiac output in man under physiological conditions using the principle formulated by Fick (1870) in the now self-evident conclusion that the quantity of oxygen absorbed by the body per minute must be equal to that taken up at the lungs, which would in turn be equal to the total pulmonary blood flow multiplied by the difference in oxygen concentration between the blood entering and leaving the lungs. That principle had also been applied by Smith (1943) and by Bradley and associates (1945) to the measurement of renal and hepatic blood flow, using, instead of oxygen, substances specifically excreted by those organs.

The brain, however, unlike the kidney and liver, does not specifically and selectively remove foreign substances from the blood and excrete them for accurate measurement. Furthermore, although it does consume large quantities of oxygen, that consumption cannot independently be measured or even assumed to be constant since it would be expected to vary with activity and disease. The brain does, however, absorb by physical solution an inert gas, such as nitrous oxide, which reaches it by way of the arterial blood. The accumulation of such a gas in the brain should be independent of the state of mental activity and determined instead by relatively simple physical principles, such as diffusion and solubility, which would be quite constant in the brain whether asleep or awake, working out a complex problem, or suffering from schizophrenia. It was found that an arteriovenous difference did exist across the brain for inert gases as for oxygen, but in the case of the former, the difference gradually decreased as the brain approached equilibrium with the tension of the gas in arterial blood (Fig. 1). At such a point near equilibrium, the tension of gas in the brain as a whole should be close to its tension in the venous blood draining the brain. From the tension and solubility of the gas in brain, the quantity of gas taken up could be calculated; this quantity, divided by the integrated arteriovenous difference over the time of equilibration, would yield the cerebral blood flow per minute for unit weight of brain, in an adaptation of the Fick principle to a process of varying uptake rather than a steady state.

Determination of the solubility of nitrous oxide in various samples of blood and brain indicated that the partition coefficient for this gas be-

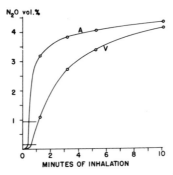

FIG. 1. Concentration of nitrous oxide in arterial (A) and cerebral venous (V) blood over a 10 minute period of inhalation of 15% nitrous oxide.

tween brain and blood was close to unity, that it was the same in the brain of dog and man, in living brain and in dead brain, and was unaffected by a variety of diseases. Measurement of the concentration of nitrous oxide in the brains of dogs exposed to a low concentration of this gas for varying lengths of time indicated that at the end of 10 minutes the brain was essentially in equilibrium with the venous blood that drained it (Kety et al., 1948a). This finding was eventually confirmed in man with the use of a radioactive inert gas (^{79}Kr), which permitted measurement of its concentration in living human brain by means of an externally placed detector.

After additional studies, which indicated that the blood draining the brain via the internal jugular was relatively free of extracerebral contamination (Shenkin et al., 1948) and that there was no systematic difference between the two sides, the new technique was used to obtain normal values. The predictions of Lawrence (1823) from astute deductive reasoning were confirmed: The brain, which comprises only 2% of the body weight of man, receives for its nutrition one-sixth of the heart's output of blood and consumes one-fifth of the oxygen utilized by the body at rest (Kety and Schmidt, 1948a).

The next several years saw the technique applied to a number of problems in physiology, medicine, neurology, and psychiatry. The importance of carbon dioxide and oxygen tensions in the regulation of cerebral circulation was confirmed (Kety and Schmidt, 1948b), but a clue to the overriding importance of hydrogen ion concentration was also obtained (Kety et al., 1948b). The studies in essential hypertension (Kety et al., 1948c) revived the concept of regional homeostasis or autoregulation (Lassen, 1959) that Roy and Sherrington (1890) had developed, since cerebral blood flow was normal in the face of a markedly elevated perfusion pressure. The obvious extrinsic neurogenic regulation by way of the cervical sympathetics did not appear to be involved (Harmel et al., 1949), leaving humoral or local chemical factors as the probable mediators of the homeostasis.

Studes on cerebral oxygen consumption revealed a marked reduction in that function associated with coma or anesthesia. The demonstration by Sokoloff and associates (1953) that the brain did not participate in the increased metabolism of hyperthyroidism led eventually to his demonstration of an important effect of thyroxine on protein synthesis (Sokoloff, 1961a). The finding that sleep was associated with no diminution in cerebral oxygen consumption (Mangold *et al.*, 1955) laid to rest the prevailing notion shared by Sherrington and Pavlov that this state represents a generalized depression of neuronal activity, and anticipated the neurophysiological evidence that sleep is a highly active process (Evarts, 1961). Studies of the aging process permitted the conclusion that cerebral circulation and oxygen consumption are not diminished in the normal elderly individual, but show a significant reduction, highly correlated with the degree of intellectual impairment, in senile dementia (Freyhan *et al.*, 1951; Dastur *et al.*, 1963). In severe, chronic schizophrenia, no reduction was found in the circulation, oxygen consumption, or energy utilization by the brain as a whole (Kety *et al.*, 1948d).

In coma, anesthesia, and dementia, the altered consciousness and mental function could be related to a significant reduction in energy metabolsim, sometimes as great as 50% (Kety, 1957). But there were other states of profoundly altered mental function, such as sleep, the performance of mental arithmetic, toxic psychosis, and schizophrenia, that occurred without any perceptible alteration in the total energy utilized by the brain. Thus, the neuronal oxidative metabolsim that represented the power supply of the brain could affect mental function when it was the limiting factor, but in most normal states and in a wide range of abnormality, changes in functional state could be brought about without any measurable alteration in total energy utilization. It was possible that such mental changes depended on how the energy was directed by the countless number of switches and the circuits they controlled. To begin to understand these complexities would require techniques capable of measuring the nutrition and the energy metabolism at functionally demarcated regions of the brain without disturbing their physiological activity.

In the course of measuring the cerebral blood flow in various clinical states, changes in the shape of the arterial and venous curves of nitrous oxide were observed that appeared to reflect physiological processes such as ventilation, cardiac output, and rate of perfusion through the various tissues of the body. This had stimulated an attempt to derive theoretical expressions relating these variables (Kety, 1951). An expression that described the uptake of an inert gas at the lung found a strong inverse relationship between solubility of the gas in blood and the rate at which the arterial blood achieved equilibrium with the inspired partial pressure. This appeared to be capable of accounting for the different rates of induction and recovery for various volatile anesthetics. Analysis of the process of exchange between a tissue and its capillaries for a nonmetabolized substance found a dependency on either capillary permeability or rate of perfusion when the other factor was limiting and permitted the measurement of each by appropriate choice of tracer (Renkin, 1955; Landau et al., 1955). The derivation leaned upon the earlier work of Bohr (1909) and Krogh (1919), who had described the exchange of oxygen at lung and tissue. In a steady state oxygen gradients are constant, but in the case of a nonmetabolized substance these would change with time as blood and tissue approached equilibrium. With a few simplifying assumptions, the concentration of a diffusible, inert substance in a particular tissue could be related to the past history of the arterial concentration, properties of the tissue capillaries (i.e., intercapillary distance, capillary area available for diffusion), relative solubility of the substance in blood and tissue, and blood flow through the tissue. For lipid soluble substances that could diffuse through the entire capillary wall, diffusion should not be limiting and local blood flow could be ascertained from levels of the substance in the tissue and in the arterial blood.

Experimental validation of the theory came eventually from studies indicating that substances as diverse in their molecular weights and diffusion rates as hydrogen, xenon, or trifluoroiodomethane yielded similar values for blood flow in various parts of the brain. Experimental approaches that applied autoradiography in animals or external monitoring in man of a radioactive tracer have adduced changes in regional blood flow that accompany sleep (Reivich et al., 1968), anesthesia, or photic stimulation in animals (Sokoloff, 1961b), and cerebrovascular disease (Lassen and Ingvar, 1963), mental activity or schizophrenia in man (Ingvar, 1975). If it was a safe assumption that blood flow was altered locally to meet metabolic demand, it was possible to infer rate of energy metabolism and functional activity from such measurements. Recently, Sokoloff and his associates (1977) have taken a major step forward, measuring local energy metabolism via glucose utilization with labeled 2-deoxyglucose and demonstrating a remarkably close coupling between the utilization of that substrate and neuronal activity in well-demarcated structures of the brain (Sokoloff, 1977). That technique has demonstrated its usefulness in precisely mapping functionally active regions in the brain of animals, and recent developments indicate that it will be possible to do so by means of noninvasive techniques in man (Reivich *et al.*, 1977). The deoxyglucose technique can be expected to contribute greatly to an understanding of the important interface between structure and function in the brain.

Although coma of various types and anesthesia were found to be associated with and partially explained by a profound depression of overall cerebral energy utilization, it was not until chemical transmisison at central synapses became established, and certain of the neurotransmittors identified, that a plausible role could be conceptualized for chemical processes in mood, emotions, cognition, and memory and in the disturbances of these functions that are the cardinal features of the mental illnesses. By 1953, norepinephrine, dopamine, and serotonin had been identified in the brain, as had acetylcholine and γ-aminobutyric acid earlier. Two of these substances were regarded as neurotransmitters at peripheral synapses: acetylcholine at the skeletal myoneural junction, and norephinephrine at sympathetic nerve terminals.

The implications of these substances in the brain to normal and disturbed behavior and mental function were as yet unrealized, although studies on blood levels and urinary excretion of catecholamines as reflections of sympathetic and adrenal medullary activity had revealed significant correlations with emotional state. There was also a highly speculative hypothesis that adrenochrome or other abnormal metabolites of circulating epinephrine, were responsible for the mental dysfunctions of schizophrenia. A difficulty in identifying abnormal metabolites of epinephrine in schizophrenia was that the normal metabolism of the hormone was largely unknown. One strategy would be to administer labeled epinephrine in pharmacologically insignificant amounts and compare the urinary chromatographic profiles of radioactivity. The ^{14}C-labeled material available would not provide sufficient specific activity, but it was possible that a tritium-labeled epinephrine could be prepared with the requisite stability and activity. Another approach was to work out the normal metabolism of epinephrine. Julius Axelrod became interested in the problem and, even before the tritium-labeled compound could be synthesized, had discovered the enzymic catabolism of catecholamines via O-methylation, characterized the enzyme responsible, predicted the major catecholamine metabolites, and then went on to identify them in the urine (Axelrod, 1959). This made it possible for some of his colleagues to examine the metabolism of circulating catecholamines in normal man and in schizophrenic patients (LaBrosse *et al.*, 1961a,b). No evidence was found for the existence of abnormal epinephrine metabolites in that disorder; instead, the products were the same in type and quantity as those that occurred in normal volunteers.

The adrenochrome hypothesis was one of many heroic attempts to explain schizophrenia in biological terms that were based upon an inadequate background of basic biological knowledge and were therefore premature (Kety, 1959). Axelrod's fundamental contributions, on the other hand, did not immediately solve a particular psychiatric problem, nor were they designed to do so; yet, there is little doubt that ultimately they will be of great importance to our understanding of the nature of mental illness.

Probably the most important change that occurred in the biological knowledge of the brain and mental state in this century is the recognition that transmission across the synapse in the brain as well as the periphery was, with few exceptions, mediated by a number of chemical neurotransmitters and modulators of synaptic activity, which now include, in addition to acetylcholine and the biogenic amines, a number of amino acids and polypeptides. The concept of the synapse has changed to that of a chemical switch rather than an electrical junction, and the brain has become a unique kind of computer, the functions and output of which are determined by biochemical and physicochemical processes regulating the synthesis of neurotransmitters, their release and inactivation, and their action on postsynaptic receptors. Genetic factors, nutritional state, hormones, and drugs should affect these chemical processes and, through them, mental state and behavior. Many heuristic hypotheses have been developed, and there has been considerable research on the possible roles that neurotransmitters may play in mood, particular types of behavior, and memory (Kety, 1976). It now seems clear that a psychological function represents not the activity of one transmitter, but the resultant of many in concert. Among the interactions at synapses would also be expected to lie the biochemical contributions to disorders in thought, mood, and behavior.

Beginning in 1950, the development of new drugs began which, for the first time, specifically affected the symptoms of particular mental disorders while only minimally altering normal processes. Chlorpromazine suppresses hallucinations and delusional thinking in most schizophrenics, without disturbing normal cognition. The antidepressant drugs restore normal mood in many depressed patients, but in the same dose do not produce euphoria in normal individuals. Lithium relieves the runaway thought processes and wild behavior of the manic patient, but does not suppress normal activity. In the past decade or two, understanding of the pharmacology of these drugs has increased remarkably so that their mechanism of action is in many cases as well understood as that of other drugs in medicine. All the medications that relieve the schizophrenic of abnormal thinking and disturbed behavior have potent suppressor activity on dopamine synapses, in most cases by blocking the dopamine receptors (Snyder *et al.*, 1975). The antidepressant drugs, by inhibiting monoamine oxidase or presynaptic reuptake mechanisms, enhance the concentration of certain neurotransmitters at their synapses (Glowinski and Axelrod, 1966). Even electroconvulsive shock, which has a demonstrable therapeutic effect in depression, was found to be associated in rats with a persistent increase in cerebral norepinephrine turnover (Kety *et al.*, 1967) and in tyrosine hydroxylase activity (Musacchio *et al.*, 1969). The evidence is good that neurotransmitter mechanisms are crucially involved in the actions of the various psychoactive drugs. That, of course, does not mean that the chemical disturbances peculiar to these mental disorders will also be found where these drugs act, since we know many instances where drugs may act on normal processes to correct a disturbance elsewhere. Nor need there always be a biological abnormality present to account for a therapeutic benefit from the administration of a chemical substance. Severe anxiety can be produced in a biologically normal individual by a psychosocial interaction and yet be relieved by certain drugs. Thus, the therapeutic effects of the newer drugs in the major psychoses are compatible with, but not proof of, the existence of biological alterations in their etiology.

If there were evidence that genetic factors played an important role in schizophrenia or in other psychoses of unknown nature, there would be reason to believe that biological mechanisms were involved in their etiology and pathogenesis, since the genes can express themselves only through such processes. There is much that we know about schizophrenic illness that is compatible with the etiological importance of genetic factors. Ever since the first description of the syndrome it has been known to cluster in families. That observation is not, in itself, very compelling, since family members share environmental influences as well as their genetic endowment. Pellagra also had a familial tendency, and, in the case of kuru, distribution in families even presented a pseudo-Mendelian pattern. The familial nature of both of these disorders has now been explained in terms of nutritional, infectious, and cultural factors shared by members of a family. More compelling have been the results of studies on the occurrence of schizophrenia in twins, where its concordance in monozygotic twins is approximately 50%, or five times higher than that in dizygotic pairs (Gottesman and Shields, 1972).

Even the most systematic and thorough of the twin studies, however, do not definitively test the importance of genetic factors. Since the concordance rate for schizophrenia in the genetically identical pairs is considerably less than 100%, nongenetic factors must clearly be of etiological importance in a substantial segment of patients, and, since monozygotic twins share more of their environment than do dizygotic twins, the higher concordance rate in the former is not necessarily the result of their shared genetic endowment.

The process of adoption appeared to offer a means of separating the confounding variables and minimizing many of the sources of error. Since an adopted individual receives his genetic contribution from one family but his life experience as a member of another, it seemed possible to disentangle genetic and environmental factors by studies that were based upon such individuals and their families. If a total population of adopted individuals could be compiled where the mental status of the biological relatives and the adoptees were largely unknown to each other and where independent diagnoses in each population could be made without that information, it should be possible to avoid many types of selective and diagnostic bias as well as the confounding of genetic and environmental influences (Kety, 1959).

In 1962, David Rosenthal, Paul Wender, Fini Schulsinger, and I began to collect such a sample. Because of the remarkable system of records in Denmark, to which we were given access with our assurances of confidentiality, we were able to compile a total national sample of individuals who are now between 25 and 50 years of age, and were legally adopted at an early age by people not biologically related to them. We began with all adoptions granted in Greater Copenhagen and eventually extended this to all of Denmark. For the purposes of the study we included three subtypes of the schizophrenic syndrome defined in the diagnostic manual of the American Psychiatric Association: chronic schizophrenia, latent (ambulatory or borderline) schizophrenia, and acute schizophrenic reaction. Among the 5483 adoptees in the Greater Copenhagen Sample, 33 schizophrenic "index" adoptees were selected by independent review of the abstracts of the institutional records of the 507 who had ever been admitted to a mental institution. Unanimous agreement on a diagnosis of chronic, latent, or acute schizophrenia was arrived at among four raters. A control group of 33 was selected from the adoptees who had never been admitted to a psychiatric facility by matching with each index case on the basis of age, sex, socioeconomic class of the rearing family, time spent with biological relatives, child-care institutions, or foster home before transfer to the adopting family.

Our first report of the prevalence and type of mental illness in the relatives was based simply on an examination of institutional records that were available for the biological and adoptive parents, siblings and half-siblings, of the index and control adoptees. These were identified through the adoption records and the Folkeregister, a comprehensive population register. Abstracts of the hospital records were made, translated into English, edited to remove any information that would suggest whether a subject was a biological or adoptive relative of an index case or a control, and then independent diagnoses were made by each of the four raters. A consensus diagnosis was then arrived at by conference among the raters.

We had previously developed the concept of a "schizophrenia spectrum" of disorders presumably related to schizophrenia and including, besides the three forms of schizophrenia we had accepted in the selection of index cases, a category of "uncertain schizophrenia," where schizophrenia seemed to be the best diagnosis although we could not be certain because the symptoms described were insufficient or atypical, and a category of "schizoid or inadequate personality" which appeared to have certain characteristics related to schizophrenia, but to a milder extent. A statistically significant concentration of "schizophrenia spectrum" disorders was found among the biological relatives of index cases as compared with those of the control; the adoptive relatives showed a low incidence of schizophrenia spectrum disorders for both the index and the control group with no difference between them (Kety et al., 1968). The number of these diagnoses that we made on the basis of institutional records was too small to permit a further breakdown of the schizophrenia spectrum. Furthermore, we had secured little information about the environment of the probands other than the presence or absence of mental illness in their adoptive families. One of our other studies (Rosenthal *et al.*, 1968) had also suggested that there were many more schizophrenics and individuals within the schizophrenia spectrum than those who had ever been hospitalized.

For these reasons we felt that it would be important to carry out complete psychiatric interviews with these relatives, which might permit a more exhaustive survey of the population with regard to schizophrenia and other psychiatric diagnoses and more information about life experience. We secured the collaboration of Dr. Bjørn Jacobsen, a Danish psychiatrist, who agreed to carry out the interviews and spent the greater part of the next two years in doing so.

A total of 512 relatives were identified through the population registers. Of these, 119 had died and 29 had emigrated or disappeared. There was an interesting and highly significant difference in the death rate between the biological relatives of index cases (of whom 35 had died by February 1973 as compared with only 13 dead among the biological relatives of controls, $p = 0.0004$). That difference is accounted for mainly by suicide, accidental and other traumatic deaths. Of the 364 relatives still alive and residing in Denmark, Norway, or Sweden, more than 90% participated in an exhaustive psychiatric interview conducted by Dr. Jacobsen, who was not informed of the relationship of any subject to a proband. In practically all the biological relatives, the subject himself did not know of that relationship or did not mention it during the interview. Extensive summaries of these interviews were then prepared, edited to remove any clues to the type of relationship of a subject to a proband, and were then read by three raters. Each rater independently recorded his best psychiatric diagnosis for each subject from a list of possible diagnoses covering the entire range listed in the diagnostic manual (DSM-II) of the American Psychiatric Association, ranging from no mental disorder to chronic schizophrenia. After that a consensus was arrived at among the three raters, the code was broken, and the subjects were allocated to their respective four groups: biological or adoptive relatives of schizophrenic index adoptees and biological or adoptive relatives of control adoptees (Kety *et al.*, 1975).

Of these four populations, one is different from the rest in being genetically related to a schizophrenic adoptee with whom they have not lived, i.e., the biological relatives of the index cases. With regard to mental illness other than schizophrenia, these relatives do not differ from the rest (Table I).

In the case of the schizophrenia spectrum of disorders and for the individual components with the single exception of "schizoid or inadequate personality," however, there is a concentration in the biological relatives of index cases in contrast to the persons who are not genetically related to a schizophrenic. For definite schizophrenia. chronic or latent, the prevalence in the biological relatives of index cases is 6.4% compared with 1.7% in the control biological relatives; for uncertain schizophrenia it is 7.5% compared with 1.7%. (Table II) The difference between the group genetically related to the schizophrenic index cases and those not so related is highly significant statistically and speaks for the operation of genetic factors in the transmission

TABLE I

PSYCHIATRIC DIAGNOSES OUTSIDE THE SCHIZOPHRENIA SPECTRUM
IN RELATIVES OF SCHIZOPHRENIC AND CONTROL ADOPTEES[a]

	Biological relatives				Adoptive relatives			
	Index	%[b]	Control	%	Index	%	Control	%
Total identified	172		174		74		91	
Alive and in Scandinavia	124		149		39		52	
Interviewed	118		140		35		48	
Without spectrum diagnosis	81		121		31		41	
Psychiatric diagnosis								
None	30	37.0	49	40.5	11	35.5	11	26.8
Organic disorders	7	8.6	6	5.0	5	16.1	6	14.6
Neuroses	4	4.9	6	5.0	3	9.7	2	4.9
Affective disorders	2	2.5	11	9.1	1	3.2	3	7.3
Personality disorders	27	33.3	39	32.2	8	25.8	15	36.6
Total psychiatric diagnoses outside schizophrenia spectrum	40	49.4	62	51.2	17	54.8	26	63.4

[a] Consensus diagnoses based on interviews.

[b] Calculated as percentage of interviewed relatives without schizophrenic spectrum diagnosis.

TABLE II

SCHIZOPHRENIA SPECTRUM DIAGNOSES IN RELATIVES OF SCHIZOPHRENIC AND CONTROL ADOPTEES[a]

	Biological relatives				Adoptive relatives			
	Index	%[b]	Control	%	Index	%	Control	%
Total identified	172		174		74		91	
Alive and in Scandinavia	124		149		39		52	
Interviewed	118		140		35		48	
Psychiatric diagnoses								
Chronic schizophrenia	5	2.9*[c]	0	0	1	1.4	1	1.1
Latent schizophrenia	6	3.5	3	1.7	0	0	1	1.1
Uncertain schizophrenia	13	7.5**	3	1.7	1	1.4	3	3.3
Schizoid or inadequate personality	13	7.5	13	7.5	2	2.7	2	2.2
Schizophrenia or uncertain schizophrenia	24	14.0***	6	3.4	2	2.7	5	5.5
Total spectrum diagnoses	37	21.5**	19	10.9	4	5.4	7	7.7

[a] Consensus diagnoses based on interviews.
[b] Expressed as percentage of identified relatives.
[c] Fischer's exact probability, one-tailed, index vs control: *p = 0.03; **p = <0.01; ***p = <0.001.

of schizophrenia. The diagnosis of schizoid or inadequate personality was made rather frequently among biological relatives of both index and control adoptees (7.5%). The adopted-away offspring of a schizophrenic parent also showed a higher prevalence of schizophrenia spectrum disorders and an indication that schizoid traits in the coparent tended to increase the risk (Rosenthal *et al.,* 1968).

The evidence thus far presented is compatible with genetic transmission in schizophrenic illness, but it is not entirely conclusive, since there are possible environmental factors such as *in utero* influences, birth trauma, and early mothering experiences, that have not been ruled out. However, there are 127 biological paternal half-siblings of index cases and controls among the relatives of the adoptees who can help to settle that question, since the biological paternal half-siblings of the adoptees had different mothers and therefore did not share the same uterine or early mothering experience nor the postnatal environment of their adopted half-siblings. What they shared was the same father and a certain amount of genetic overlap. The number of paternal half-siblings was almost identical for index cases and controls, but the number of those diagnosed as having definite or uncertain schizophrenia was quite different, with 14 among the half-siblings of the index cases and only 2 among the half-siblings of controls ($p = 0.001$). There was a similar concentration if we restrict the diagnosis to definite schizophrenia (Table III). We regard this as compelling evidence that genetic factors operate significantly in the transmission of schizophrenia.

TABLE III

SCHIZOPHRENIC ILLNESS (SZ) IN THE BIOLOGICAL PATERNAL HALF-SIBLINGS OF SCHIZOPHRENIC AND CONTROL ADOPTEES

Adoptees	N	Definite Sz: chronic or latent		Definite or uncertain Sz	
Schizophrenic	63	8	(13%)	14	(22%)
Control	64	1	(2%)	2	(3%)
		$p < 0.02$		$p < 0.001$	

Biological paternal half-siblings

The three types of schizophrenia included in the initial characterization of the schizophrenic adoptees are apparently not part of a
homogeneous syndrome. There is considerably more schizophrenic illness in the biological relatives of the adoptees with classical schizophrenia than of those with latent or acute schizophrenia (Table IV).
Furthermore, classical chronic schizophrenia appears to occur only in
the biological relatives of the adoptees with chronic schizophrenia. But
those probands also have biological relatives with milder forms of illness described by latent or uncertain schizophrenia, suggesting that
these milder or atypical syndromes are also genetically related to classical schizophrenia. We found practically no acute schizophrenia, however, in these biological relatives and, in fact, no definite cases of
schizophrenia among the biological relatives of a larger sample of adoptees in whom we had made the diagnosis of acute schizophrenia. Since
the original syndrome was thought to be a chronic illness, psychiatrists
in this country may have been too hasty in attaching a schizophrenic
label to an acute psychosis of unknown etiology unless it were known to
be an acute phase of a chronic schizophrenic illness.

The tabulation also indicates that while schizophrenia is not limited to
only a few of the biological families, neither is it uniformly distributed
among them. In fact, only half of the probands had schizophrenia in
their biological relatives. Of course many of the latter families were too
small to rule out a genetic contribution to the proband's illness, but
others were sufficiently large that the genetic risk in the proband was
low or negligible. Thus, it is likely that there are at least two groups of
schizophrenic disorders, those in which the genetic contribution is substantial and others in which environmental influences are playing the
major role. The distribution of schizophrenia in kinships has not provided clear evidence for one mode of genetic transmission rather than
another when the illness is assumed to be unitary; on the other hand, an
assumption of genetic heterogeneity would recognize the existence of a
particular mode in certain families or subgroups. In the half-siblings of
schizophrenic adoptees whose shared parent is also affected, the prevalence of schizophrenic illness is 50% (Table IV), compatible in this
subsample with a dominant monogenic transmission.

The assumption of heterogeneous etiology has been employed in an
ingenious search for environmental variables important in schizophrenia
(Kinney and Jacobsen, 1978). On the premise that the environmental
contribution would be greater in those probands with low genetic risk,

TABLE IV

CONSENSUS DIAGNOSES OF CLASSICAL CHRONIC SCHIZOPHRENIA (S), LATENT
SCHIZOPHRENIA (L), ACUTE SCHIZOPHRENIC REACTION (A), OR UNCERTAIN
SCHIZOPHRENIA (U) IN SCHIZOPHRENIC ADOPTEES AND THEIR BIOLOGICAL FAMILIES[a]

Adoptees		Biological relatives					
Index No.	Adoptee diagnosis	Total identified	Mother	Maternal 1/2-sibs	Father	Paternal 1/2-sibs	Full sibs
3	S	6	(1)S	(1)S	(1)	(3)U	(0)
5	S	6	(1)	(1)	(1)	(2)	(1)L
6	S	9	(1)	(2)	(1)U	(4)	(1)
8	S	4	(1)	(0)	(1)	(2)U	(0)
9	S	3	(1)	(0)	(1)	(1)L	(0)
18	S	14	(1)	(6)	(1)L	(6)SSL	(0)
22	S	18	(1)L	(2)SU	(3)	(12)	(0)
25	S	4	(1)U	(1)U	(1)	(1)L	(0)
31	S	3	(1)	(2)U	(0)	(0)	(0)
32	S	4	(1)	(0)	(1)	(2)UU	(0)
1	S	2	(1)	(0)	(1)	(0)	(0)
7	S	2	(1)	(0)	(1)	(0)	(0)
12	S	2	(1)	(0)	(1)	(0)	(0)
15	S	2	(1)	(0)	(1)	(0)	(0)
16	S	3	(1)	(0)	(1)	(1)	(0)
30	S	17	(1)	(10)	(1)	(5)	(0)
33	S	4	(1)	(1)	(1)	(1)	(0)
4	L	3	(1)	(0)	(1)U	(1)L	(0)
11	L	5	(1)U	(0)	(1)	(3)	(0)
34	L	8	(1)	(1)	(1)	(4)LU	(1)
13	L	2	(1)	(1)	(0)	(0)	(0)
20	L	5	(1)	(1)	(1)	(2)	(0)
21	L	4	(1)	(0)	(1)	(2)	(0)
23	L	5	(1)	(1)	(1)	(2)	(0)
26[b]	L	2	(1)	(0)	(1)	(0)	(0)
27[b]	L						
29	L	4	(1)	(2)	(1)	(0)	(0)
2	A	6	(1)	(2)	(1)	(2)U	(0)
14	A	7	(1)	(0)	(1)	(5)U	(0)
17	A	1	(1)U	(0)	(0)	(0)	(0)
28	A	7	(1)	(4)U	(1)	(1)	(0)
10	A	2	(1)	(0)	(1)	(0)	(0)
19	A	4	(1)	(1)	(1)	(1)	(0)
24	A	4	(1)	(2)	(1)	(0)	(0)

[a] Numbers in parentheses indicate number of identified family members.

[b] Monozygotic twins.

they have examined a number of environmental influences described in the interviews, comparing their incidence in probands with a high and a low genetic background. The findings to date are interesting. The probands with a low genetic risk have significantly more evidence of brain damage as exemplified by birth complications, encephalitis, concussion, or EEG abnormalities, than those who became schizophrenic with a strong genetic background. The probands with low genetic risk were different from the others in being born predominantly in the first four months of the year. A number of epidemiological studies employing large samples have indicated a small excess of births in the first third of the year for schizophrenics compared with the rest of the population (Dalen, 1975), but a significant difference found among only 34 probands is remarkable and likely to reflect an important variable. Although the risk of birth trauma is higher in the cold winter months, it is equally possible that some virus may have a peak incidence in that season or, alternatively, in the warm summer months that would coincide with the first trimester of such pregnancies. Some personality characteristics have also been found that appear to be more common in the adoptive parents of probands with a low genetic risk, which this technique is especially suitable for pursuing. Since all of the adoptive parents in the sample have reared a schizophrenic individual, the possibility of feedback from the child to parental personality is controlled.

The greater prevalence of schizophrenia that has with some consistency been found in lower social classes has suggested social stress as an etiological factor, but there is an alternative hypothesis that should be examined. There are viral agents known to attack the nervous system that have properties that may be relevant (Torre and Peterson, 1973). The prevalence of schizophrenia does not show a simple negative correlation with socioeconomic class, but, according to Kohn (1968), is primarily concentrated in the lower socioeconomic classes of large cities. It is also known that schizophrenia has a higher recognized prevalence in urban, in contrast with rural, populations. These characteristics would be compatible with a virus whose propagation is favored by congestion, poor living conditions, and less than optimal hygiene. A number of bacterial and viral diseases show similar predilections (Fenner, 1971), and very recently a central neurotropic cytomegalovirus has been found to have twice the prevalence in lower socioeconomic groups than in middle class populations (Hanshaw *et al.,* 1976). Evidence was also adduced that this agent was congenitally transmitted and adversely affected central nervous system development, although it was associated with deafness and school failure rather than schizophrenia.

If a virus is involved in some forms of schizophrenia, it would be a different virus from those now known to affect the nervous system, or at least to have a different type of interaction with the host. Although an unusually high incidence of childhood autism has been reported in children with congenital rubella infection (Chess, 1971), the disorders of the nervous system where a viral etiology has been most clearly demonstrated are characterized by obvious neuropathological changes and neurological deficits that have not been seen in typical schizophrenia. I find it interesting, however, that many of these disorders involve a psychosis often misdiagnosed as schizophrenia, in their early phases. The same is true for other neurological disorders in which a virus has not been implicated, i.e., Wilson's disease, Huntington's chorea, the adult form of metachromatic leukodystrophy, among others. This suggests that there are particular regions or pathways in the central nervous system which, when affected by one of several disease processes, produce a schizophrenic syndrome, which may then become more neurologically obvious as the disease extends to other regions. If there were a virus that affected those initial regions and did not spread beyond them, the disorder it produced might resemble typical schizophrenia very closely. This hypothetical schizophrenogenic virus would also be required to produce a lesion that would not be obvious on traditional neuropathological examination. But a virus or an immune reaction that merely involved the active site of an enzyme or a receptor necessary for neurotransmission could produce profound and specific dysfunctions, yet not be detectable by neuropathological techniques that have hitherto been applied (Matthysse and Matthysse, 1978).

The clusters of psychological symptoms that constitute the schizophrenic or affective disorders do not imply that these are unitary diseases. It is more likely that each is comprised of several disorders of differing etiology, but with common manifestations by virtue of common neuronal dysfunction. In a substantial number, genetic factors play an important role although their mode of transmission and the biological processes of their expression remain to be identified. Environmental influences must also be of etiological importance although their nature has not been established. In addition to psychological factors that affect the information stores of the brain, there are infectious, dietary, toxic, and traumatic influences that may alter its biological function. All of these and their interactions have become the province of psychiatric research and the basis for an understanding of mental disorder.

REFERENCES

Axelrod, J. (1959). *Physiol. Rev.* **39,** 751–776.

Bohr, C. (1909). *Skand. Arch. Physiol.* **22,** 221–280.

Bradley, S. E., Ingelfinger, F. J., Bradley, G. P., and Curry, J. J. (1945). *J. Clin. Invest.* **24,** 890.

Chess, S. (1971). *J. Autism Childhood Schiz.* **1,** 33–47.

Cournand, A. (1945). *Fed. Proc., Fed. Am. Soc. Exp. Biol.* **4,** 207.

Dalen, P. (1975). "Season of Birth: A Study of Schizophrenia and Other Mental Disorders." Am. Elsevier, New York.

Dastur, D. K., Lane, M. H., Hansen, D. B., Kety, S. S., Butler, R. N., Perlin, S., and Sokoloff, L. (1963). *In* "Human Aging: A Biological and Behavioral Study," pp. 59–76. Public Health Service Publication No. 986, U.S. Government Printing Office, Washington, D.C.

Dumke, P. R., and Schmidt, C. F. (1943). *Am. J. Physiol.* **138,** 421–428.

Evarts, E. V. (1961). *In* "The Nature of Sleep" (G. E. N. Wolstenholme and M. O'Connor, eds.), pp. 171–182. Churchill, London.

Fenner, F. (1971). *Med. J. Aust.* **2,** 1099–1102.

Fick, A. (1870). *Sitzungsber. Phys. Med. Ges. Wurzberg,* July 9.

Freyhan, F. A., Woodford, R. B., and Kety, S. S. (1951). *J. Nerv. Ment. Dis.* **113,** 449–456.

Glowinski, J., and Axelrod, J. (1966). *Pharmacol. Rev.* **18,** 775–785.

Gottesman, I. I., and Shields, J. (1972). "Schizophrenia and Genetics: A Twin Study Vantage Point." Academic Press, New York.

Hanshaw, J. B., Scheiner, A. P., Moxley, A. W., Gaev, L., Abel, V., and Scheiner, B. (1976). *N. Engl. J. Med.* **295,** 468–470.

Harmel, M. H., Hafkenschiel, J. H., Austin, G. M., Crumpton, C. W., and Kety, S. S. (1949). *J. Clin. Invest.* **28,** 415–418.

Ingvar, D. H. (1975). *In* "Brain Work" (D. H. Ingvar and N. A. Lassen, eds.), pp. 397–413; 478–492. Munksgaard, Copenhagen.

Kety, S. S. (1951). *Pharmacol. Rev.* **3,** 1–41.

Kety, S. S. (1957). *In* "Metabolism of the Nervous System" (D. Richter, ed.), pp. 221–237. Pergamon, Oxford.

Kety, S. S. (1959). *Science* **129,** 1528–1532; 1590–1596.

Kety, S. S. (1961). *Science* **132,** 1861–1870.

Kety, S. S. (1976). *In* "Neural Mechanisms of Learning and Memory" (M. R. Rosenzweig and E. L. Bennett, eds.), pp. 321–326. MIT Press, Cambridge, Massachusetts.

Kety, S. S., and Schmidt, C. F. (1948a). *J. Clin. Invest.* **27,** 476–483.

Kety, S. S., and Schmidt, C. F. (1948b). *J. Clin. Invest.* **27,** 484–492.

Kety, S. S., Harmel, M. H., Broomell, H. T., and Rhode, C. B. (1948a). *J. Biol. Chem.* **173,** 487–496.

Kety, S. S., Polis, B. D., Nadiler, C. S., and Schmidt, C. F. (1948b). *J. Clin. Invest.* **27,** 500–510.

Kety, S. S., Hafkenschiel, J. H., Jeffers, W. A., Leopold, I. H., and Shenkin, H. A. (1948c). *J. Clin. Invest.* **27,** 511–514.

Kety, S. S., Woodford, R. B., Harmel, M. H., Freyhan, F. A., Appel, K. E., and Schmidt, C. F. (1948d). *Am. J. Psychiat.* **104,** 765–770.

Kety, S. S., Javoy, F., Thierry, A. M., Julou, L., and Glowinski, J. (1967). *Proc. Natl. Acad. Sci. U.S.A.* **58,** 1249–1254.

Kety, S. S., Rosenthal, D., Wender, P. H., and Schulsinger, F. (1968). *In* "The Transmission of Schizophrenia" (D. Rosenthal and S. S. Kety, eds.), pp. 345–362. Pergamon, Oxford.

Kety, S. S., Rosenthal, D., Wender, P. H., Schulsinger, F., and Jacobsen, B. (1975). *In* "Genetic Research in Psychiatry" (R. Fieve, D. Rosenthal, and H. Brill, eds.), pp. 147–165. Johns Hopkins Press, Baltimore, Maryland.

Kinney, D., and Jacobsen, B. (1978). *In* "The Nature of Schizophrenia" (L. Wynne, R. Cromwell, and S. Matthysse, eds.), pp. 38–51. Wiley, New York.

Kohn, M. L. (1968). *In* "The Transmission of Schizophrenia" (D. Rosenthal and S. S. Kety, eds.), pp. 155–173. Pergamon, Oxford.

Krogh, A. (1919). *J. Physiol. (London)* **52,** 391–408.

LaBrosse, E. H., Axelrod, J., Kopin, I. J., and Kety, S. S. (1961a). *J. Clin. Invest.* **40,** 253–260.

LaBrosse, E. H., Mann, J. D., and Kety, S. S. (1961b). *J. Psychiat. Res. 1,* 68–75.

Landau, W. M., Freygang, W. H., Rowland, L. P., Sokoloff, L., and Kety, S. S. (1955). *Trans. Am. Neurol. Assoc.* **80,** 125–129.

Lassen, N. A. (1959). *Physiol. Rev.* **39,** 183–238.

Lassen, N. A., and Ingvar, D. H. (1963). *Arch. Neurol.* **9,** 615–622.

Lawrence, W. (1823). "Lectures on Comparative Anatomy, Physiology and Zoology." Smith, London.

Mangold, R., Sokoloff, L., Conner, E., Kleinerman, J., Therman, P. G., and Kety, S. S. (1955). *J. Clin. Invest.* **34,** 1092–1100.

Matthysse, S., and Matthysse, A. G. (1978). *In* "Psychopharmacology: A Generation of Progress" (M. S. Lipton, A. DiMascio, and K. F. Killam, eds.), pp. 1125–1129. Raven Press, New York.

Musacchio, J. M., Julou, L., Kety, S. S., and Glowinski, J. (1969). *Proc. Natl. Acad. Sci. U.S.A.* **63,** 1117–1119.

Quastel, J. H. (1939). *Physiol. Rev.* **19,** 135–183.

Reivich, M., Jehle, J., Sokoloff, L., and Kety, S. S. (1968). *J. Neurochem.* **15,** 301–306.

Reivich, M., Kuhl, D., Wolf, A., Greenberg, J., Phelps, M., Ido, T., Casella, V., Fowler, J., Gallagher, B., Hoffman, E., Alavi, A., and Sokoloff, L. (1977). *In* "Cerebral Function, Metabolism and Circulation" (D. H. Ingvar and N. A. Lassen, eds.). Munksgaard, Copenhagen.

Renkin, E. M. (1955). *Am. J. Physiol.* **183,** 125–136.

Rosenthal, D., Wender, P. H., Kety, S. S., Schulsinger, F., Welner, J., and Ostergaard,

L. (1968). *In* "The Transmission of Schizophrenia" (D. Rosenthal and S. S. Kety, eds.), pp. 377–391. Pergamon, Oxford.

Roy, C. S., and Sherrington, C. S. (1890). *J. Physiol. (London)* **11**, 85–108.

Schmidt, C. F., Kety, S. S., and Pennes, H. H. (1945). *Am. J. Physiol.* **143**, 33–52.

Shenkin, H. A., Harmel, M. H., and Kety, S. S. (1948). *AMA Arch. Neurol. Psychiat.* **60**, 240–252.

Smith, H. (1943). "Lectures on the Kidney." University of Kansas, Lawrence, Kansas.

Snyder, S. H., Creese, I., and Burt, D. R. (1975). *Psychopharmacol. Commun.* **1**, 663–673.

Sokoloff, L. (1961a). *In* "Chemical Pathology of the Nervous System" (J. Folch-Pi, ed.), Pergamon, Oxford.

Sokoloff, L. (1961b). *In* "Regional Neurochemistry" (S. S. Kety and J. Elkes, eds.). Pergamon, Oxford.

Sokoloff, L. (1977). *J. Neurochem.* **29**, 13–26.

Sokoloff, L., Wechsler, R. L., Mangold, R., Balls, K., and Kety, S. S. (1953). *J. Clin. Invest.* **32**, 202–208.

Sokoloff, L., Reivich, M., Kennedy, C., Des Rosiers, M. H., Patlak, C. S., Pettigrew, K. D., Sakurada, O., and Shinohara, M. (1977). *J. Neurochem.* **28**, 897–916.

Thudichum, J. W. L. (1884). "A Treatise on the Chemical Constitution of the Brain." Ballière, London.

Torre, E. F., and Peterson, M. R. (1973). *Lancet* **2**, 22–24.

THE IMMUNOGENETICS OF DIFFERENTIATION IN THE MOUSE*†

EDWARD A. BOYSE and LLOYD J. OLD

Memorial Sloan-Kettering Cancer Center,
New York, New York

A s students of immunogenetics, we shall try to illustrate ways in which immunogenetics is useful in studying some popular aspects of biology that involve differentiation. This absolves us from dealing with anything so tangible as data, but, unfortunately, we must touch on subjects like embryology and so forth in which we are by no means widely read. However, we are consoled by the thought that the tide seems to be running against scholarship. Perhaps there is no time for it these days. In popular literature, one sees the conventional hero declining in favor of the anti-hero. Perhaps the scholar will likewise give way to the anti-scholar. Although the reading of books is not yet reckoned an actual vice, it may come to that (Fig. 1).

This paper is concerned entirely with cell surfaces—that is, with the façades that cells present to their environment and to each other. One can view the entire development of an organism as a series of steps in which cells pass from one compartment of differentiation into the next. For any such transition from one compartment to another we may ask: Is the *cell surface* thereby changed, and can one recognize any *new display of molecules* in the form of newly expressed antigens? If so, can one identify the *origin, nature,* and *mechanism* of the inductive signal?

These are vital issues in developmental embryology and morphogenesis, for they bear on the programming of the branching pathways of differentiation that generate a complete organism from a single cell. We shall concentrate on the differentiation of one class of cells—the "thymus-derived" lymphocyte, or T cell, population—for three reasons: (1) We know much more about the surface composition

*Lecture delivered October 16, 1975.

†This work was supported by grants CA-08748, CA-16889 and CA-16599 from the National Institutes of Health.

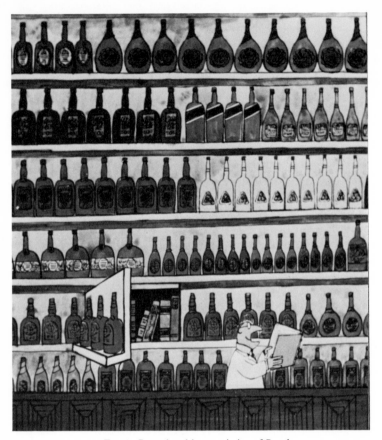

FIG. 1. Reproduced by permission of *Punch*.

of T cells than of any other cell type. (2) We believe the lessons learned will prove widely applicable. (3) We remember that the thymus has already accomplished essential functions by about the time of birth. Only if the thymus is removed at birth is immunocompetence severely affected, and then only in animals like mice, which are born in an immature state (Archer and Pierce, 1961; Miller, 1961; Good *et al.*, 1962; Good, 1973).

So one can think of the thymus as an organ of late embryogenesis, and not yield to any prejudice that T-cell differentiation should be unlike that of other cell types whose development might seem to be the exclusive province of embryology. Thus, for example, the migration of adult bone marrow cells to the thymus, where a new phenotype is induced, is not exceptional; this is commonplace in embryology.

The great value of immunogenetics, in the context of this lecture, is its role as all-purpose instrument for recognizing molecules of the plasma membrane and pinpointing the genes responsible. So we shall begin by briefly reviewing the history of what we have called "cell surface immunogenetics" (Boyse and Old, 1969).

An early discovery that brought immunology and mendelian genetics together was that of the ABO human blood groups, about 1900 (see Race and Sanger, 1958), and for many years the field was dominated by the investigation of blood group antigens. Not until Gorer's work on the H-2 system of mice, from the 1930s to the 1950s, were serological methods applied extensively to cells other than erythrocytes (Gorer and Mikulska, 1959). Gorer studied with Haldane and set out systematically to delineate blood groups in mice, the only vertebrate species that had been extensively inbred to provide genetically uniform stocks.

When mice of an inbred strain, say B on the right in Fig. 2, are immunized with any of a variety of tissues from an unrelated inbred mouse, strain A on the left, antibodies are generated that agglutinate the red cells of the donor. Exhaustive analysis of such antisera over several years identified two closely linked H-2 loci shown in the bottom left on

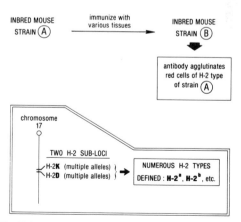

Fig. 2. The H-2 system of alloantigens demonstrated by hemagglutination.

chromosome 17, and labeled H-2K and H-2D. We can call them K and D for short. Each is highly polymorphic, determining a wide range of antigens, and the collective profile of H-2 antigens, for a given inbred strain, is denoted H-2^a or H-2^b and so forth (see Klein, 1975). Note the sketch of chromosome 17 in Fig. 2, because it will appear twice again, with other loci added. It became obvious that these H-2 blood group antigens would more aptly be termed tissue antigens because they occurred on at least most cell types and are the major determinants of histoincompatibility.

Gorer's thoughts turned to ways in which surface antigens could be demonstrated on nucleated cells by some direct serological method. He achieved this in 1956 with the cytotoxicity assay (Gorer and O'Gorman, 1956). This is the counterpart of the hemolytic test in which red cells are lysed by antibody and complement. When a living cell is incubated with H-2 antibody in the presence of complement, the plasma membrane is disrupted, permitting the entry of trypan blue into the dead cell (Fig. 3). At the end of the test, the living unstained cells and the dead blue cells are enumerated in a counting chamber. In the lower diagram of Fig. 3 is a typical titration of an H-2 antiserum in which the percentage of dead cells is plotted against the dilution of H-2 antiserum. As shown, an anti-H-2^a antiserum lyses virtually 100% of H-2^a lymphocytes to a titer

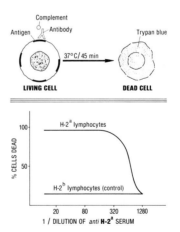

Fig. 3. The H-2 system of alloantigens demonstrated by the cytotoxicity test.

exceeding 1:320, the control H-2^b lymphocytes being unaffected. This simple yet immensely important technical advance presaged applications extending far beyond blood-typing and tissue transplantation, and it underlies all the work to be described herein.

All we knew around 1960 was that the same H-2 antisera that agglutinated red cells would lyse nucleated cells in the presence of complement. We needed to choose some plentiful supply of homogeneous living nucleated cells suitable for analysis by this new method. Among normal cells of the mouse, thymocytes are an obvious choice, and our own interest in thymocytes began with these practical considerations of availability, rather than because they happen to belong to the immune system. When molecular biologists discussed models for the study of metazoan organisms, a popular question used to be: *Which* beast should we choose? An alternative view is that one might think in terms not so much of a particular organism, as of one particular class of cells. And we came to regard T cells somewhat in that light, namely as a discrete population of cells that can be studied in different phases of development, and on which it seemed profitable to focus the same sort of undivided attention that molecular biologists had devoted to *Escherichia coli*. Much of this paper concerns the several systems of surface components peculiar to mouse T cells that are now known.

The technical details of how these thymocyte surface components were defined are not important, but it is appropriate to say something about the basic principles.

The successful discovery and analysis of each new thymocyte surface component has usually followed the course shown in Fig. 4. We begin by immunizing one strain against another, as before, but in this case only with thymocytes. And in this case the donor and recipient are selected to be of the same H-2 type. In some of many such immunizations, antibody is generated that is selectively cytotoxic for thymocytes of the donor strain. Step 2 consists in typing the thymocytes of all inbred strains available for the new thymocyte antigen. In step 3, reverse immunizations are performed to identify reciprocal alleles and antigens of the new system. Step 4 consists in typing appropriate backcross populations to ascertain whether we are dealing with a single mendelian locus. If that hurdle can be surmounted, then other standard genetic markers, such as coat color and H-2, can be included in order to locate the new gene by formal linkage. In the meantime, step 5, the representa-

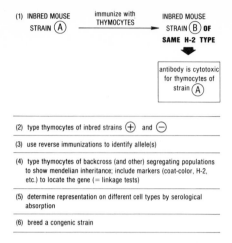

FIG. 4. Definition of a thymocyte alloantigen system (general method).

tion of the new component on cells of different types will have been established by serological absorption. Finally, if all has gone well, we must breed a congenic strain.

Congenic mice deserve very special emphasis, for generally speaking no system can be finally analyzed without them. A congenic stock is a strain of mouse that differs from a selected inbred base strain for only one character. Figure 5 shows the basic procedure for producing most of the congenic strains that are playing such an essential part in T-cell immunogenetics. Let us call the alleles and thymocyte types of any new system a and b. First, we cross some selected base strain of thymocyte type a with some donor strain of thymocyte type b. This F_1 hybrid is backcrossed to the base strain to produce a first backcross generation of which 50% will carry the allele b. These we select by typing thymocytes obtained by thymic biopsy (Boyse *et al.*, 1971b), and these b^+ mice are bred again to the base strain to generate mice of the second backcross, which are similarly typed. And so on for a minimum of eight generations. At that point, as shown in the lower right box in Fig. 5, we cross male and female backcross segregants bearing the b allele, and select from their progeny males and females that are homozygous for the b allele. These are the foundation mice from which the congenic strain is generated.

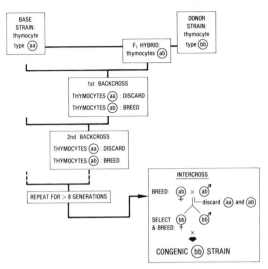

FIG. 5. Derivation of a congenic strain for a thymocyte alloantigen.

Figure 6 illustrates at a glance what we have achieved. The mouse has 20 pairs of chromosomes, of which only three are illustrated here. In the left column is shown the base strain bearing the allele *a,* with thymocytes of type *a.* In the right column is shown the donor strain, with the allele *b,* and with thymocytes of type *b.* In the center column is shown the congenic strain, whose chromosomes are now identical with those of the base strain, with the exception of a small chromosomal segment bearing the allele *b*, and thymocytes of type *b.* Thus the base strain and congenic strain approach the ideal of two strains that differ only in respect of one particular thymocyte type.

Just as we suggested a parallel between bacteria as raw material for molecular biology, and T cells as one raw material for the molecular biology of metazoan cells, so the use of congenic strains of mice might be likened to the use of mutants in bacterial genetics.

We can now look at the present inventory of thymocyte surface systems, our knowledge of which comes largely from Miyazawa, Itakura, Stockert, and others who have worked with us throughout the years; Boyse and Old (1969), Old and Boyse (1973), and Shen *et al.* (1975) have provided keys to the relevant literature). Table I shows the

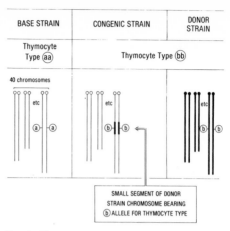

FIG. 6. The genomic constitution of congenic mice.

six systems that are expressed selectively or exclusively on T cells. The first, G_{IX}, is governed by two independent genes whose locations we have not found, except to say that they are not close to any of the others named here. Second, the TL gene is on chromosome 17, close to the H-2D locus, and this should be noted for reference later. Third, the gene for Thy-1 is on chromosome 9. There remain the three Ly loci, with genes on chromosomes 19 and 6, and another (for Ly-5) in a different but unknown position.

TABLE I

SIX SYSTEMS OF ALLOANTIGENS EXPRESSED EXCLUSIVELY OR SELECTIVELY[a] ON THYMIC LYMPHOCYTES

System	Location of genes
$G_{IX}{}^a$	Two unlinked genes (locations unknown) required for expression of G_{IX}
TL	Chromosome 17; *close to H-2D*
Thy-1[a]	Chromosome 9
Ly-1	Chromosome 19
Ly-2/Ly-3	Chromosome 6 (may be a single locus, or two closely linked loci)
Ly-5	Unknown (not linked to any of the above)

[a] G_{IX} and Thy-1 participate in other differentiative programs.

Note particularly that the first two systems, G_{IX} and TL, are not represented in all mice. Some mice express no thymocyte components referable to G_{IX} or TL genes. Also, with reference to the systems G_{IX} and Thy-1, these are expressed on some cell types other than T cells and so must participate in more than one differentiative program. Finally, for present purposes we shall treat the Ly-2 and Ly-3 systems as a single unit, because their genetic determinants are so closely linked that they may even constitute different regions of the same cistron (Boyse *et al.*, 1971a; Itakura *et al.*, 1972).

Consider first that all six systems are represented either solely or selectively on thymocytes, and that they were all discovered by immunizing mice of one strain with the thymocytes of another unrelated strain. Yet in no case did we uncover a system like H-2, in which the components identified would be shared by all cells. The implication is that much of the thymocyte surface may be composed of components specified by genes whose expression is exclusively or selectively limited to T cells, because these appear to form the prominent features to which the immunized recipient responds. An important question arises: Are T cells peculiar in having a special set of genes for their plasma membranes, or may this apply to all cells? It is a far-reaching thought, for if the latter is true, then a very large number of genes must be allocated for composing the surfaces of cells in accordance with their types and phases of differentiation. This is no trivial matter, because most of the great expansion of the genome that has accompanied the evolution of higher organisms is unexplained. That is why we shall digress to show you how we sought an answer for another tissue—skin. An apparent obstacle to the generalization that each differentiated cell type may have its own surface elements was the phenomenon of acquired tolerance described by Medawar and his colleagues (Billingham *et al.*, 1953), illustrated in Fig. 7. Experiments like this, illustrating acquired tolerance, are so famous that little comment is needed. In short, when hemopoietic cells from an adult mouse of say the CBA strain are inoculated into newborn mice of, say, the A strain, the recipient is colonized by the donor cells, and in adult life will permanently accept skin grafts from the donor strain.

Now if such absolute tolerance were the rule, we might be forced to conclude that epidermal cells cannot possess surface components absent from hemopoietic cells, for these would doubtless show antigenic varia-

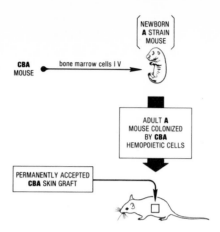

Fig. 7. Chimerism with tolerance of donor skin grafts.

tion, like blood groups and the thymocyte systems, in which case colonization by hemopoietic cells would not confer absolute tolerance of donor skin, which could be rejected by homograft reactions against alloantigens expressed selectively on epidermal cells. But there were already hints that hemopoietic chimerism does not characteristically entail absolute and permanent tolerance of skin (Boyse *et al.,* 1970; source reference). For example, most people know the classical experiments in which nonidentical cattle twins, which are commonly chimeric because they shared their placental circulations *in utero,* accepted skin grafts from one another in later life (Anderson *et al.,* 1951). But fewer people remember that many such interchanged skin grafts are ultimately rejected, although chimerism persists (Stone *et al.,* 1965).

For a long time therefore we searched for an experimental model in the mouse in which donor skin grafts would be invariably and promptly rejected by some type of chimera, and in which we might prove the existence of specific epidermal cell surface components serologically. We eventually found one (Boyse *et al.,* 1970), and it is illustrated in Fig. 8. Here we used chimeras formed by restoring lethally irradiated adult C57BL mice with bone marrow or spleen from hybrid donors carrying a different H-2 type for use as a marker for the donor cells. Radiation chimeras are especially favorable because virtually the whole

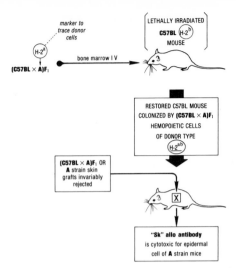

FIG. 8. Chimerism without tolerance of donor skin grafts.

hemopoietic system is replaced by donor cells, making it particularly easy to prove persistent chimerism. In these experiments, the red cells and lymphocytes of the chimeras were invariably and permanently of donor type, as indicated very simply by their reactions with antiserum against the foreign H-2 haplotype (H-2^a) of the donor. The use of a hybrid as the donor is dictated by the need to avert graft-versus-host reactions. In the system shown in Fig. 8, donor skin grafts were always promptly rejected. Finally, using enzymically dissociated epidermal cells, Margrit Scheid proved that the serum of such chimeras, after they had rejected several donor grafts, contained antibody specifically cytotoxic for the epidermal cells of the donor (Scheid *et al.*, 1972). Thus it was proved serologically that epidermal cells have a distinctive surface component, referable to what we call the Sk system of antigens, which happens to be shared with brain (Table II), and our colleague Wachtel has since found evidence of a second Sk system.

Thus the regulation of cell-surface composition by selective gene action is not an idiosyncrasy of thymocytes. All subsequent evidence points to the same conclusion for other cell types.

TABLE II

THE SK SYSTEM OF DIFFERENTIATION
ALLOANTIGENS ON EPIDERMAL CELLS

Sk-positive	Sk-negative
Epidermal cells	All hemopoietic cells
Brain	

Now we return to the thymocyte systems which constitute the special coat of this cell. Each of these deserves extensive treatment, but we can include only one or two comments on each, to put them in some sort of biological perspective.

The G_{IX} system (Stockert *et al.*, 1971) is illustrated in Fig. 9. On the right is mouse leukemia virus. The major constituent of its coat is a glycoprotein called gp70 because it has a molecular weight of around 70,000 (Nowinski *et al.*, 1972; August *et al.*, 1974). On the left is a thymocyte bearing G_{IX} antigen. Some strains of mice express G_{IX} antigen on their thymocytes, and other strains do not. Among the G_{IX}^+ strains of mice are all those, like AKR, that have a high incidence of leukemia and produce abundant leukemia virus throughout life. The G_{IX}^+ thymocyte in Fig. 9 is not from such a mouse, but is representative of several other mouse strains which express G_{IX} but do not produce abundant leukemia virus. What our colleagues have shown is that G_{IX}

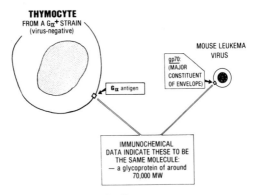

FIG. 9. The G_{IX} system.

and gp70 are one and the same molecule (Obata *et al.*, 1975; Tung *et al.*, 1975). This tells us three things: (1) that this constituent of leukemia virus can be incorporated in the thymocyte plasma membrane independently of virus production; (2) that it may be inherited as a mendelian character; (3) that the expression of this leukemia virus obeys the physiological thymic controls that govern the surface phenotype of thymocytes.

The TL system (Boyse *et al.*, 1966) is illustrated in Fig. 10. As in the case of G_{IX}, some strains of mice express TL components on their thymocytes, and others do not. The TL system was used to gain information about molecular organization within the plasma membrane. First, at the bottom on the left in Fig. 10, note the diagram of chromosome 17 with the *Tla* locus added, next to the H-2D and H-2K loci, the order being K—D—TL. The illustrations at the top in Fig. 10 indicate the quantities of K, D, and TL expressed on the thymocytes of TL^- mice (on the left), and TL^+ mice (on the right). The thymocytes of TL^- mice manifest double the amount of D, but the same amount of K (Boyse *et al.*, 1968a), so the linked D and TL loci are interrelated. This was later supported by immunochemical evidence that they produce similar glycoproteins (Davies *et al.*, 1969; Vitetta *et al.*, 1972; Muramatsu *et al.*, 1973) that also have in common the incorporation of a subunit similar or identical to β-2 microglobulin (Vitetta *et al.*, 1975a;

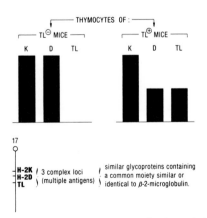

FIG. 10. The TL system—the H-2D/TL interrelation.

Ostberg *et al.*, 1975), which itself, by analogy with man, is probably coded by a gene on another chromosome (Goodfellow *et al.*, 1975; Faber *et al.*, 1976).

The fact that D and TL appear as interchangeable molecules suggests one of two things: either (1) the D and TL genes are coordinately controlled at the chromosomal level, or (2) there are sites in the plasma membrane that can be occupied alternatively by D or TL. If the latter is true, we should expect D and TL to occupy adjacent positions when both are expressed. Stockert tested this by a new technique (Boyse *et al.*, 1968b) illustrated in Fig. 11. As shown at the top, thymocytes from TL$^+$ mice are first saturated with excess anti-TL antibody. Then precise measurements are made of their capacity to take up anti-D antibody. This was reduced by nearly 50%. The reciprocal experiment is shown at the bottom. Thus D and TL are neighboring molecules.

Stockert then made an extensive study to decide whether other components of the thymocyte surface, which are not related by genetic linkage, might also have defined topographical positions. Using the same principle of interference between different antibodies competing for adjacent antigens, she tested all possible pairs representing the thymocyte components then known. For every given pair she invariably found either interference, indicated in this hypothetical pattern by placing the symbols side by side, or no interference, illustrated in Fig. 12 by an intervening span of one or more boxes. Thus every component known was shown to have a defined position in the total display. No one

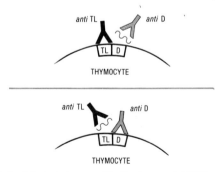

Fig. 11. Principle of the technique used by Stockert *et al.* (1968) to demonstrate that a given pair of antigens occupy adjacent sites in the plasma membrane.

	Thy-1	Thy-1	Thy-1	Thy-1	Thy-1	Thy-1		
TL-3	TL-2	TL-1	H-2D	Ly-2 Ly-3			Ly-1	H-2K

FIG 12. The thymocyte "map"; a hypothetical pattern that accommodates the "antibody-blocking" data (see Fig. 11).

should be misled into thinking that present evidence that components of the cell surface can be displaced in such phenomena as capping is contrary to this evidence of molecular patterning; we are speaking of the natural configurations of the resting undisturbed plasma membrane (see Stackpole, 1976).

The importance we attach to these findings is the likelihood that certain properties of cell surfaces, among which mutual recognition occupies much of our thoughts, may depend not only on what gene products the cell surface contains, but also upon the configurations in which these are displayed; this must be included in our concepts of differentiation.

Little need be said about the Thy-l system (Reif and Allen, 1964), briefly noted in Table III, except to comment that because it is represented on cell types other than T cells it is unlikely to have a specific immunological function. And, second, that it is absent from B lymphocytes, and (to be noted for further reference) also from the "prothymocyte," or immediate precursor of the thymocyte.

We are left with the group of Ly systems. The outstanding finding here is that when thymocytes undergo further differentiation they generate a population of peripheral T cells that includes subclasses expressing

TABLE III

THE THY-1 SYSTEM

Positive	Negative
T lymphocytes	B lymphocytes
Epidermal cells	Prothymocytes
Fibroblasts	
Brain cells	

only one or two of the Ly systems, rather than the complete set found on thymocytes (Fig. 13). We must return to this in detail later.

So much for the Joseph's coat of the thymocyte. Next let us consider how the thymus engineers the manifestation of this intricate surface phenotype.

The three columns in Fig. 14 represent three compartments of T-cell differentiation. The first contains the prothymocyte of bone marrow and spleen. On reaching the thymic cortex, this is induced to enter the second compartment and become a thymocyte, exhibiting all the components of column 2 (the top two lines, representing G_{IX} and TL, are hatched to signify that only some mice express these particular components). Last, in the thymic medulla and peripheral lymphoid tissues we meet only T cells of the third compartment. They have lost G_{IX} and TL; Thy-1 is greatly diminished; and the population has diversified in regard to Ly phenotypes. H-2 has greatly increased. The three compartments can also be represented as shown in Table IV, reading downward, where the ($+$) and ($-$) signs stand for selective expression of the respective genes, or for conditional exhibition of their products at the cell surface.

We shall now deal with the first transition, of prothymocyte to thymocyte. Our first hint as to how this might be analyzed came about somewhat obliquely as follows: We have made hundreds of antisera, and sometimes this has required immunizing TL^- mice with cells from TL^+ mice in cases where we want to avoid the production of TL antibody. It was our habit to obviate this by omitting thymocytes from the inoculum, on the grounds that only these cells have TL antigens. But we repeatedly found that TL antibody was produced, notwithstanding. This is illustrated here in Fig. 15. As shown in the left-hand box, we are here using only bone marrow and spleen cells for immunization. Nevertheless, as shown in the top right-hand boxes, normal TL^- recipients respond by producing TL antibody just as though we had included TL^+

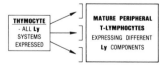

FIG. 13. The Ly systems.

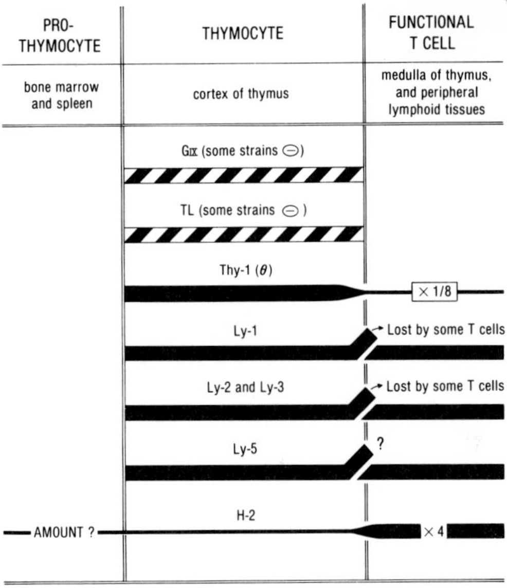

FIG. 14. Three compartments of T-cell differentiation.

thymocytes. The lower-right boxes give the answer, for if we first thymectomize the recipients they produce no TL antibody, although their capacity to produce other antibodies is not impaired (Komuro *et al.*, 1973). We concluded that thymocyte precursors, in the inoculated bone marrow and spleen, are very readily induced by the host's thymus

TABLE IV

THREE COMPARTMENTS OF T-CELL DIFFERENTIATION

Compartments	G_{IX}	TL	Thy	Ly-1	Ly-2 Ly-3	Ly-5	H-2
Prothymocyte (bone marrow and spleen)	−	−	−	−	−	−	+
Thymocyte (thymic cortex)	+	+	+	+	+	+	+
Functional T cell (thymic medulla, and periphery), 3 subclasses	−	−	+↓	+ + −	+ − +	? ? ?	+ ↑

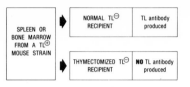

FIG. 15. Induction of prothymocytes *in vivo*.

to differentiate into thymocytes that express TL and so provoke the formation of TL antibody.

This prompted the idea of a simple test system in which the conversion of prothymocytes to thymocytes might be observed and studied *in vitro,* and in 1972 Komuro devised the prothymocyte induction assay (Komuro and Boyse, 1973a,b) (Fig. 16). The first step is to fractionate spleen or bone marrow cells to obtain layers rich in inducible prothymocytes. This population is then incubated with an inducer for 2 hours, after which the appearance of TL and the other thymocyte surface components is demonstrable by cytotoxicity tests in the usual way.

The mechanism of this transformation of the phenotype is of great interest. The first point to note is that its very complexity, involving as it does the manifestation of so many diverse gene products, suggests that the prothymocyte is already programmed to manifest this set of genes and that induction consists in an instruction for fulfillment of the program, rather than in transmission of the information contained in the program. This is substantiated by the nature of the agents that can act as inducers *in vitro* (Scheid *et al.,* 1973).

Three of the most informative inducers are shown in Table V. In the first column is thymopoietin, which has been found only in thymus. It is

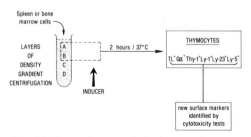

FIG. 16. The prothymocyte induction assay *in vitro*.

TABLE V

THREE AGENTS THAT INDUCE PROTHYMOCYTES *in Vitro*

Thymopoietin	Ubiquitin	Cyclic AMP
Source: thymus	Source: most living cells; strictly intracellular	
Physiological function: natural thymic inducer of prothymocytes	Physiological function: unknown	Presumed secondary mediator, generated by the action of primary inducers
Structure: single polypeptide chain of 49 amino acids; sequence known; MW 5562	Structure: single polypeptide chain of 74 amino acids; sequence known; MW 8451	

a polypeptide whose amino acid sequence has been established by Schlesinger (1975) and is, we believe, the natural prothymocyte inducer. In the next column is a second fully sequenced polypeptide; it is called ubiquitin because it has been found in all nucleated living cells (Goldstein *et al.*, 1975) and, under normal circumstances, is strictly intracellular. And third there is the "second messenger"—cyclic AMP.

Thymopoietin and ubiquitin require further introduction: Thymopoietin was isolated from thymus by Goldstein during studies related to the neuromuscular disorder myasthenia gravis in man (Goldstein, 1974), which is always accompanied by pathological changes in the thymus (Goldstein and MacKay, 1969). Goldstein assayed it by its capacity to cause a neuromuscular block in mice (Goldstein, 1974), its ability to induce prothymocytes being then unknown. Accordingly, the neuromuscular disability of myasthenia is ascribed by Goldstein to escape of thymopoietin from the diseased thymus (Goldstein and Schlesinger, 1975). Thymopoietin's pathological action in causing neuromuscular block can be interpreted as an evolutionary accident whereby it happens to cross-react with acetylcholine receptors of some kind (Goldstein, 1974).

Goldstein studied ubiquitin from thymus because it was so abundant, and he incorrectly guessed that it might be a prohormone. Its widespread occurrence and its ability to induce prothymocytes were discovered only later. Like thymopoietin, it induces prothymocytes in minute amounts (Scheid *et al.,* 1975a). Its normal function is totally mysterious, but it evidently must be vital, because ubiquitins from extremely diverse sources show a high degree of conservation of amino acid sequence (Goldstein *et al.,* 1975).

The third inducing agent, cyclic AMP, speaks for itself. Evidently prothymocyte induction belongs to the category of cellular responses that utilize this common mediator. Therefore it can scarcely be doubted that prothymocyte induction represents fulfillment of a predetermined program by committed cells. The most profound question is *the form in which information is stored.* But unfortunately this is merely to restate perhaps the most fundamental enigma of embryonic development (see Balinsky, 1970). For naturally the facts of prothymocyte induction invite comparison with past studies of induction of embryonic tissues *in vitro,* in which attempts to identify specific inducers were foiled because the uninduced tissues were already programmed for particular options, and so could be triggered in culture by incongruous agents of no physiological relevance. Figure 17 will serve as an example. Normally, the optic vesicle induces neurula ectoderm to form a lens, but

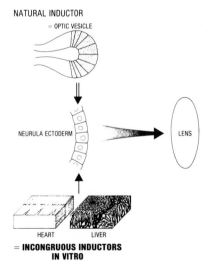

FIG. 17. An example of the induction of embryonic tissue.

under the abnormal conditions of isolation *in vitro* such incongruous tissues as heart or liver can supply an inductive signal (Holtfreter, 1934).

It follows that if we wish to propose prothymocyte induction as a general model, we must overcome the bugbear of nonspecific induction. Otherwise how can we tell whether a given agent is the natural inducer, or a mimic like ubiquitin? One approach we have adopted is to devise a parallel induction assay for two kinds of preprogrammed cells, assuming that a nonspecific inducer will trigger both types of primed cells, whereas the specific inducer will induce only the cognate cell. For this purpose the obvious companion for the prothymocyte is a prolymphocyte of the B type. The latter are abundant in bone marrow and spleen. These two cell populations, prothymocytes and pro-B cells, are the basis of this dual induction assay, elaborated by Hammerling and Scheid. At the top in Fig. 18, thymopoietin and ubiquitin are seen to induce the prothymocyte to express TL, etc. At the bottom, ubiquitin is shown also to induce immature B cells to express the characteristic surface marker, CR, or complement receptor, which is a convenient readily demonstrable surface component that B lymphocytes acquire

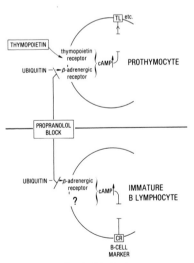

FIG. 18. The dual induction assay.

during differentiation. Thus ubiquitin can induce both these cell types. It probably does so by reacting with the β-adrenergic receptors that are found on many cell types, because the β-adrenergic antagonist propranolol blocks induction of both cell types by ubiquitin. Thymopoietin, in contrast, triggers only the prothymocyte, and propranolol does not interfere with this (Scheid *et al.*, 1975a). This implies that thymopoietin triggers the prothymocyte by engaging a receptor which only prothymocytes possess, as befits a *specific* inducer.

These various considerations resolve the otherwise obscure finding that mice that lack a thymus, notably the congenitally athymic nude mouse, often have some circulating cells that express T-cell surface components (Raff, 1973). These are most numerous in our experience when such mice succumb to severe infections, where dying cells may release potent inducing agents like ubiquitin (discussed by Scheid *et al.*, 1975b). But the fact that mice that never had a thymus, despite the fact that they may harbor such cells, are nonetheless immunologically crippled, emphasizes that there is more to T-cell differentiation than is revealed by prothymocyte induction, and one must assume that prothymocyte induction does not autonomously generate the complete range of immunocompetent T lymphocytes. Otherwise we should be faced with the embarrassing conclusion that the thymus is superfluous, which is not to be taken lightly at an Institute headed by Robert Good. So we must turn to the less clearly comprehended transition from thymocyte to functional T cell, compartments 2 and 3. First we put forward the possible general view of induction illustrated in Fig. 19.

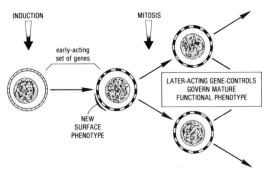

Fig. 19. A hypothesis for premitotic and postmitotic phases of differentiation.

According to this scheme, which we can refer to as compartments 1, 2, and 3 of T-cell differentiation, induction of an early-acting set of genes first reconstitutes the cell surface; this is followed by mitoses leading to inauguration of function by a later-acting set of genes. The first transition is admirably illustrated by prothymocyte induction, and one suspects that phenotypic transformation without cell division may be a general feature of induction, whatever the cell type. Such initial reconstitution of the cell surface, ensuing on induction, would make excellent sense in embryological settings, where induced cells must undertake strictly regulated morphogenetic movements, which doubtless involve surface discrimination, before manifesting their destined functions (see Boyse and Abbott, 1975). The generation of functionally primed T cells very probably involves mitosis corresponding to the second phase.

Peripheral T lymphocytes belong to one of two or more functionally distinct subclasses. First, there are helper T cells which collaborate with B lymphocytes in the production of antibody. Second, there are cytotoxic or "killer" T cells, best known for their capacity to destroy foreign cells. Third, there is evidently another T-cell subclass that suppresses the immune response. We shall now see how these functional subclasses may be related to the differential expression of the Ly systems mentioned earlier.

First, as illustrated in Table VI (based on Cantor and Boyse, 1975), we can take a suspension of peripheral T cells and eliminate cells bearing a particular Ly component by lysing them with the relevant Ly antibody and complement, as in the cytotoxicity assay. Then we can take the remaining unlysed cells and see whether there remain any that are susceptible to a different Ly antiserum in a second cytotoxicity assay. This will establish the existence of any T cells expressing the latter Ly component, but not the former. Let me remind you that Ly-2 and Ly-3 can *provisionally* be regarded as a single system, since they are specified by subregions of the same locus, or even of the same gene (Boyse *et al.*, 1971a). Ly-1 is a separate system coded by a locus on another chromosome (Itakura *et al.*, 1972). Ly-5 (Komuro *et al.*, 1975), the third Ly system, is omitted from now on because we do not yet have a congenic mouse strain for Ly-5, and therefore little has been done with it. Reading from left to right in Table VI, the upshot is that lysis with anti-Ly-1 leaves some cells susceptible to anti-Ly-2 or -3, which identifies a 1^-23^+ cells, denoted the Ly-23 cell, and reversely, lysis with

TABLE VI

Ly Phenotypes of Peripheral T Cells[a,b]

Lysis with	leaves cells susceptible to	which identifies
Anti-Ly-1	*Anti*-Ly-2 or -3	An Ly-1⁻ Ly-23⁺ subclass ("Ly-23" cell)
Anti-Ly-2 or -3	*Anti*-Ly-1	An Ly-1⁺ Ly-23⁻ subclass ("Ly-1" cell)

[a] Based on Cantor and Boyse (1975).

[b] Frequency of subclasses $\begin{cases} \text{Ly-123} = 50\% \\ \text{Ly-1} = 30\% \\ \text{Ly-23} = 7\% \end{cases}$ of peripheral T cells.

anti-Ly-2 or -3 leaves some cells susceptible to anti-Ly-1, which identifies a 1^+23^- cell, denoted the Ly-1 cell. Simple arithmetic demands a third subclass expressing all three, the Ly-123 cell. Now we can find out whether these selected T cell populations have restricted functions.

The most informative experimental design is summarized in Fig. 20, together with the conclusions reached mainly by Cantor and Boyse (1975), Shiku *et al.*, (1975), and Kisielow *et al.* (1975). The initial procedure at the top is the same as before. Peripheral T cells are treated either with anti-Ly-1 serum and complement (at the top left), or with anti-Ly-2 or -3 serum and complement (at the top right). As before, this yields the selected populations Ly-23 and Ly-1, respectively. Each population is now presented with appropriate antigen and is later tested for helper and killer functions. As shown at the bottom, cells of the Ly-23 subclass develop killer but not helper function. For cells of the Ly-1 subclass, the opposite is true.

In interpreting these findings, a point of crucial importance has been emphasized and established especially by Cantor (1975). Note that in the design shown in Fig. 20, antigen is presented to the two populations only after they have been isolated. Thus the two subclasses Ly-1 and Ly-23 must already be programmed for helper and killer functions,

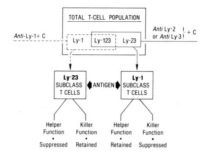

Fig. 20. Concordance of T-cell functions with the Ly phenotypes.

respectively, *before* they meet antigen. This tells against a formidable alternative hypothesis according to which functional subclasses would be generated only after a hypothetically indifferent T-cell population meets antigen (Cantor and Boyse, 1975). Therefore it seems we must postulate separate differentiative programs for helper T cells and killer T cells. And we surmise that these involve different sets of the hypothetical late-acting genes for function, postulated in Fig. 19.

Thus the proposition confronting us in regard to compartments 2 and 3 is that divergent functional programs are an autonomous feature of T-cell differentiation, independent of antigen, and that Ly-1 cells and Ly-23 cells are as decisively committed to helper and killer functions as, for example, are erythroblasts to the production of hemoglobin. This hypothesis may well represent the frontier of contemporary research on how the thymus achieves a balanced output of harmonious sets of functionally discrete T lymphocytes.

But first it should be stressed that the experimental evidence for separate autonomous pathways, namely the restricted capabilities of the isolated Ly subclasses, is as yet slender. Consider, for example, that (1) the functional correlates of the Ly-5 system are not yet known; (2) the Ly-123 subclass has not yet been physically isolated; (3) there are probably yet other Ly systems, which we do not know about, that would add further discriminations; and (4) the Ly phenotype of the proposed suppressor T cell (or cells) has not yet been identified.

With those wholesome reservations, let us focus on the critical question of where and how these subclasses are generated (Fig. 21). The

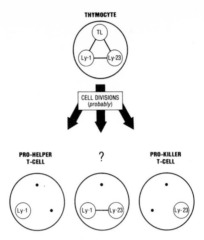

FIG. 21. Compartments two and three.

great value of the Ly phenotypes is clearly that the subclasses can be separated, and their functions studied in isolation. Thus the sheep can be separated from the goats. As a working hypothesis we shall say that at no time are there sheep in goat's clothing, or goats in sheep's clothing. Within this framework, what arguments can be adduced in support of the contention that each subclass is autonomously differentiated in the absence of antigen?

First, appropriate doses of cortisone destroy the majority of thymocytes in the thymic cortex, and leave a minor cortisone-resistant population of medullary T cells. According to Cantor (1975), these comprise Ly subclasses in proportions similar to those found in the periphery. Because we know that this cortisone-resistant population is responsible for whatever immune functions can be elicited from the thymocyte population as a whole (see Leckband and Boyse, 1971), this fits the picture of medullary cells as an already heterogeneous population of T lymphocytes that have begun to express both their functional competence and their Ly phenotypes, and it implies that commitment to function and distinctive Ly phenotype both occur within the thymus, or even earlier. This tells against any role for antigen in the process of commitment to function, for (according to our arbitrary terms of reference) commitment will have occurred before new T cells are disseminated to sites where they can encounter antigen.

Another argument applies to species that are born more immunologically mature than are mice. For if we adhere to the premise that differential immunocompetence can be equated with the acquisition of distinctive Ly phenotypes, then both must already be well advanced in embryos of species that exhibit highly developed immunocompetence at birth, and hence both should be independent of antigen.

How far the foreseeable extensions of current research will explain how this branching of pathways is governed, granted that this can be incontrovertibly substantiated, we hesitate to guess. But one prediction is worth attention, and it is this: the postulate of separate autonomous pathways implies discrete genes for each T-cell function. It follows that there should be corresponding mutations that alter or abolish that capability. This presupposes a class of hereditary immunodeficiencies comprising defects or variations in immunocompetence related specifically to one class of functional T cells, in each case, but not to the others. To pinpoint such discrete disorders or variations by exclusively biological methods might well prove too cumbersome to be rewarding. But to scan laboratory mice for variations in the representation of Ly subclasses, or for the competence of Ly subsets separated from different mouse stocks, is well within the compass of quite modest future studies.

So much for differentiation within the T-cell lineage. Finally, we return briefly to the broader theme that this may be a valid general model for differentiation. Figure 22 shows chromosome 17 as you saw it before, but with the T locus added. The notation "T" is apt to be confusing, because the T locus has nothing to do with T cells. Genes at

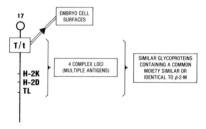

FIG. 22. A family of loci with a common ancestry?

the T locus mediate a series of essential steps in the formation of the embryo. Each is responsible for a single embryogenetic event. For example, one T gene mediates a very early step, the formation of blastula from the morula, and another a late step resulting in the differentiation of brain stem and forebrain from neural ectoderm. Each T gene has been pinpointed by a corresponding mutation that arrests embryogenesis at that precise phase of development (reviewed by Bennett, 1975).

Using essentially the same immunogenetic methods described above, Bennett *et al.* (1972) and Yanagisawa (1974) have shown that each of these T locus genes determines its own cell-surface component, identified as a specific antigen. We think it likely that each component is expressed on the relevant embryo cells at the corresponding phase of development. The neighboring H-2 loci likewise are subject to selective expression, because H-2 components do not appear until cleavage and early embryogenesis are under way (see Bennett, 1975); and finally there is TL, which enters the field at a late stage of the embryo's history. Bennett proposes that these four linked loci are evolutionary descendants of a single common ancestral locus, most likely concerned with surface recognition. The evidence includes the finding of Vitetta *et al.* (1975b) that all four loci code for glycoproteins that are similar in composition and incorporate a moiety similar or identical to β-2-M.

It is but a step to the notion that they share common control mechanisms, and hence that the details of the thymic differentiative program that includes TL will apply to embryonic differentiation governed by the T locus.

We venture to close on a note of personal reflection. Even this fragmentary account may suffice to indicate the remarkable penetration of immunogenetics into the maze of biology, leading us into embryology, oncology, virology, and immunology proper. What is the secret of the success of immunogenetics? We believe it has to do with the remarkable simplicity of the basic approach, which when all is said and done amounts to little more than juggling with the endless detective possibilities of the antigen–antibody reaction, often coupled with no more than the sort of beanbag genetics that can be picked up from a high-school primer. Of course, the sophisticated techniques of, say, biochemistry and molecular biology are called for now as never before, but no doubt the essential spadework will continue to be provided by rudimentary immunogenetics.

In attaining our personal research goals we have all had our crosses to bear. One of us endured a spell in a Public Health Laboratory. It was mercifully brief, but the recollection remains of such things as the use of bacterial typing antisera to determine which genetic variant of *Salmonella* was ravaging the bowels of schoolchildren in this or that outbreak of food poisoning. This did not lead to entertaining any vision that the principles involved in even so humble an immunogenetic system are enough for one to start probing into metazoan biology. If it had, this might seem appropriate, because the elaborate devices that we may be glimpsing must have originated when primitive cells first joined forces, and so had to set up the administrative machinery for mutual identification that living in society requires.

REFERENCES

Anderson, D., Billingham, R. E., Lampkin, G. H., and Medawar, P. B. (1951). *Heredity* **5,** 379–397.

Archer, O., and Pierce, J. C. (1961). *Fed. Proc., Fed. Am. Soc. Exp. Biol.* **20,** 26.

August, J. T., Bolognesi, D. P., Fleissner, E., Gilden, R. V., and Nowinski, R. C. (1974). *Virology* **60,** 595–600.

Balinsky, B. I. (1970). "An Introduction to Embryology." Saunders, Philadelphia, Pennsylvania.

Bennett, D. (1975). *Cell* **6,** 441–454.

Bennett, D., Goldberg, E., Dunn, L. C., and Boyse, E. A. (1972). *Proc. Natl. Acad. Sci. U.S.A.* **69,** 2076–2080.

Billingham, R. E., Brent, L., and Medawar, P. B. (1953). *Nature (London)* **172,** 603–606.

Boyse, E. A., and Abbott, J. (1975). *Fed. Proc., Fed. Am. Soc. Exp. Biol.* **34,** 24–27.

Boyse, E. A., and Old, L. J. (1969). *Annu. Rev. Genet.* **3,** 269–290.

Boyse, E. A., Old, L. J., and Stockert, E. (1966). *Immunopathol. Int. Symp. 4th 1965,* pp. 23–40.

Boyse, E. A., Stockert, E., and Old, L. J. (1968a). *J. Exp. Med.* **128,** 85–95.

Boyse, E. A., Old, L. J., and Stockert, E. (1968b). *Proc. Natl. Acad. Sci. U.S.A.* **60,** 886–893.

Boyse, E. A., Lance, E. M., Carswell, E. A., Cooper, S., and Old, L. J. (1970). *Nature (London)* **227,** 901–903.

Boyse, E. A., Itakura, K., Stockert, E., Iritani, C. A., and Miura, M. (1971a). *Transplantation* **11,** 351–352.

Boyse, E. A., Old, L. J., and Iritani, C. A. (1971b). *Transplantation* **12,** 93–95.

Cantor, H., and Boyse, E. A. (1975). *J. Exp. Med.* **141,** 1376–1389.

Davies, D. A. L., Alkins, B. M., Boyse, E. A., and Stockert, E. (1969). *Immunology* **16,** 669–676.

Faber, H. E., Kucherlapati, R. S., Poulik, M. D., Ruddle, F. H., and Smithies, O. (1976). *Somatic Cell Genetics.* **2,** 141–154.

Goldstein, G. (1974). *Nature (London)* **247,** 11–14.

Goldstein, G., and MacKay, I. R. (1969). "The Human Thymus." Heinemann, London.

Goldstein, G., and Schlesinger, D. H. (1975). *Lancet* **2,** 256–259.

Goldstein, G., Scheid, M., Hammerling, U., Boyse, E. A., Schlesinger, D. H., and Niall, H. D. (1975). *Proc. Natl. Acad. Sci. U.S.A.* **72,** 11–15.

Good, R. A. (1973). *Harvey Lect.* **67,** 1–107.

Good, R. A., Dalmasso, A. P., Martinez, C., Archer, O. K., Pierce, J. C., and Papermaster, B. W. (1962). *J. Exp. Med.* **116,** 773–795.

Goodfellow, P. N., Jones, E. A., van Heyningen, V., Solomon, E., Dobrow, M., Miggiano, V., and Bodmer, W. F. (1975). *Nature (London)* **254,** 267–269.

Gorer, P. A., and Mikulska, Z. B. (1959). *Proc. R. Soc. London Ser. B* **151,** 57–69.

Gorer, P. A., and O'Gorman, P. (1956). *Transplant. Bull.* **3,** 142–143.

Holtfreter, J. (1934). *Wilhelm Roux' Arch. Entwicklungsmech. Organismen* **133,** 367.

Itakura, K., Hutton, J. J., Boyse, E. A., and Old, L. J. (1972). *Transplantation* **13,** 239–243.

Kisielow, P., Hirst, J., Shiku, H., Beverley, P. C. L., Hoffmann, M. K., Boyse, E. A., and Oettgen, H. F. (1975). *Nature (London)* **253,** 219–220.

Klein, J. (1975). "Biology of the Mouse, Histocompatibility," Vol. 2 Springer Publ., New York.

Komuro, K., and Boyse, E. A. (1973a). *Lancet* pp. 740–743.

Komuro, K., and Boyse, E. A. (1973b). *J. Exp. Med.* **138,** 479–482.

Komuro, K., Boyse, E. A., and Old, L. J. (1973). *J. Exp. Med.* **137,** 533–536.

Komuro, K., Itakura, K., Boyse, E. A., and John, M. (1975). Immunogenetics **1,** 452–456.

Leckband, E., and Boyse, E. A. (1971). *Science* **172,** 1258–1260.

Miller, J. F. A. P. (1961). *Lancet* **2,** 748–749.

Muramatsu, T., Nathenson, S. G., Boyse, E. A., and Old, L. J. (1973). *J. Exp. Med.* **137,** 1256–1262.

Nowinski, R. C., Fleissner, E., Sarkar, N. H., and Aoki, T. (1972). *J. Virol.* **9,** 359–366.

Obata, Y., Ikeda, H., Stockert, E., and Boyse, E. A. (1975). *J. Exp. Med.* **141,** 188–197.

Old, L. J., and Boyse, E. A. (1973). *Harvey Lect.* **67,** 273–315.

Ostberg, L., Rask, L., Wigzell, H., and Peterson, P. A. (1975). *Nature (London)* **253,** 735–736.

Race, R. R., and Sanger, R. (1958). "Blood Groups in Man." Thomas, Springfield, Illinois.

Raff, M. C. (1973). *Nature (London)* **246,** 350–351.

Reif, A. E., and Allen, J. M. V. (1964). *J. Exp. Med.* **120,** 413–433.

Scheid, M., Boyse, E. A., Carswell, E. A., and Old, L. J. (1972). *J. Exp. Med.* **135,** 938–955.

Scheid, M. P., Hoffmann, M. K., Komuro, K., Hammerling, U., Abbott, J., Boyse, E. A., Cohen, G. H., Hooper, J. A., Schulof, R. S., and Goldstein, A. L. (1973). *J. Exp. Med.* **138,** 1027–1032.

Scheid, M. P., Goldstein, G., Hammerling, U., and Boyse, E. A. (1975a). *Ann. N. Y. Acad. Sci.* **249,** 531–540.

Scheid, M., Goldstein, G., and Boyse, E. A. (1975b). *Science* **190,** 1211–1213.

Schlesinger, D. H., and Goldstein, G. (1975). *Cell* **5,** 361–365.

Shen, F. W., Boyse, E. A., and Cantor, H. (1975). *Immunogenetics* **2**, 591–595.

Shiku, H., Kisielow, P., Bean, M. A., Takahashi, T., Boyse, E. A., Oettgen, H. F., and Old, L. J. (1975). *J. Exp. Med.* **141**, 227–241.

Stackpole, C. (1977). *Prog. Surface Membrane Sci.* **12.**

Stockert, E., Old, L. J., and Boyse, E. A. (1971). *J. Exp. Med.* **133**, 1334–1355.

Stone, W. H., Cragle, R. G., Swanson, E. W., and Brown, D. C. (1965). *Science* **148**, 1335–1336.

Tung, J. S., Vitetta, E. A., Fleissner, E., and Boyse, E. A. (1975). *J. Exp. Med.* **141**, 198–205.

Vitetta, E., Uhr, J. W., and Boyse, E. A. (1972). *Cell. Immunol.* **4**, 187–191.

Vitetta, E. S., Uhr, J. W., and Boyse, E. A. (1975a). *J. Immunol.* **114**, 252–254.

Vitetta, E. S., Artzt, K., Bennett, D., Boyse, E. A., and Jacob, F. (1975b). *Proc. Natl. Acad. Sci. U.S.A.* **72**, 3215–3219.

Yanagisawa, K., Bennett, D., Boyse, E. A., Dunn, L. C., and Dimeo, A. (1974). *Immunogenetics* **1**, 57–67.

EARLY STUDIES ON GENE AMPLIFICATION*

JOSEPH G. GALL

Department of Biology, Yale University, New Haven, Connecticut

I. Introduction

T HE term *gene amplification* as applied to eukaryotic cells refers to the selective extrachromosomal replication of specific genes. The only fully documented cases involve the genes coding for ribosomal RNA. These genes (rDNA) are amplified in the oogonia and oocytes of many animals, both vertebrate and invertebrate (reviewed in Gall, 1969; Macgregor, 1972; Tobler, 1975), and in the vegetative nuclei of several primitive eukaryotes, including the protozoan *Tetrahymena* (Yao *et al.,* 1974; Gall, 1974), the slime mold *Physarum* (Vogt and Braun, 1976), and probably the green alga *Acetabularia* (Trendelenburg *et al.,* 1974). In oocytes the extrachromosomal rDNA is usually associated with multiple nucleoli located around the periphery of the enlarged nucleus. The multiple nucleoli were described nearly a century ago, but the presence of DNA in them was first reported in the early 1940s. Proof that the nucleolar DNA was specifically rDNA and that it was amplified relative to the amount in the chromosomes came from biochemical studies on the African clawed toad, *Xenopus* (Brown and Dawid, 1968; Gall, 1968). In this sense it can be said that gene amplification was first demonstrated about 10 years ago. However, the biochemical studies merely culminated a long series of cytological observations extending back to the turn of the century, studies which suggested that some of the DNA in the nucleus resided outside the chromosomes. Certain observations, such as those of Giardina (1901) on oogenesis in the beetle *Dytiscus,* could not be correctly interpreted given the state of genetics and biochemistry at the time. Others, like Painter and Taylor's (1942) observations on the toad *Bufo,* would have been more influential had they come a few years later when the idea was more firmly established that DNA was the genetic material.

*Lecture delivered November 20, 1975.

During the past 10 years much has been learned about the molecular and cytological details of amplification in several organisms. Several summaries of the recent work are available (Gall, 1969; Macgregor, 1972; Tobler, 1975). Here I will concentrate on studies before the mid-1960s. My purpose is to show that the idea of amplification was firmly established in the cytological literature and served as a guide for the later biochemical studies. The history of the subject shows, as do many similar histories, that certain observations had to await a theoretical framework before they could be understood, and that the theoretical framework, when it came, fell at first on unreceptive ears.

II. STUDIES ON VERTEBRATE OOCYTES

During the 1870s improvements in microscopes and microscopical techniques ushered in the modern era of cytology. Within a few years, cells of many types were accurately described for the first time and all major cell components resolvable by light microscopy were detected. It was only natural that germ cells should receive much attention, since they were known to provide the physical link between generations. Amphibian oocytes were readily available; several investigators (e.g., Flemming, 1882) described their giant nucleus or "germinal vesicle" with its unusual lampbrush chromosomes and multiple, peripheral nucleoli (Figs. 1 and 2). During succeeding years multiple nucleoli were observed in a variety of vertebrate and invertebrate animals (Montgomery, 1898; Jörgensen, 1913). Observations were usually made on sections of fixed material stained in various ways. In such sections the multiple peripheral nucleoli were frequently the most prominent component of the germinal vesicle.

Nearly all observers discussed the significance of oocyte nucleoli. Since essentially nothing was known about cellular physiology at the time, the suggestions were seldom of much value. One very wrong hypothesis was that put forward by Carnoy and Lebrun (1897, 1898, 1899) based on their observations of amphibian oocytes. Because the lampbrush chromosomes became exceedingly diffuse during later stages of oogenesis, Carnoy and Lebrun concluded that they disappeared entirely, to arise *de novo* from nucleoli at a later stage. Although they were wrong about the conversion of nucleoli into chromosomes, their description of "nucléoles en anneaux" from the salamander *Pleurodeles*

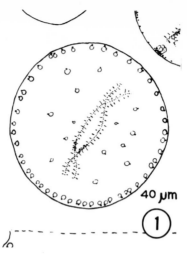

FIG. 1. Diagram of the oocyte nucleus of the toad *Bufo*. Most of the multiple nucleoli are located peripherally just beneath the nuclear membrane. Each is associated with a small Feulgen-positive granule represented as a dot between the nucleolus and the membrane. Painter and Taylor identified these granules as extrachromosomal nucleolar organizers. From Painter and Taylor (1942).

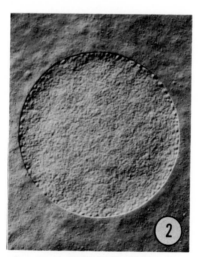

FIG. 2. The nucleus from an immature oocyte of the newt *Triturus*, showing the multiple peripheral nucleoli. The Feulgen-positive organizers are barely demonstrable in this species and cannot be seen in this photograph. Nomarski interference optics. × 190.

was probably the first mention of circular nucleoli. Such circular nucleoli were noted from time to time in later studies (Jörgensen, 1913;
Guyénot and Danon, 1953). We now know that they owe their form to
the circular rDNA molecule that constitutes their core and to which
rRNA transcripts are attached (Figs. 3 and 4).

Few early workers, or even later ones, concerned themselves with the
origin of the multiple nucleoli during early prophase in the oocyte. An
exception was Helen King (1908), who examined these stages in the
American toad *Bufo lentiginosus* (= *B. americanus*). King used a double staining procedure, safranin and gentian violet, which stained the
nucleoli vivid red and the chromosomes deep blue. She showed that
blue-staining fibers arose during the pachytene stage in association with
the first red-staining nucleoli (Fig. 5). These fibers moved with the
nucleoli to the periphery of the nucleus and eventually lay in close
contact with the multiple nucleoli just under the nuclear membrane.
Speaking of such compound nucleoli, she said: "It is evident that they

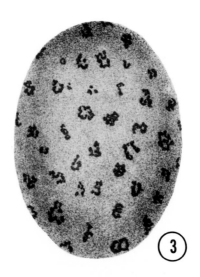

FIG. 3. Surface view of an oocyte nucleus from a deep-sea teleost fish, *Melamphaes,*
figured by Jörgensen (1913). Although circular and linear nucleoli had been seen before
by Carnoy and Lebrun (1897), this is an especially striking example.

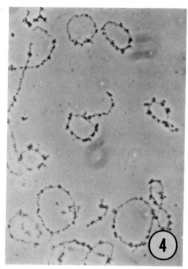

FIG. 4. Nucleolar cores in circular form derived from *Triturus* oocyte nucleoli by isolation in low-molarity saline. Miller (1964, 1966) and Kezer and Peacock (Peacock, 1965) showed that such circles are fragmented by DNase, thus providing the first evidence that amplified rDNA molecules are circular. Photograph kindly provided by O. L. Miller. Phase contrast. × 240.

contain two different substances; fine fibres which are doubtless composed of chromatin not used for the chromosomes, and rounded bodies which are nucleoli.'' It is clear that King saw the accumulation of amplified rDNA during pachytene and its subsequent migration to the nuclear periphery. Her accurate observations were seldom cited and probably had little influence on subsequent work.

Studies on nucleoli assumed added significance with the demonstration by Heitz (1931) and others that the nucleolus in somatic cells was regularly associated with a particular locus on one or more chromosomes. McClintock (1934) in a beautiful cytogenetic analysis of maize defined the *nucleolar organizer* as the chromosome region responsible for the production of the nucleolus. She examined a translocation involving a break through the organizer on chromosome 6 and found that both parts of the split organizer could produce nucleoli. She concluded

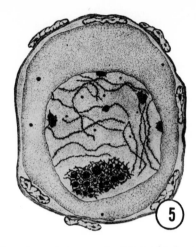

FIG. 5. Section through a pachytene oocyte of the toad *Bufo,* stained with safranin and gentian violet, from the study of Helen King (1908). In the lower part of the nucleus one can see a cluster of red-staining nucleoli associated with blue-staining fibers. Because the fibers stained the same as the chromosomes, King concluded that they consisted of a special nucleolar chromatin.

that the organizer could be subdivided without loss of function, foreshadowing later work that demonstrated the repetitive nature of the ribosomal RNA genes in the organizer.

The introduction of the Feulgen reaction (Feulgen and Rossenbeck, 1924) provided the first opportunity to identify DNA at the cellular level. This cytochemical test quickly became a great favorite among cytologists. Here at last was a stain that not only delineated chromosomes in a striking fashion in both plants and animals, but also had a firm basis in biochemistry. It was soon found that DNA was limited almost exclusively to the chromosomes within the nucleus. Nucleoli, despite their very dense structure and strong staining with various basic dyes, were Feulgen negative. Later studies showed that the basophilic nature of nucleoli was due to a high concentration of RNA (reviewed by Brachet, 1950; Caspersson, 1950).

Sections of frog and salamander oocytes were also stained with Feulgen's reagent. As anyone knows who has looked at such material, there is little stain in mature or half-grown oocytes. Indeed, most of the color is in the follicle nuclei closely appressed to the surface of the oocyte, whereas the large germinal vesicle appears at first sight to be unstained. Koltzoff (1938) maintained that the lampbrush chromosomes within the germinal vesicle completely lost their stainability and therefore contained no DNA. He argued from this that genes could not be made of DNA, since oocyte chromosomes were the carriers of the genes through the female germ line. Later workers were at pains to point out Koltzoff's error and to affirm the Feulgen-positive nature of lampbrush chromosomes.

Among those who disputed Koltzoff was Brachet (1940), who published an extensive and important account of Feulgen staining during oogenesis in frogs and salamanders. Brachet studied the frogs *Rana fusca* (= *R. temporaria*) and *R. esculenta* and the salamanders *Triton* (= *Triturus*) *alpestris* and *T. cristatus*. He obtained a positive Feulgen reaction in the chromosomes of salamanders during all stages of oogenesis, but was not able to see coloration during the most extended lampbrush stage in the frogs. He argued that the negative reaction in the frogs was due to the small size of their chromomeres. More important for the present account, Brachet found Feulgen-positive material associated with the nucleoli of *Rana*. He stated that each nucleolus adhered to a small mass which stained strongly with the Feulgen reagent and that Feulgen-positive material was detectable even in nucleoli from the most mature oocytes.

Brachet's observations on nucleolar DNA in *Rana* were confirmed and extended in a remarkable paper by Theophilus Painter and A. N. Taylor (1942) entitled "Nucleic acid storage in the toad's egg." Painter and Taylor described oocytes of the toad *Bufo valliceps* stained by the Feulgen reaction. They confirmed Brachet's observation of DNA granules associated with the peripheral nucleoli (independently, since Brachet's paper did not reach them until after their study had been completed). They also traced the origin of the nucleolar DNA granules in the earliest oocytes, showing that the extrachromosomal DNA was present even in pachytene before the oocyte had begun its growth phase. They accurately depicted the granular rDNA localized as a "cap" on the side of the nucleus opposite the free ends of the chromosomes (Fig. 6). They showed that the cluster of granules broke up and spread out along the inner border of the nuclear membrane, and stated, "About this

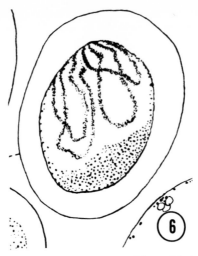

FIG. 6. Section through a pachytene oocyte of the toad *Bufo*, stained by the Feulgen reaction. A cluster of Feulgen-positive granules, identified as extrachromosomal nucleolar organizers, forms a characteristic cap on the nucleus on the side opposite to the free ends of the chromosomes. From Painter and Taylor (1942).

time small nucleoli begin to arise in association with the granules'' (Fig. 1). Painter and Taylor repeated Brachet's observations with RNase in conjunction with methyl green–pyronin staining, finding high concentrations of RNA both in the egg cytoplasm and in the multiple nucleoli. On this point they commented, ''Obviously then, the heterochromatic granules and the nucleoli associated with them are part of a mechanism for the laying down of ribonucleic acid in the cytoplasm of the toad's or frog's egg.'' No more accurate statement of the case could be made today. Painter and Taylor clearly recognized that the DNA of the nucleoli was of special importance and that an amplification of genes had taken place: ''If these nucleolar organizers are genetically the same as those which form nucleoli in ordinary somatic cells, then we may say that the germinal vesicle of the toad is highly polyploid in nucleolar organizers but otherwise lampbrush chromosomes are normal meiotic structures. Perhaps the most important aspect of the present study is the striking demonstration that chromatin can exist and function within the nucleus apart from the chromosomes.''

Occasional references were made to Brachet's and Painter and Taylor's studies during succeeding years, and later Guyénot and Danon (1953) confirmed the existence of Feulgen-positive granules in nucleoli of the frog *Rana temporaria*. Nevertheless, the subject of amplification effectively disappeared from the cytological literature for nearly a quarter of a century. In the meantime, studies on the lampbrush chromosomes made good progress following Duryee's (1937) demonstration that germinal vesicles and their chromosomes could be isolated and manipulated quite easily by hand. In unfixed preparations the nucleoli were even more prominent than the chromosomes, and they were described by several investigators (e.g., Gersch, 1940; Gall, 1954; Callan and Lloyd, 1960). In this way the stage was set for studies on the chemical composition of isolated nucleoli. Simultaneously but independently, Miller (1964, 1966) and Kezer and Peacock (Peacock, 1965) examined the effect of DNase on amphibian nucleoli. Miller studied germinal vesicles of the newt *Triturus viridescens,* whose usually spherical nucleoli can be separated into a cortex and a circular core ("beaded necklace") when isolated into low-molarity saline (Fig. 4). Kezer and Peacock studied the normally ring-shaped nucleoli of the salamander *Plethodon*. In both cases the ring nucleoli were fragmented by DNase but not by RNase or proteases. In addition to providing a new kind of evidence for DNA in oocyte nucleoli, these observations raised the possibility that the DNA might exist as a circular molecule. At about the same time studies by Brown and Gurdon (1964) and by Ritossa and Spiegelmen (1965) had established that the nucleolus organizer in somatic tissue contained the genes coding for rRNA. Both Miller and Kezer and Peacock recognized that the DNA in the multiple nucleoli might well be that which coded for rRNA. Miller introduced the term "amplification" to describe the extrachromosomal DNA, and this term has been used ever since.

Final proof of the amplification hypothesis came with the demonstration that the extra DNA in oocytes was, indeed, rDNA and was synthesized early in oogenesis as extrachromosomal copies. While examining ovaries from recently metamorphosed *Xenopus* toadlets I was struck by the massive Feulgen-positive "cap" in the pachytene nuclei (Fig. 7), and I realized immediately that Painter and Taylor had been right all along. Moreover, it was clear that the extrachromosomal DNA synthesis should be easily demonstrable by labeling young oocytes with

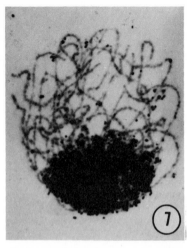

FIG. 7. Autoradiograph of a squashed pachytene oocyte nucleus of the toad *Xenopus,* hybridized *in situ* with ³H-labeled RNA complementary to rDNA. The cap of amplified rDNA hybridizes strongly and is obscured in the autoradiograph by a mass of silver grains. Note similarity to the drawings of King (Fig. 5) and Painter and Taylor (Fig. 6). Giemsa stain. × 1020.

[³H]thymidine. The labeling experiments were completed within a few weeks (Gall, 1967). The more detailed buoyant density and hybridization experiments followed soon afterward, establishing that the newly synthesized DNA in the young ovaries had the known characteristics of rDNA (Gall, 1968). At the same time Brown and Dawid (1968) independently demonstrated that *Xenopus* oocyte nuclei contained a large amount of rDNA. This they did by isolating many thousands of nuclei manually, extracting the DNA from them, and examining its buoyant density by analytical ultracentrifugation. They noted the characteristic high density of the extra rDNA, and they established its identity by showing that it hybridized with rRNA. Following these initial biochemical studies, subsequent papers have dealt with various aspects of the amplification process, both cytological and biochemical (see reviews by Gall, 1969; Macgregor, 1972; Tobler, 1975).

III. STUDIES ON INSECT OOGENESIS

Just as the first inklings of gene amplification in vertebrate oocytes can be traced back to the turn of this century, so can similar descriptions from insect oocytes be found at an early date. The most notable of these is the beautiful study by Giardina (1901) of oogenesis in the diving water beetle, *Dytiscus marginalis*. If a water beetle seems an unlikely object of study to modern workers, it should be recalled that *Dytiscus* is the most massive European insect and for years was the "standard" insect for classroom dissection; a two-volume treatise on the biology of *Dytiscus* was published by the zoologist Korschelt in 1924.

Giardina followed oogenesis in *Dytiscus* from the earliest oogonia to the fully mature oocytes. He discovered and accurately described the curious oogonial divisions in which a large mass of extrachromosomal chromatin surrounds the chromosomes at metaphase and is segregated into only one of the two division products (Figs. 9 and 10, cf. Fig. 8, which shows the corresponding stage in *Xenopus*). He showed that the four oogonial divisions produce sixteen cells, an oocyte containing the extrachromosomal chromatin and 15 nurse cells without such material. Even the most casual inspection of the ovary shows that "Giardina's ring" or Giardina's body" is a supplement to the basic chromatin content of the nucleus. It grows to enormous size during the oogonial divisions, and the nucleus that contains it stains much more intensely than adjacent nuclei. Nevertheless, Giardina interpreted his observations in terms of chromatin diminution. That is, he felt that the oocyte *retained* the total chromatin content of the organism, whereas the nurse cells *lost* the material represented by the extrachromosomal chromatin. This incorrect interpretation was repeated in Wilson's book, "The Cell in Development and Heredity" (1928), whence it was absorbed by many students over the years. The misinterpretation arose by supposing that Giardina's body in the oogonia was equivalent to the eliminated chromatin of *Ascaris* eggs, made famous by the observations and speculations of Boveri (1888) and Weismann (1892). In their scheme of development the germ line retained the full complement of hereditary determinants. The somatic cells, on the other hand, received only a part of the chromatin, the rest being eliminated during the cleavage divisions or later. To analogize the cases of *Ascaris* and *Dytiscus*, it was neces-

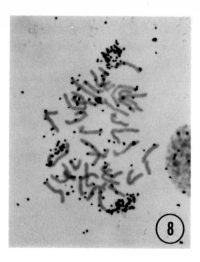

FIG. 8. Autoradiograph of an oogonial mitosis of the toad *Xenopus* hybridized *in situ* as in Fig. 7. Amplification is present in these oogonia, but the amount of extra-chromosomal rDNA is not nearly so great as in the oogonia of the beetle *Dytiscus* (Figs. 9 and 10). The small clumps of amplified rDNA can be detected among the chromosomes by staining, but they are more convincingly shown by autoradiography after *in situ* hybridization with rRNA. Giemsa stain. × 1100.

sary to suppose that for some reason chromatin elimination in *Dytiscus* was delayed, occurring not in the cleavage stages of the embryo, but in the oogonial divisions of the adult. These divisions would be much later in time, but, as so neatly diagrammed by Wilson, they would be only a few cell divisions later in *Dytiscus* than in *Ascaris,* since in both cases the presumptive germ cells were sequestered early in embryogenesis. Undoubtedly Wilson's repetition of Giardina's error hindered later workers from recognizing the essential similarity of gene amplification in insects and vertebrates.

The next important step in understanding amplification in insects was made by Bauer (1933), who studied several different species using the Feulgen reaction. Bauer showed that Giardina's body in *Dytiscus* contained DNA, thereby establishing the existence of extrachromosomal nuclear DNA for the first time. In the same paper Bauer described the prominent DNA body in oocytes of the crane fly *Tipula* and the somewhat less striking body in two species of mosquito.

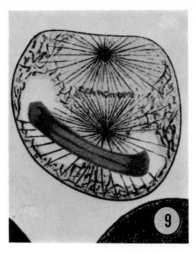

FIG. 9. A section through a dividing oogonium of the beetle, *Dytiscus,* redrawn by Jörgensen (1913) from the original of Giardina (1901). The chromosomes on the metaphase spindle are dwarfed by the massive ring of rDNA (Giardina's body). Only one of the two daughter cells receives the rDNA. Giardina's original figure was unfortunately available to me only in a copy not suitable for reproduction.

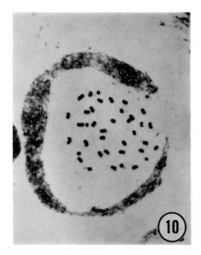

FIG. 10. A squash preparation of a dividing oogonium of the beetle *Dytiscus.* The tiny chromosomes are surrounded by a nearly complete ring of rDNA. *Dytiscus* has a much greater amount of rDNA in its oogonia than other investigated organisms (cf. Fig. 8). Giemsa stain. × 640.

Several studies were made on the extrachromosomal DNA of insect oocytes during the next three decades (Johnson, 1938; Bayreuther, 1956; Lima-de-Faria, 1962; Urbani and Russo-Caia, 1964), but the significance of this material was not guessed until the mid-1960s. Work on three organisms, the beetle *Dytiscus,* the cricket *Acheta,* and the crane fly *Tipula,* converged to produce a coherent picture of gene amplification. In each case morphological and cytochemical studies showed that the extra DNA was associated with nucleolus-like material and that RNA was being synthesized in association with the DNA body (Lima-de-Faria and Moses, 1966; Nilsson, 1966; Bier *et al.,* 1967; Heinonen and Halkka, 1967; Kunz, 1967a,b, 1969; Lima-de-Faria *et al.,* 1968). It was concluded that the extra DNA was involved with the synthesis of nucleolar RNA. Since other studies had shown that nucleoli contained primarily ribosomal RNA precursors, it was postulated that the extra DNA was rDNA. It should be noted that this conclusion was drawn before it was shown biochemically that the RNA and DNA under consideration were ribosomal.

Biochemical evidence was not long in coming. Gall *et al.* (1969) showed by nucleic acid hybridization that the ovary of the water beetle *Colymbetes* contained a large excess of rDNA, and the same was suggested for *Dytiscus.* In *Dytiscus* the situation was confused by the existence of a large satellite DNA of nearly the same buoyant density in CsCl as the rDNA. This led to the mistaken interpretation that the satellite and rDNA were physically related, a mistake corrected in a later study (Gall and Rochaix, 1974). Lima-de-Faria *et al.* (1969) showed that oocytes of the cricket *Acheta* contained an excess of rDNA compared to testis and somatic tissue.

Thus studies on rDNA amplification in insects followed much the same course as those in vertebrates. Morphological papers at the turn of the century provided evidence that something unusual was happening in oocytes. Next the Feulgen reaction was applied, and it was realized that extrachromosomal DNA occurred in association with nucleoli. The correct interpretation was then enunciated—in 1942 for amphibian oocytes, but not until the early 1960s for the insects. Finally, the extra DNA was studied biochemically and was shown to have the properties of rDNA. Clearly the exact time when gene amplification was "discovered" is hard to pinpoint.

REFERENCES

Bauer, H. (1933). *Z. Zellforsch. Mikrosk. Anat.* **18,** 254–298.

Bayreuther, K. (1956). *Chromosoma* **7,** 508–557.

Bier, K., Kunz, W., and Ribbert, D. (1967). *Chromosoma* **23,** 214–254.

Boveri, T. (1888). Zellen-Studien 2: "Die Befruchtung und Teilung des Eies von *Ascaris megalocephala.*" Fischer, Jena.

Brachet, J. (1940). *Arch. Biol.* **51,** 151–165.

Brachet, J. (1950). "Chemical Embryology." Wiley (Interscience), New York.

Brown, D. D., and Dawid, I. B. (1968). *Science* **160,** 272–280.

Brown, D. D., and Gurdon, J. B. (1964). *Proc. Natl. Acad. Sci. U.S.A.* **51,** 139–146.

Callan, H. G., and Lloyd, L. (1960). *Philos. Trans. R. Soc. London Ser. B* **243,** 135–219.

Carnoy, J. B., and Lebrun, H. (1897). *Cellule* **12,** 191–295.

Carnoy, J. B., and Lebrun, H. (1898). *Cellule* **14,** 113–200.

Carnoy, J. B., and Lebrun, H. (1899). *Cellule* **16,** 303–401.

Caspersson, T. (1950). "Cell Growth and Cell Function." Norton, New York.

Duryee, W. R. (1937). *Arch. Exp. Zellforsch. Besonders Gewebezuecht.* **19,** 171–176.

Feulgen, R., and Rossenbeck, H. (1924). *Hoppe-Seyler's Z. Physiol. Chem.* **135,** 203–248.

Flemming, W. (1882). "Zellsubstanz, Kern, und Zelltheilung." Vogel, Leipzig.

Gall, J. G. (1954). *J. Morphol.* **94,** 283–351.

Gall, J. G. (1967). *J. Cell Biol.* **35,** 43A.

Gall, J. G. (1968). *Proc. Natl. Acad. Sci. U.S.A.* **60,** 553–560.

Gall, J. G. (1969). *Genetics* **61,** Suppl., 121–132.

Gall, J. G. (1974). *Proc. Natl. Acad. Sci. U.S.A.* **71,** 3078–3081.

Gall, J. G., and Rochaix, J.-D. (1974). *Proc. Natl. Acad. Sci. U.S.A.* **71,** 1819–1823.

Gall, J. G., Macgregor, H. C., and Kidston, M. E. (1969). *Chromosoma* **26,** 169–187.

Gersch, M. (1940). *Z. Zellforsch. Mikrosk. Anat.* **30,** 483–528.

Giardina, A. (1901). *Int. Monatsschr. Anat. Physiol.* **18,** 418–484.

Guyénot, E., and Danon, M. (1953). *Rev. Suisse Zool.* **60,** 1–129.

Heinonen, L., and Halkka, O. (1967). *Ann. Med. Exp. Biol. Fenn.* **45,** 101–109.

Heitz, E. (1931). *Planta* **15,** 495–505.

Johnson, M. W. (1938). *J. Morphol.* **62,** 113–139.

Jörgensen, M. (1913). *Arch. Zellforsch. Mikrosk. Anat.* **10,** 1–126.

King, H. D. (1908). *J. Morphol.* **19,** 369–438.

Koltzoff, N. K. (1938). *Biol. Zh.* **7,** 3–46. (In Russian with English summary.)

Korschelt, E. (1924). "Bearbeitung Einheimischer Tiere. Der Gelbrand *Dytiscus marginalis* L." Engelmann, Leipzig.

Kunz, W. (1967a). *Chromosoma* **20,** 332–370.

Kunz, W. (1967b). *Chromosoma* **21,** 446–462.

Kunz, W. (1969). *Chromosoma* **26,** 41–75.

Lima-de-Faria, A. (1962). *Chromosoma* **13,** 47–59.

Lima-de-Faria, A., and Moses, M. J. (1966). *J. Cell Biol.* **30,** 177–192.

Lima-de-Faria, A., Nilsson, B., Cave, D., Puga, A., and Jaworska, H. (1968). *Chromosoma* **25,** 1–20.

Lima-de-Faria, A., Birnstiel, M., and Jaworska, H. (1969). *Genetics* **61,** Suppl., 145–159.

McClintock, B. (1934). *Z. Zellforsch. Mikrosk. Anat.* **21,** 294–328.

Macgregor, H. C. (1972). *Biol. Rev. Cambridge Phil. Soc.* **47,** 177–210.

Miller, O. L. (1964). *J. Cell Biol.* **23,** 60A.

Miller, O. L. (1966). *Natl. Cancer Inst. Monogr.* **23,** 53–66.

Montgomery, T. H. (1898). *J. Morphol.* **15,** 266–560.

Nilsson, B. (1966). *Hereditas* **56,** 396–398.

Painter, T. S., and Taylor, A. N. (1942). *Proc. Natl. Acad. Sci. U.S.A.* **28,** 311–317.

Peacock, W. J. (1965). *Natl. Cancer Inst. Monogr.* **18,** 101–131.

Ritossa, F. M., and Spiegelman, S. (1965). *Proc. Natl. Acad. Sci. U.S.A.* **53,** 737–745.

Tobler, H. (1975). *In* "Biochemistry of Animal Development" (R. Weber, ed.), Vol. 3, pp. 91–143. Academic Press, New York.

Trendelenburg, M., Spring, H., Scheer, U., and Franke, W. F. (1974). *Proc. Natl. Acad. Sci. U.S.A.* **71,** 3626–3630.

Urbani, E., and Russo-Caia, S. (1964). *Rend. Ist. Sci. Univ. Camerino* **5,** 19–50.

Vogt, V. M., and Braun, R. (1976). *J. Mol. Biol.* **106,** 567–587.

Weismann, A. (1892). "Das Keimplasma. Eine Theorie der Vererbung." Fischer, Jena.

Wilson, E. B. (1928). "The Cell in Development and Heredity." Macmillan, New York.

Yao, M.-C., Kimmel, A., and Gorovsky, M. (1974). *Proc. Natl. Acad. Sci. U.S.A.* **71,** 3082–3086.

CONTROL OF ADENOHYPOPHYSIAL FUNCTIONS BY PEPTIDES OF THE CENTRAL NERVOUS SYSTEM*

ROGER GUILLEMIN

*Laboratories for Neuroendocrinology,
The Salk Institute, La Jolla, California*

T HE text of this review borrows heavily from several specific papers as well as reviews written over the last few years either by me alone or with several of my senior collaborators. There should be, after all, only one way to describe a scientific object. This text should provide the reader uninitiated in the field with a solid appraisal of the various concepts involved, with descriptions of the progression of the mind (an inadequate anglicization of the hard-to-translate ''démarche de l'esprit'') from the humble beginnings in the 1950s to the extraordinary current expansion of these concepts as well as that of the results they have generated of clinical relevance. The text does not, however, attempt to be fully descriptive of methodology, even when entirely new scientific instruments had to be devised to answer one question or another; that is handled simply by referring to the pertinent papers of description and validation.

I. THE EXISTENCE OF BRAIN PEPTIDES CONTROLLING ADENOHYPOPHYSIAL FUNCTIONS. ISOLATION AND CHARACTERIZATION OF THEIR MOLECULAR STRUCTURES

In the early 1950s, based on the anatomical observations and physiological experimentation from several groups in the United States and Europe, it became abundantly clear that the endocrine secretions of the anterior lobe of the hypophysis—well known by then to control all the functions of all the target endocrine glands (thyroid, gonads, adrenal cortex) plus the overall somatic growth of the individual—were some-

---

*Lecture delivered January 8, 1976.

how entirely regulated by some integrative mechanism located in neuronal elements of the ventral hypothalamus. Because of the peculiar anatomy of the junctional region between ventral hypothalamus (floor of the 3rd ventricle) and the parenchymal tissue of the anterior lobe of the pituitary (Fig. 1), the mechanisms involved in this hypothalamic control of adenohypophysial functions were best explained by propos-

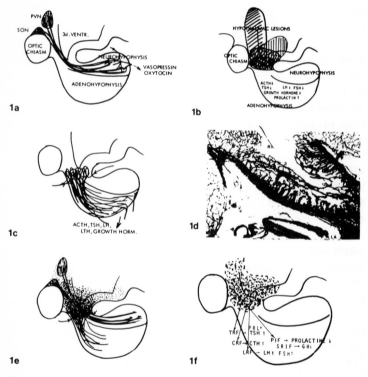

Fig. 1. (a) Diagrammatic representation of the pituitary gland and the innervation of the neurohypophysis by nerve fibers from the n. paraventricularis (PVN) and supraopticus (SON). (b) Localized lesions in the hypothalamus produce changes in the pituitary secretion of the various adenohypophysial hormones (increase ↑, or decrease ↓). (c) Diagrammatic representation of the hypothalamohypophysial portal system. (d) Photomicrograph of the hypothalamohypophysial portal system after injection with an opaque dye. (e) Diagrammatic representation of the hypophysiotropic area. (f) Changes in pituitary secretion of various adenohypophysial hormones (increase ↑, or decrease ↓).

ing the existence of some secretory product(s) by some (uncharacterized) neuronal elements of the ventral hypothalamus; these products would somehow reach the adenohypophysis by the peculiar capillary vessels observed, as if to join the floor of the hypothalamus to the pituitary gland.

That concept was definitely ascertained in 1952 by simple experiments using combined tissue cultures of fragments of the pituitary gland and of the ventral hypothalamus (Guillemin and Rosenberg, 1955). The search for means of characterizing the hypothetical hypothalamic hypophysiotropic factors started then. Simple reasoning and early chemical confirmation led to the hypothesis that these unknown substances would be small peptides. After several years of pilot studies involving both biology and relatively simple chemistry in several laboratories in the United States, Europe, and Japan, it became clear that characterizing these hypothalamic hypophysiotropic substances would be a challenge of (originally) unsuspected proportions. Entirely novel bioassays would have to be devised for routine testing of a large number of fractions generated by the chemical purification schemes; more sobering still was the realization in the early 1960s that enormous amounts of hypothalamic fragments (from slaughterhouse animals) would have to be obtained to have available a sufficient quantity of starting material to attempt a meaningful program of chemical isolation. The early pilot studies has indeed shown the hypothalamic substances to be extremely potent and, on the basis of simple assumptions, to be present in each hypothalamic fragment only in a few nanogram quantities. Essentially one laboratory, then two, both in the United States, approached the problem with enough constancy and resolution to stay with it for the 10 years that it took to provide the first of its definitive solution, i.e., the primary structure of one of the hypothalamic hypophysiotropic factors: My own laboratory, then at Baylor College of Medicine in Houston, Texas, organized the collection over several years of more than 5 million sheep brains, handling in the laboratory more than 50 tons of hypothalamic fragments. Schally's group, in the Tulane University School of Medicine in New Orleans after he had left my laboratory at Baylor, collected also very large numbers of porcine hypothalamic fragments. Late in 1968, from 300,000 sheep hypothalami, Burgus and I isolated 1.0 mg of the first of these hypothalamic hypophysiotropic peptides, the thyrotropin-releasing factor (TRF), the molecule by which the hypothalamus regulates through the pituitary the functions of the thyroid gland.

The following year, after more technical difficulties were overcome, the primary structure of ovine TRF was established by my group as that of the deceivingly simple tripeptide pGlu-His-Pro-NH$_2$. The material of porcine origin was shown later by Schally and his collaborators to be identical. The synthetic replicate, rapidly available in unlimited quantities, was shown to be highly potent in all vertebrate species, particularly in man; it is now widely used throughout the world in a highly sensitive test of pituitary function, an early means of detection of pituitary tumors in man.

The isolation and characterization of TRF was the result of an enormous effort. It was also the turning point that separated doubt—and often confusion—from unquestionable knowledge. It was of such heuristic significance that I can say that neuroendocrinology became an established science on that event. Because of this unique significance of the characterization of TRF, I will describe in some detail in this review, how it was done. I will be brief to the point of laconism in the description of the isolation of LRF, somatostatin, and the endorphins.

A. Purification, Isolation, and Characterization of TRF

Despite earlier claims based on questionable methodology, which proved to be incorrect in their conclusions as to the chemical characterization of TRF but turned out also to be (unwittingly) correct in much of their physiological conclusions (what we term in this laboratory "the prophetic literature"), the first incontrovertible evidence for the existence and early purification of a hypothalamic TSH-releasing factor (TRF) appeared in 1962 (Guillemin *et al.*, 1962). A 2 *N* acetic acid extract of several hundred sheep hypothalamic fragments was filtered on Sephadex G-25, and in the bioassay animals (Yamazaki *et al.*, 1962a,b) two zones of activity were found in the effluent. One corresponded to nonretarded materials, thus showing that these were substances with TSH-like activity in the hypothalamic extract. The other zone, which was strongly retarded on the gel (elution volume similar to that of α-MSH, preceding that of arginine-vasopressin), was active in the assay animals with an intact pituitary, and its biological activity (release of TSH) was inhibited by pretreatment with thyroxine. Furthermore, it stimulated secretion of TSH *in vitro* when added directly to incubated fragments of rat pituitary tissues. The conclusion was drawn that the material so purified corresponded to the then hypothetical TRF of hypothalamic origin. The biological activity of this crude preparation was resistant to heating and to incubation with trypsin but was destroyed during incubation with pepsin (Jutisz *et al.*, 1963a) or by 6 *N* HCl hydrolysis (110°C, 24 hours). The material having TRF activity, obtained from gel filtration, considered to be polypeptide in nature, was rapidly further purified by ion-exchange chromatography on carboxymethyl cellulose (CMC) (Jutisz *et al.*, 1963b).

These early observations were amply confirmed by subsequent investigators using extracts of the hypothalamus of sheep, pig, beef, rats, guinea pigs, mice, rabbits, and fragments of human brain origin (reviews in Guillemin, 1964, 1967; Schally *et al.*, 1968; McCann and Porter, 1969).

Guillemin *et al.* (1965) later reported purification of ovine TRF from 2 *N* acetic acid extracts of acetone powder from 80,000 sheep hypothalamic fragments by gel filtration, countercurrent distribution (CCD), ion-exchange chromatography on IRC-50, and finally thin-layer chromatography (TLC), obtaining 400 μg of material active at approximately 100 ng per dose *in vivo*. TRF activity was found in a ninhydrin-positive, Pauly-positive zone on TLC; amino acid composition after 6 *N* HCl hydrolysis was Lys, His 4, Thr, Ser, Glu 3, Pro 3, Gly, Ala, Met, Leu, Tyr. However, a final quantitative analysis was not claimed because of the small quantities of peptide available, and it was noted that a much larger quantity of brain fragments would be needed to approach the amino acid sequence.

Partial purification of bovine TRF was described by Schally *et al.* (1966a, 1968) and by Tsuji *et al.* (1968); bovine TRF showed properties similar to those of ovine TRF on gel-filtration and CMC chromatography (Schally *et al.*, 1966a, 1968) and was reported to be retarded by Sephadex G-50 and DEAE-cellulose (Tsuji *et al.*, 1968).

In a sequence of purification reported by Schally *et al.* (1966c), which included gel filtration of 2 *N* acetic acid–glacial acetic acid extracts of 20,000 lyophilized hypothalami, phenol extraction, CMC chromatography and CCD, porcine TRF showed properties similar or identical to those obtained for bovine and ovine TRF. Free-flow electrophoresis of this material yielded 900 μg of a TRF reported to be active at 10 ng *in vivo* and 0.1 ng *in vitro,* which on hydrolysis gave the amino acid analysis: Gly 1, His 5, Pro 5, Thr 6, Leu 0.5, Ser 0.6, and Lys 0.4. After a private communication from me, Schally later revised this amino acid analysis to Glu 6 instead of Thr 6.

By that time (1966) it had become obvious (Guillemin, 1964) that huge quantities of hypothalamic tissue would have to be procured and processed in order to obtain sufficient amounts of any of the releasing factors before meaningful chemical studies could be performed. There was rather slow progress in the elucidation of the structure of TRF during the next 3–4 years; during this time, the logistics of collecting and extracting large quantities of hypothalamic fragments was organized. Our laboratory worked with tissues of ovine origin; Schally and co-workers worked primarily with tissues of porcine origin. During this period, a number of preliminary reports appeared from both laboratories reporting progress and tribulations in the development of purification schemes and observations on the chemical nature of TRF (Schally *et al.,* 1966a, 1968, 1969; Guillemin, 1964, 1968; Guillemin *et al.,* 1965, Burgus *et al.,* 1966b; Burgus and Guillemin, 1967) and describing the processing of about 3/4 million ovine hypothalamic fragments. Schally *et al.* (1968) summarized at the 1967 Laurentian Hormone Conference, and later with additional data (1969) their purification scheme for porcine TRF, and Burgus and Guillemin (1970) presented their final purification sequence for ovine TRF in early 1969. Although there were some differences in the final versions of extraction methods and the order of application of certain purification steps, the final schemes utilized by the two laboratories were essentially identical in several purification steps and very similar in others.

Schally *et al.* (1966b, 1968) described the purification of TRF from 100,000 porcine hypothalami according to the scheme published in 1966 (1966b) with an additional partition-chromatography stage, recording a yield of 2.8 mg of TRF, reported to be active at doses ≤1 ng *in vivo.* This material, which was judged to be homogeneous by TLC and thin-layer electrophoresis (TLE) contained the amino acids Glu, His, Pro in essentially equimolar ratio, accounting for 30% of the weight of the preparation. It was later subjected to additional stages of partition chromatography, adsorption chromatography on charcoal, analytical gel filtration, and finally paper chromatography (Schally *et al.,* 1969). No change in the amino acid content or specific biological activ-

ity was reported. Another batch of 165,000 porcine hypothalamic fragments was purified by the same scheme, producing essentially an identical material with a slightly higher amino acid content (33.6%), with a
reported total yield from 265,000 hypothalami of 7.2 mg of "pure
TRF."

The final scheme for purification of ovine TRF described by Burgus
and Guillemin (1970) utilized an organic solvent extraction; the extract
was then further purified by ultrafiltration through an ion-exchange
membrane, gel filtration, partition chromatography, adsorption
chromatography on charcoal, and finally partition chromatography in a
second system. Each of the chromatographic steps was repeated before
proceeding to the next step.

The alcohol–chloroform extraction procedure, including a glacial
acetic acid–ether precipitation step as in the Kamm procedure (Kamm *et
al.*, 1928), had the advantage over procedures used previously in that a
considerable weight reduction was achieved in a batch process; together
with the ultrafiltration step, it yielded a material of sufficiently high
specific activity so that the extract from over a quarter million
hypothalamic fragments could be applied to a single preparative column
(15×150 cm) for gel filtration, whereas 20–25 columns of this size
would have been required otherwise (Guillemin *et al.*, 1965, 1968;
Schally *et al.*, 1966b). However, these two steps introduced some difficulties that arose from rather interesting properties of the crude materials. The solvent extraction procedure yielded a TRF-active material
that was not as firmly bound to CM-Sephadex as material derived from
$2 N$ acetic acid extraction and gel filtration (Guillemin, 1968; Guillemin
et al., 1968; Burgus *et al.*, 1966a; Burgus and Guillemin, 1967). It was
also observed that the TRF activity which passed through the ultrafiltration membrane was not retarded to the same extent as the original
extract on refiltration; the same observation appeared to hold true for
material that had passed unadsorbed through the CM-Sephadex columns. These were the first observations indicating that the molecular
weight of TRF could be much below 1000. Second, it is tempting to
speculate that the apparent changes in behavior observed in the early
stages of purification of the hypothalamic factor may have resulted from
binding of the low molecular weight materials to a larger molecule
whose size and/or charge governed the behavior of the complex. Such a
hypothesis would also explain the retention of TRF on anion-exchange

columns observed by Tsuji *et al.* (1968), an observation that is not consistent with the structure of isolated TRF (see below) since the molecule has no free anionic groups.

The yield from 270,000 sheep hypothalamic fragments was 1 mg of TRF having a biological activity of 57,000 ± 9900 TRF U/mg [see Guillemin and Sakiz (1965) for a definition of the TRF unit]; it was active at ≤15 ng *in vivo* in a mouse assay described by Redding *et al.* (1966) identical in design to the rat assay described by Yamazaki *et al.* (1963a,b), but of greater sensitivity because it used a much smaller animal, and less than 0.1 ng *in vitro* (see Guillemin and Vale, 1970). Although the last steps of purification of ovine TRF indicated a constant specific biological activity by statistical criteria and the material appeared to be homogeneous as assessed by TLC in four different systems at 5-µg loads using a variety of visualization tests, we did not claim "isolation" or homogeneity of the material at that time because of the difficulties of proving this point without wasting precious supplies; we pointed out that, as proof of homogeneity, such simple methods as multiple TLC should be considered with caution—a view that we were happy to see shared later by others working in the field (Folkers *et al.*, 1969; Bøler *et al.*, 1969).

Total recovery of ovine TRF in terms of units of biological activity based on 4-point bioassays was about 20% for nine steps of purification (about 85% average recovery per step). Schally *et al.* (1969) claimed a recovery of porcine TRF of over 90% during each purification step for eleven steps of purification (theoretical overall recovery at 90% per step is calculated to be about 30% for 11 steps); however it is unclear upon what these figures were based: if we calculate total number of minimal effective doses *in vivo* based on the weights, and the minimal effective dose reported for porcine TRF at each step, there appears to be a fluctuation between 2 million and 18 million total doses throughout the purification scheme, with an overall recovery of 115%.

For some time there were reasons to question whether ovine TRF was a simple homomeric polypeptide: the low content of amino acids (5–8%) in HCl hydrolyzates of ovine TRF preparations which had been carried through several purification steps and were apparently homogeneous in TLC and TLE with a variety of visualization tests, together with the observation that amino acids did not appear to concentrate during the last few stages of purification (Guillemin *et al.*, 1968), had led us to question the long-held hypothesis that TRF was a simple polypeptide. Subsequent observations that pepsin, trypsin, Pronase, carboxypeptidases A and B, and leucineaminopeptidase failed to inactivate TRF (Burgus *et al.,* 1966b), that the biological activity always accompanied a Pauly-positive, but ninhydrin-negative zone on TLC or TLE, that dansylation followed by two-dimensional chromatoelectrophoresis gave no evidence of free amino groups, and finally that an apparently constant specific biological activity was maintained in the last stages of purification (Burgus *et al.,* 1966b; Burgus and Guillemin, 1967) did nothing to shake this hypothesis. However, infrared (IR) and high-resolution nuclear magnetic resonance (NMR) spectra suggested an alicyclic or heterocyclic structure and were still compatible with a polypeptide, as clearly stated in several notes reporting these results (Guillemin, 1967; Burgus *et al.,* 1966a,b; Burgus and Guillemin, 1967).

Schally *et al.* (1966b, 1968) made similar observations finding that all the enzymes that had been tested for ovine TRF (Burgus *et al.,* 1966b), plus papain, subtilisin, and Nagarse, failed to inactivate porcine TRF (Schally *et al.,* 1969). Porcine TRF activity was also associated with a ninhydrin-negative, Pauly-positive zone in all chromatographic and electrophoretic systems tested (Schally *et al.,* 1966b, 1968, 1969). Schally *et al.* thus *concluded* that TRF was not a simple polypeptide; the material which they considered to be homogeneous consistently yielded approximately 30% total amino acid content as Glu, His, and Pro in equimolar ratio. They thus reasoned that these three amino acids were part of the TRF molecule, since on TLC or TLE, TRF activity was always associated with a Pauly-positive zone that yielded the three amino acids on hydrolysis; moreover, they observed that treatment of porcine TRF with Pauly reagent (Schally *et al.,* 1966b, 1968, 1969) or *N*-bromosuccinimide (Schally *et al.,* 1968, 1969) resulted in loss of biological activity. [The loss of biological activity of ovine TRF after treatment with Pauly reagent in solution (Guillemin, 1968; Burgus and Guillemin, 1970) had also been observed.] Schally *et al.* (1968, 1969) further observed that 8 synthetic tripeptides containing Glu, His, Pro, or Gln in equimolar ratios were inactive in doses up to 10,000 times greater than doses of natural porcine TRF, and thus they concluded that the "nonpeptide moiety which formed up to 70% of the TRF molecule was necessary for biological activity."

In January 1969, with the new supply of highly purified ovine TRF available (Burgus and Guillemin, 1970), amino acid analysis of $6 N$ HCl hydrolyzates of this preparation revealed only the amino acids Glu, His, and Pro, which occurred in exactly equimolar ratios and accounted for 81% of the preparation (theoretical contribution of His, Pro, and Glu for a tripeptide monoacetate calculates to 86%). Furthermore the ultraviolet (UV), IR, and NMR spectra obtained with that preparation of TRF were consistent with those of a polypeptide, and upon close examination most of the characteristics of those spectra could be accounted for by the structural features of the amino acids found in the hydrolyzates of TRF. Moreover, the solubility properties and the lack of volatility observed in attempts to obtain mass spectra or to perform gas chromatography (Burgus *et al.*, 1969b), as well as other analytical data, were consistent with those of a polypeptide; also, the lack of effect of proteolytic enzymes could be related to the particular amino acids observed. With the analyses of the more highly purified material unmistakably showing the amino acids to account for the total weight of the preparation, the hypothesis that TRF could be a heteromeric polypeptide was therefore abandoned in favor of the possibility that it might be a cyclic or a protected peptide, a view compatible with failure to detect an N-terminus (Schally *et al.*, 1966b, 1968, 1969; Burgus *et al.*, 1966b; Burgus and Guillemin, 1967, 1970; Guillemin, 1968) or a C-terminus (Schally *et al.*, 1969; Burgus and Guillemin, 1970) as well as the resistance of the biological activity to proteases.

The knowledge that the amino acids His, Pro, and Glu not only occurred in equimolar ratio in porcine and ovine TRF but indeed accounted for almost the theoretical total weight of the molecule in the case of ovine TRF, along with the previous knowledge of a lack of an N-terminal amino acid, led us to reexamine derivatives of polypeptides containing equimolar ratios of these amino acids to serve at least as possible models for the methodology to be used in the characterization of ovine TRF. We tested for TRF activity 6 tripeptide isomers containing L-His, L-Pro, and L-Glu synthesized upon our request by Gillessen *et al.* (1970) (containing only the peptides involving the α-carboxyl group of glutamic acid). The tripeptides proved to be devoid of TRF activity, confirming the earlier results of Schally *et al.* (1968, 1969). Following treatment of each of the six tripeptides by acetic anhydride in an effort to protect the N-terminus as in natural TRF, the acetylation mixture from one, and only one, of the peptides, namely H-Glu-His-Pro-OH, showed biological activity qualitatively indistinguishable from that of natural TRF. It was active in *in vivo* and *in vitro* assays specific for TRF, and its action *in vivo* was blocked by prior injection of the animals with thyroxine (Burgus *et al.*, 1969a). The specific activity of the material obtained (15 TRF U/mg) was lower than that of purified natural TRF (ca. 50,000 TRF U/mg), and preliminary experiments with TLC of the acetylation mixture of Glu-His-Pro demonstrated several zones, Pauly-positive or -negative, having TRF activity. The nature of several possible reaction products was considered: monoacetyl or diacetyl derivatives, polymers of Glu-His-Pro, and cyclic peptide derivatives or derivatives containing pyroglutamic acid (pGlu) as the N-terminus. Subsequently we reported (Burgus et al., 1969b) that the major product, by weight, of this procedure was indeed pGlu-His-Pro-OH. The material was isolated from the reaction mixture, and its structure was confirmed by mass spectrometry of the methyl ester and by its identity to authentic pGlu-His-Pro-OH (Gillessen *et al.*, 1970) on TLC, the IR spectrum as well as similarity of specific biological activity *in vivo* (7–15 TRF U/mg). This represented the first demonstration of a fully characterized synthetic molecule, based on the known composition of natural TRF, to reproduce the biological activity of a releasing factor.

Several other products present in the acetylation mixture, some possibly having higher specific activity than pGlu-His-Pro-OH, were not characterized. It is of interest that acetyl-Glu-His-Pro-OH obtained by total synthesis (Gillessen *et al.*, 1970) was devoid of TRF activity in the *in vivo* assay at doses up to 250 μg (Burgus *et al.*, 1969a,b).

Because of the differences between the specific biological activities of pGlu-His-Pro-OH and natural ovine TRF and the different behavior of these two compounds in various chromatographic systems, it was evident that TRF was not pGlu-His-Pro-OH as such. It was the proposal of Burgus based on knowledge of the primary structures of other biologically active polypeptides (vasopressin, oxytocin, gastrin, etc.) that a likely candidate for the structure of the natural material would be pGlu-His-Pro-NH$_2$, and its synthesis was approached through the simple procedure of methanolysis of the methyl ester, pGlu-His-Pro-OMe (Burgus *et al.*, 1969b, 1970a,b). The ester, prepared by treatment of the pure synthetic pGlu-His-Pro-OH with methanolic HCl, was purified by partition chromatography and identified as pGlu-His-Pro-OMe on the

basis of its behavior on TLC, its IR spectrum, and by mass spectrometry
(Burgus *et al.*, 1969b). It had biological activity *in vivo* (28,600 ± 6700
TRF U/mg) approaching half of the specific activity of isolated ovine
TRF (57,000 ± 9900 TRF U/mg); the compound was active *in vivo* at
≤10 ng and *in vitro* at 1.0 ng. Ammonolysis of the methyl ester in
methanol produced a material that upon partition chromatography gave
a small yield of a substance, presumably pGlu-His-Pro-NH$_2$, occurring
in a Pauly-positive zone separated from the starting material, which had
a higher specific activity *in vivo* (44,000 ± 1000 TRF U/mg) with a
minimum active dose *in vivo* at ≤5 ng/animal and *in vitro* at ≤1.0 ng.
The properties of pGlu-His-Pro-OMe and pGlu-His-Pro-NH$_2$ were
compared to the totally synthetic compounds (see also Gillessen *et al.*,
1970) pGlu-His-Pro-OH and pGlu-His-Pro-NH$_2$. Among the derivatives
tested, the properties of ovine TRF most closely matched that of the
amide, failing to separate from the synthetic compound in four different
systems of TLC when run in mixtures. The IR spectra of several of the
more highly purified preparations of the amide, including pGlu-His-
Pro-NH$_2$ prepared by total synthesis, were almost identical to that of
ovine TRF, showing only minor differences in two regions of the
spectra. These new observations, together with the demonstration that
the specific activity of the pGlu-His-Pro-NH$_2$ was not statistically different from that of natural ovine TRF, led us to reconsider (Burgus *et
al.*, (1969c, 1970a) an earlier hypothesis (Burgus *et al.*, 1969b) that
ovine TRF may have a secondary or tertiary amide on the C-terminal
proline, rather than correspond to the primary amide of the tripeptide
pGlu-His-Pro. Folkers *et al.* (1969) and Bowers *et al.* (1969) reported
that they had demonstrated biological activity in a mixture of derivatives
of a synthetic peptide H-Glu-His-Pro-OH. The synthetic preparation,
judged by the authors to be not over 80% pure, was treated in a manner
very similar to that previously described by Burgus *et al.* (1969a,b),
i.e., ammonolysis of the methyl ester, with the exception that the ammonolysis was carried out at a lower temperature. The conditions used
were expected to produce both the pyroglutamyl N-terminus and the
amide derivative at the carbonyl terminus. The material obtained, called
"preparation A," was ninhydrin negative and Pauly positive, indicating
that closure of Glu to pGlu had indeed occurred. Samples of "preparation A" were subjected directly to biological tests without purification;
doses of 6–54 ng were claimed to be active *in vivo,* 2–18 ng of porcine

TRF giving similar responses (Folkers *et al.*, 1969; Bowers *et al.*, 1970). The activity of the synthetic reaction mixture appeared to be inhibited by triiodothyronine and by incubation with human plasma in agreement with the results obtained by Burgus *et al.* (1969a). The reported lack of response by oral administration (Folkers *et al.*, 1969; Bowers *et al.*, 1969) was in disagreement with the results of Vale *et al.* (1970) using pure tripeptide-OMe or amide, which showed activity at ≤1 mg/dose. Probably, the doses administered by Folkers *et al.* (1969) and Bowers *et al.* (1969) of the crude material were too low to give a response; indeed Bowers *et al.* later (1970) reported oral activity of pGlu-His-Pro-NH$_2$ at doses essentially similar to those used by us. Similar reactions carried out by Folkers *et al.* (1969) on the derivatives of Glu-Pro-His, Pro-His-Gln, and Pro-His-Glu, gave no TRF activity, confirming the results obtained with acetylation mixtures of the various tripeptides (Burgus *et al.*, 1969a–c) and in accord with the sequence "Glu-His-Pro" for porcine TRF, reported by Schally *et al.* (1969). "Preparation A" was not subjected to any form of purification, which is unfortunate; the yield of amide prepared according to this procedure would be expected to be low, and the methyl ester, pGlu-His-Pro-OMe, may have been the major component of the mixture (Burgus *et al.*, 1969a, 1970a,b). Moreover, the specific biological activity of the methyl ester being about half that of pGlu-His-Pro-NH$_2$ (Burgus *et al.*, 1970a), the bioassay used by Bowers *et al.* (1969) would not have allowed Folkers *et al.* (1969) to distinguish between the methyl ester or the amide in their "preparation A" on the basis of biological activity.

Shortly after the publication of these preliminary communications, evidence was presented (Burgus *et al.*, 1969) based primarily on low- and high-resolution mass spectrometry, that the ovine TRF preparation originally obtained in late 1968 had been all along essentially homogeneous and had unquestionably the structure pGlu-His-Pro-NH$_2$: Both synthetic pGlu-His-Pro-NH$_2$ (Burgus *et al.*, 1969c, 1970a) and the highly purified ovine TRF (Burgus and Guillemin, 1970) were introduced by direct probe into a low-resolution mass spectrometer after treatment with diazomethane or trifluoroacetic anhydride–trifluoroacetic acid to give the methyl or trifluoroacetyl (TFA) derivatives, respectively. All preparations gave volatile materials in the temperature range of 150°–200°C ($\leq 10^{-6}$ torr). Several mass spectra taken throughout the range of the thermal gradient (7 in the case of the isolated ovine TRF) showed fragmentation patterns corresponding to a single component. Although none of the spectra revealed a molecular ion, fragments arising from the structures pGlu, methyl-pGlu, His, methyl-His, Pro, Pro-NH$_2$, CONH$_2$, pGlu-His, and His-Pro-NH$_2$ were observed. The low-resolution mass spectra of the corresponding derivatives of synthetic pGlu-His-Pro-NH$_2$ and TRF were essentially identical. Fragments arising from unsubstituted pGlu or His were observed in the spectra of both types of derivatives.

The elemental composition of all the fragments, except m/e 221, the intensity of which was too weak for it to be observed on the photoplate used, were confirmed by high-resolution mass spectroscopy of the methyl derivatives. The methyl derivatives of natural TRF, as well as pGlu-His-Pro-NH$_2$, presented a rather interesting problem in the interpretation of the mass spectra. Since no molecular ion was present, the proof of the sequence of the tripeptides required presence of ions unique to the pGlu-His and the His-Pro-NH$_2$ sequences. However, as examination of the structure will show, a form of symmetry about the α-carbon atom of His exists such that the combinations of methylated or unmethylated fragments of either dipeptide would produce fragments of the same nominal masses and in some cases the same elemental compositions. Thus the fragments m/e 234, 235, 248, and 249 could arise from pGlu-His-Pro-NH$_2$, or as another combination, as Schally et $al.$ (1968, 1969) had reported for porcine TRF, the diketopiperazine of His,Pro. The strength of high-resolution mass spectroscopy as a tool is illustrated by the fact that the nominal mass m/e 248 was shown by exact mass measurement to have the elemental composition $C_{11}H_{14}N_5O_2$, which distinguishes it as arising from His-Pro-NH$_2$ (-2H) resulting from a cleavage between the α-carboxyl carbon of pGlu and the α-amino group of His. This fragment, together with others, such as pGlu-His, m/e 221, considered with the identity of the mass spectra of the two types of derivatives of ovine TRF with those of the synthetic material, established without doubt the structure of ovine TRF as pGlu-His-Pro-HN$_2$.

More evidence obtained shortly thereafter by our group confirmed this structure. We repeatedly observed the molecular ions of ovine TRF (m/e 361) in mass spectrometry by the use of chemical ionization probes or modified electron impact probes. Chromatographic analysis of the hydrolyzate of ovine TRF showed no basic constituents other than His separating from the ammonia peak (Burgus et $al.,$ 1969b, 1970a). The amino acid analysis of 6 N HCl hydrolyzates of ovine TRF corrected for contamination by ammonia in the reagents and atmospheric sources gave essentially a 1:1 ratio of ammonia to His; in the same series of experiments, methylamine, ethylamine, and dimethylamine could be distinguished from the ammonia peak on the basis of their retention values. The presence of both methylated and unsubstituted pGlu and His in the diazomethane-treated materials provides strong evidence that the α-amino group in pGlu and the imidazole nitrogen of His are unsubstituted in the isolated TRF. The positive Pauly reaction had already essentially ruled out substitution of the imidazole group. Furthermore the NMR spectrum of ovine TRF (obtained by time averaging in D_2O) is essentially identical to that of synthetic pGlu-His-Pro-NH_2.

In addition, a pyroglutamyl peptidase isolated by Fellows and Mudge (1970) destroyed the biological activity of ovine TRF. The enzyme had been shown to be specific for the cleavage of pGlu from pGlu-terminal peptides; it released a similar fragment, presumably His-Pro-NH_2, as determined by TLC (Pauly reagent) and by the dansyl method (Burgus et al., 1970a).

Therefore, the structure of ovine TRF as *isolated* from the hypothalamus was established as pGlu-His-Pro-HN_2. However, we did point out (Burgus et al., 1969b) that the possibility was not excluded that, as opposed to the isolated material, the *native* molecule of TRF may occur as Gln-His-Pro-NH_2 either free or conjugated to another structure, such as protein, which would not be necessary for biological activity *in vivo* or *in vitro;* there were such precedents in the chemistry of the eledoisins (Schröder and Lübke, 1965) and in the case of the prohormones for insulin, parathyroid hormones, etc. At the time of this lecture, we and others are still looking for a hypothetical prohormone of TRF.

Bøler et al. (1969) compared the properties of porcine TRF with those of a synthetic preparation which they considered to be characterized as pGlu-His-Pro-NH_2 by "its hydrolysis to the 3 amino acids," by its NMR spectrum, and by paper and thin-layer chromatography employing 17 different systems of solvent and adsorbents using Pauly reagent for visualization. Unfortunately, the authors refer only to their "preparation A as in Folkers et al. (1969)" and no details of purification of that mixture were given; it would appear that the data presented were inadequate to distinguish pGlu-His-Pro-NH_2 from other constituents in the mixture, such as Glu-His-Pro, pGlu-His-Pro-OH, pGlu-His-Pro-OMe, and up to 20% impurities in the starting material.

Indeed, in subsequent reports the preparation of porcine TRF used for structural studies, prepared as described by Schally *et al.* (1969) was acknowledged to contain 50–70% impurities by weight including what appeared to be myristoleic acid and dioctylphthalate and therefore was judged to have been 30–50% pure. Mass spectra were obtained and reported although neither the natural nor the synthetic product showed a molecular ion in mass spectrometry. The synthetic "preparation A" as well as a sample of pGlu-His-Pro-NH$_2$ synthesized by Flouret (Abbott Laboratories) and the natural produce were reported to have essentially identical R_f values (Pauly color) in the 17 chromatographic systems; data were presented representing graded responses of biological activity *in vivo* over a dose range of 1–18 ng/dose with no significant difference between responses of the natural or synthetic products. Possibilities of structures other than pGlu-His-Pro-NH$_2$ for TRF were considered, as we had done earlier, including substitution of the pGlu or a Gln residue by hydrolyzable groups on the nitrogen atom, or modification of the Pro-NH$_2$ groups, in other words as in a secondary or tertiary amide group. The possibility of substitution of the imidazole ring of His was ruled out because of the positive Pauly reaction. It was further reasoned (Bøler *et al.*, 1969) that "any structural modification of (Pyro)Glu-His-Pro-(NH$_2$) would necessitate another compound having identical R_f values to those of (Pyro)Glu-His-Pro-(NH$_2$) in all seventeen [chromatographic] systems" and that a "certain lack of structural specificity and potency [would have to exist] for the hormonal activity of TRH." On the basis of the mass spectrometric data, IR, NMR spectroscopy and all the above observations, Nair *et al.* (1970) finally concluded that porcine TRF had indeed the structure of pGlu-His-Pro-NH$_2$.

It is most interesting that TRF from two widely different species of mammals should have the same structure and apparently the same specific (biological) activity in similar assays. TRF shows no evidence of species specificity for its biological actions, pGlu-His-Pro-NH$_2$ being readily active in humans.

B. Purification, Isolation, and Characterization of LRF

In the early 1960s, several investigators reported experimental results that were best explained by proposing the existence in crude aqueous extracts of hypothalamic tissues, of substances that specifically stimulated the secretion of luteinizing hormone, and that were probably polypeptides (McCann et al., 1960; Campbell et al., 1961; Courrier et al., 1961). The active substance was named LH-releasing factor, or LRF. Rapidly following these early observations, preparations of LRF, active at 1 μg per dose in animal bioassays, were obtained by gel filtration and ion-exchange chromatography on CMC (Guillemin et al., 1963) an observation that was confirmed with similar methods by several investigators (Schally et al., 1968; Burgus et al., 1971). In spite of the vagaries of the various bioassay methods available, several laboratories reported preparations of LRF of increased potency (Schally et al., 1968; Amoss et al., 1970). Several of these early publications led, however, to contradictory statements regarding purification and separation of LH-releasing factor (LRF), from a follicle-stimulating hormone releasing factor (Schally et al., 1968; Dhariwal et al., 1967).

Two laboratories independently reported in 1971 the isolation of porcine LRF (Schally et al., 1971a) and ovine LRF (Amoss et al., 1971). Both groups concluded that LRF from either species was a *nonapeptide* containing, on the basis of acid hydrolysis, 1 His, 1 Arg, 1 Ser, 1 Glu, 1 Pro, 2 Gly, 1 Leu, 1 Tyr. Earlier results with the pyrrolidone-carboxylylpeptidase prepared by Fellows and Mudge (1970) had led us to conclude (Amoss et al., 1970) that the N-terminal residue of LRF was Glu in its cyclized pyroglutamic (pGlu) form, as in the case of hypothalamic TRF (pGlu-His-Pro-NH$_2$). The total amount of the highly purified ovine LRF that we had isolated from side fractions of the TRF program, and that was available for amino acid sequencing, was 30 nmol (as measured by quantitative dansylation) or 40 μg.

While our studies on the amino-acid sequence of ovine LRF were in progress, Matsuo et al. (1971b) reported that porcine LRF contained one residue of tryptophan (Trp), in addition to the other amino acids earlier observed by acid hydrolysis. On the basis of a series of experiments including enzymic hydrolysis with chymotrypsin and thermolysin and analysis of the partial sequences of their decapeptide by Edman degradation-dansylation and selective tritiation of C-termini, Matsuo et al. (1971b) proposed the sequence pGlu-His-Trp-Ser-Tyr-Gly-Leu-Arg-Pro-Gly-NH$_2$ for porcine LRF as that best compatible with the partial sequence data. Their studies were carried out with ca. 200 nmol of peptide. They also stated that synthesis of that particular sequence had given a material with biological activity. A few weeks later, we reported the synthesis by solid-phase methods of the decapeptide pGlu-His-Trp-Ser-Tyr-Gly-Leu-Arg-Pro-Gly-NH$_2$; after isolation from the reaction mixture it had quantitatively the full biological activity *in vivo* and *in vitro* of ovine LRF (Monahan *et al.*, 1971).

Later that year, we reported the amino-acid sequence of ovine LRF obtained by analysis of hydrolysis products of LRF after digestion with chymotrypsin or pyrrolidone-carboxylylpeptidase, using Edman degradation followed by determination of N- and C-termini by a quantitative dansylation technique. Confirmation of the positions of some of the amino-acid residues obtained by combined gas chromatographic–mass spectrometric analysis of phenylthiohydantoin (PTH) derivatives (Fales *et al.*, 1971; Hagenmaier *et al.*, 1970) resulting from Edman degradations was described; we also reported results obtained by degradation of the synthetic decapeptide, since they confirmed and clarified some peculiarities observed upon enzymic cleavage of the native peptide.

Determination by ^{14}C dansylation of amino acids in ovine LRF after hydrolysis with 6 N HCl in the presence of thioglycolic acid confirmed the presence of His, Arg, Ser, Glu, Pro, Gly, Leu, and Tyr, as reported earlier by Amoss *et al.* (1971) and Schally *et al.* (1971) for ovine and porcine LRF, respectively, plus the presence of Trp, as originally reported by Matsuo *et al.* (1971b) for porcine LRF.

Chymotryptic digestion of ovine LRF gave four major peptide fragments having as C-termini: Gly, His, Trp, Tyr, and possibly a small amount of a peptide with C-terminal Ser. Hydrazinolysis-dansylation showed C-terminal Gly in untreated ovine and synthetic LRF. Since this Gly residue is amidated in the synthetic preparation, and was shown by sequencing to be amidated in ovine LRF (see below), there was probably some deamidation of the Gly-NH$_2$ residue during the hydrazinolysis procedure. Dansylation of the chymotryptic digest of ovine LRF revealed primarily N-terminal Ser and Gly, plus some Trp and Arg. The major N-termini observed after the first Edman cycle were Tyr and Leu, plus some Arg and Pro; after the second cycle, Arg; the third, Pro; and the fourth, Gly-NH$_2$; Gly-NH$_2$ was determined without hydrolysis by 6 N HCl as Dns-Gly-NH$_2$ (first dimension of polyamide thin-layer chromatography, $R_f = 0.72$; second dimension, $R_f = 0.42$), and, after hydrolysis, as Dns-Gly. Total recoveries of Dns-amino acids after each cycle were in good agreement with theoretical values. Mass spectral analysis of PTH derivatives showed Gly and Ser (trace of Leu) from the first Edman cycle and Pro from the fourth Edman cycle; the extract from the second Edman cycle was accidently destroyed; to be consistent with the dansylation results the third cycle should have given Arg, which is not detectable by this method. These results were consistent with the primary structure for LRF shown in Fig. 2, the major fragments from chymotryptic digestion being Ch I, Ch II, Ch III, and Ch IV, with smaller amounts of Ch V and Ch VI. Hydrolysis of peptides by chymotrypsin at His-, Ser-, and Leu-residues is not uncommon. The same principal cleavages occurred upon digestion of synthetic decapeptide with chymotrypsin. The results of analysis of the chymotryptic digest did not rule out an alternative structure for ovine LRF, in which the Ser-4 and Gly-6 residues are interchanged; that is, pGlu-His-Trp-Gly-Tyr-Ser-Leu-Arg-Pro-Gly-NH$_2$. Moreover, the position of the His residue could be obtained only by inference, since it is not directly accounted for.

Digestion of ovine LRF with pyrrolidone-carboxylylpeptidase, followed by the Edman-dansylation analysis, however, confirmed the sequence PCA I shown in Fig. 2. Again, synthetic LRF gave similar results. Consistent with the sequence shown in Fig. 2, mass-spectral analysis revealed trimethylsilylated PTH derivatives of Trp, Ser, Tyr, Gly, and Leu in the second to sixth Edman cycles, respectively, and Pro

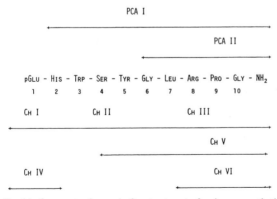

FIG. 2. Peptide fragments observed after treatment of ovine or synthetic luteinizing hormone releasing factor (LRF) with chymotrypsin (Ch I–VI) or pyrrolidone-carboxylylpeptidase (PCA I–II).

in the eighth cycle from pyrrolidone-carboxylylpeptidase-digested ovine LRF. Blanks did occur in the first and seventh cycle, as would be expected, since the determination of His or Arg is not possible by the technique described above. All the remaining degraded peptide after the eighth Edman cycle was dansylated because of the limited amount of material, so that the identity of the tenth residue could not be corroborated by our gas-chromatographic method. In contrast to the results with chymotrypsin, the total recoveries of Dns-amino acids were lower than expected after pyrrolidone-carboxylylpeptidase digestion of either ovine or synthetic LRF. Furthermore, there was some evidence for endopeptidase activity in the pyrrolidone-carboxylylpeptidase preparation used that gave rise to the fragment PCA II, similar to Ch III (Fig. 2), since there is no evidence for this fragment in the undigested LRF preparations. The batch of pyrrolidone-carboxylylpeptidase used in these experiments did show more rapid loss of enzymic activity upon storage than batches of the enzyme used in previous experiments (Amoss *et al.*, 1970) and, therefore, probably contained some endopeptidase activity (this was confirmed independently by R. Fellows, Duke University, who had prepared that particular batch of the enzyme).

Thus the amino acid sequence of ovine LRF was established to be pGlu-His-Trp-Ser-Tyr-Gly-Leu-Arg-Pro-Gly-NH$_2$. It is identical to that of the material of porcine origin.

Of considerable interest was the observation that the synthetic replicate of LRF now available in large quantities, was shown to stimulate concomitant secretion of the two gonadotropins LH (luteinizing hormone) and FSH (follicle-stimulating hormone) in all assay systems *in vivo* and *in vitro* in which it was tested. This confirmed the earlier results obtained with the minute quantities of the isolated ovine or porcine LRF (Schally *et al.*, 1971a; Amoss *et al.*, 1971). In other words, the stimulation of the release of FSH appeared to be inherent to the molecule of LRF—thus throwing considerable doubts on reports (Schally *et al.*, 1966d, 1968; Igarashi and McCann, 1964) claiming to have obtained preparations of LRF free of FSH-releasing activity.

To the day of this lecture, no solid evidence has been produced that could be interpreted to indicate the existence of an FSH-releasing factor as a specific entity, discrete from the decapeptide LRF. Statements recently published by Folkers *et al.* (1969) claiming purification of an FSH-releasing factor are difficult to appreciate in view of the paucity of data offered; to my knowledge, no other laboratory has confirmed them.

Moreover, other evidence is against the existence of an FSH-releasing factor, separate from LRF: all synthetic analogs of LRF made so far, with no exception, can be shown to release LH and FSH with the same ratio of specific activity when related to the activity of LRF in the particular assay involved. Thus none of these analogs has shown any evidence of dissociated activity for releasing FSH vs. LH.

Moreover, there is increasing evidence that the two gonadotropins (LH and FSH) can be demonstrated (immunocytochemistry) in the same pituitary cell. It is thus unlikely that one could be released without the other, as they appear to be present in the same secretory granules.

Later on, both Schally's group (1971b) and Burgus *et al.* (1971) and Ling *et al.* (1973) confirmed the primary structure, respectively, of porcine and ovine LRF using larger quantities of native material.

C. Purification, Isolation, and Characterization of Somatostatin

It has been generally accepted that the control of the pituitary secretion of growth hormone would be exerted by a hypothalamic hypophysiotropic releasing factor, as is now proved to be the case for the secretion of thyrotropin (TSH) (Burgus *et al.*, 1969c; Bowers *et al.*, 1969) and the gonadotropin, luteinizing hormone (LH) (Matsuo *et al.*, 1971b). The nature of the postulated hypothalamic releasing factor for growth hormone, however, remains elusive to this day, mostly owing to the difficulties and ambiguities of the various assay systems used so far in attempts at its characterization. For instance, there is now agreement that the growth hormone-releasing hormone (GH-RH) isolated and characterized by Schally *et al.*, (1971b) as H-Val-His-Leu-Ser-Ala-Glu-Glu-Lys-Glu-Ala-OH, was actually a decapeptide fragment of the N-terminus of the β-chain of porcine hemoglobin. The material has never been shown to be active in stimulating secretion of immunoreactive growth hormone, and there is even question of its effects on the bioassayable growth hormone activity originally reported by Schally *et al.* (1971b). Similarly, the biological activity of the tetrapeptide recently reported by Yudaev as a growth hormone releasing factor of porcine origin has not been confirmed by others including our own laboratory (see Guillemin, 1973).

Searching to demonstrate the presence of this still hypothetical somatotropin-releasing factor in the crude hypothalamic extracts used in the isolation of TRF and LRF, we regularly observed that their addition in minute doses (≤ 0.001 of a hypothalamic fragment equivalent) to the incubation fluid of dispersed rat pituitary cells in monolayer cultures (Vale *et al.*, 1972b) significantly decreased the resting secretion of immunoreactive growth hormone by the pituitary cells. [The radioimmunoassay for rat growth hormone is a double-antibody method, with NIH-rat GH-RP-1 as reference standard; for iodination, rat GH (H III-41E; courtesy of Dr. S. Ellis, Ames Research Center, Moffett Field, California); monkey antiserum to rat GH (MK 33; courtesy of Dr. J. Lewis, Scripps Research Foundation, La Jolla, California).] This inhibition was related to the dose of hypothalamic extract added and appeared to be specific. It was not produced by similar extracts of cerebellum, and the crude hypothalamic extracts that inhibit secretion of growth hormone simultaneously stimulated secretion of LH and TSH. The inhibition of growth hormone secretion could not be duplicated by addition to the assay system of [Arg^8]-vasopressin, oxytocin, histamine, various polyamines, serotonin, catecholamines, LRF, or TRF. We decided to attribute this inhibitory effect on the secretion of growth hormone to a "somatotropin-release inhibiting factor," which we later named *somatostatin*.

Inhibition of secretion of growth hormone by crude hypothalamic preparations had been reported by others (Krulich *et al.*, 1968). The active factor possibly involved in these early studies based on various types of assays for growth hormone activity had not been characterized. The results on the inhibition by the hypothalamic extracts of the secretion of immunoreactive growth hormone by the monolayer pituitary cultures (Vale *et al.*, 1972b) were so consistent and easily quantitated that we decided to attempt the isolation and characterization of the hypothalamic factor involved. We realized the possible interest of such a substance in inhibiting abnormally elevated secretion of growth hormones in juvenile diabetes; also, we considered that knowledge of the primary structure of a native inhibitor of the secretion of a pituitary hormone could be of significance in our efforts to design synthetic inhibition of the gonadotropin releasing factor LRF.

The starting material was the chloroform–methanol–glacial acetic acid extract of about 500,000 sheep hypothalamic fragments (Burgus *et al.*, 1971, 1972) used in the program of characterization of the releasing factor for the gonadotropins. The extract (2 kg) had been partitioned in two systems; the LRF concentrate was subjected to ion-exchange chromatography on CMC. At that stage, a fraction with growth hormone-release inhibiting activity was observed well separated from the LRF zone; it was further purified by gel filtration (Sephadex G-25) and liquid partition chromatography (*n*-butanol, acetic acid, water, 4:1:5). Thin-layer chromatography and electrophoresis of the final product showed only traces of peptide impurities. The yield was 8.5 mg of a product containing 75% of amino acids by weight, which is approximately 2% of that calculated on quantitative estimates of the amount of total biological activity inhibiting the secretion of growth hormone in the original extract. The low yield was not of primary concern, because the early purification stages were designed specifically for the isolation of LRF and the amount of inhibitor of the secretion of growth hormone obtained as a side fraction was considered adequate for its characterization. From now on, we will refer to this material by the name *somatostatin*, which was actually given to it only after it had been fully characterized.

Analysis of amino acids obtained from somatostatin after acid hydrolysis in 6 N HC1–0.5% thioglycolic acid gave the molar ratios Ala (0.9), Gly (1.1), Cys (0.2), Cys-SS-Cys (1.0), Lys (2.0), Asp (1.0), Phe (3.3), Trp (0.5), Thr (2.0), Ser (0.8), and NH_3 (1.1). Enzymic hydrolysis gave the ratios Ala (0.9), Gly (0.9), Lys (2.0), Phe (3.4), and Trp (0.9); Asn, Thr, and Ser were not well resolved, giving a total of about 3.6 mol per mole of peptide. Edman degradation of the carboxymethylated trypsin digests of somatostatin and mass spectrometry led finally to the proposal of the following primary structure for somatostatin (see Burgus *et al.,* 1973): H-Ala-Gly-Cys-Lys-Asn-Phe-Phe-Trp-Lys-Thr-Phe-Thr-Ser-Cys-OH in the oxidized form.

This peptide was reproduced by total synthesis using the Merrifield method (see Rivier, 1974). It had the full biological activity of native somatostatin *in vivo* and *in vitro* (Brazeau *et al.,* 1973, 1974; Vale *et al.,* 1972a). Of interest was the unexpected observation that the peptide has the full biological activity either in the oxidized (native) or reduced form.

D. The Endorphins, Opiatelike Peptides of Brain or Pituitary Origin

The concept and the demonstration a couple of years ago of the existence in the brain of mammalians of (synaptosomal) opiate receptors has led to the search of what has been termed the endogenous ligand(s) of these opiate receptors. The generic name *endorphins* (from endogenous and morphine) was proposed for these (then hypothetical) substances by Eric Simon and will be used here. In 1975 we became interested in these early observations. Besides the challenge of characterizing an endogenous substance as the ligand of the brain opiate receptors, we could not ignore that, like morphine, endorphins might stimulate the secretion of growth hormone; the nature of the growth hormone releasing factor remains unknown; endorphins might have been either releasing factors for growth hormone, or substances related to the still uncharacterized growth hormone releasing factor, or, even if none of the above, endorphins might be involved in the physiological mechanisms controlling the secretion of growth hormone and possibly prolactin. It was thus decided to engage in the isolation and characterization of the endogenous ligand(s) for the opiate receptors. As will be seen in this short review, the isolation of these endogenous ligands of the opiate receptors was a simple problem to which a solution was indeed provided in less than a couple of months of efforts.

Isolation of the Endorphins. Chemical Characterization

Dilute acetic acid–methanol extracts of whole brain (ox, pig, rat) were confirmed to contain substances presumably peptidic in nature, with naloxone-reversible, morphinelike activity in the bioassay using the myenteric-plexus longitudinal muscle of the guinea pig ileum. Evidence of such biological activity in our laboratory was in agreement with earlier results of Hughes (1975), Terenius and Wahlstrom (1975), Teschemacher *et al.* (1975), and Pasternak *et al.* (1975). Searching for an enriched source of endorphins in available concentrates from our earlier efforts toward the isolation of CRF, TRF, LRF, and somatostatin, it was recognized that acetic acid–methanol extracts of porcine hypothalamus–neurohypophysis contained much greater concentrations of the morphinelike activity, than extracts of whole brain. From such an extract of approximately 250,000 fragments of pig hypothalamus–neurohypophysis, we have isolated several oligopeptides (endorphins) with opioid activity (Guillemin *et al.,* 1976a; Lazarus *et al.,* 1976; Ling *et al.,* 1976a,b). The isolation procedure involved successively gel filtration, ion-exchange chromatography, liquid partition chromatography and high-pressure liquid chromatography (Guillemin *et al.,* 1976a,b;

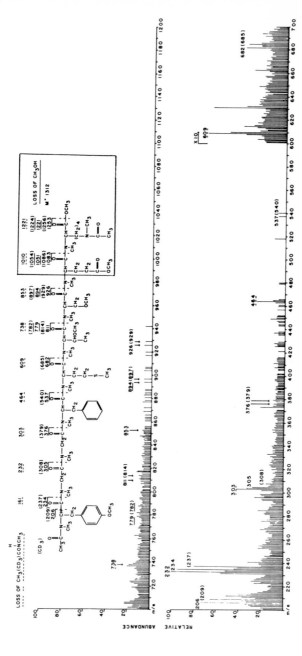

α-endorphin·NH₂ terminal fragment H-Tyr-Gly-Gly-Phe-Met-Thr-Ser

FIG. 3a. Mass spectrum of derivatized α-endorphin-1 obtained by fractional vaporization at 280°–295°. The peptide detected has the sequence H-Tyr-Gly-Gly-Phe-Met-Thr-Ser. (Modified from Ling et al., 1976b.)

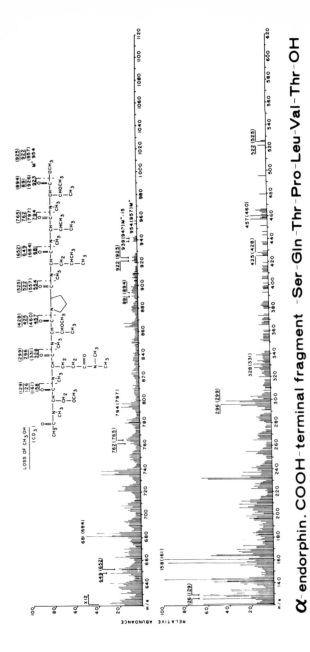

α-endorphin. COOH-terminal fragment –Ser-Gln-Thr-Pro-Leu-Val-Thr-OH

FIG. 3b. Mass spectrum of derivatized α-endorphin-1 obtained by fractional vaporization at 231°–245°. The peptide detected has the sequence H-Ser-Gln-Thr-Pro-Leu-Val-Thr-Leu-OH. (Modified from Ling et al., 1976b.)

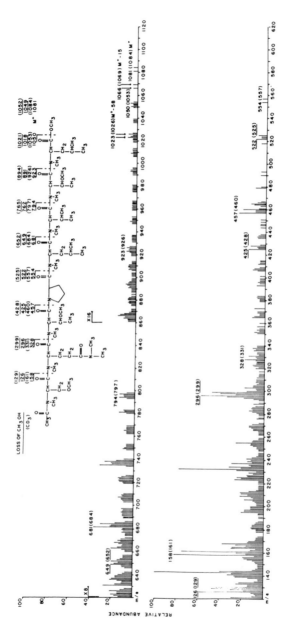

γ-endorphin. COOH-terminal fragment -Ser-Gln-Pro-Leu-Val-Thr-Leu-OH

FIG. 4. Mass spectrum of derivatized γ-endorphin obtained by fractional vaporization at 237°–246°. The peptide detected has the sequence H-Ser-Gln-Thr-Pro-Leu-Val-Thr-Leu-OH. (Modified from Ling et al., 1976b.)

Lazarus *et al.*, 1976; Ling *et al.*, 1976b). Met[5]-enkephalin and Leu[5]-enkephalin recently isolated by Hughes, Smith, Kosterlitz, Fothergill, Morgan, and Morris (1975) have not been observed in these extracts. The primary structure of *α-endorphin* was established by mass spectrometry and classical Edman degradation of the enzymically cleaved peptide and is H-Tyr-Gly-Gly-Phe-Met-Thr-Ser-Glu-Lys-Ser-Gln-Gln-Thr-Pro-Leu-Val-Thr-OH (Fig. 3a,b). The primary structure of *γ-endorphin* was similarly established by mass spectrometry and by Edman degradation: γ-endorphin has the same primary structure as α-endorphin with one additional Leu as the COOH-terminal residue in position 17 (Fig. 4). Thus Met-enkephalin is the N-terminal pentapeptide of the endorphins, which have the same amino acid sequence as β-lipotropin [61–76] and [61–77]. β-LPH[61–91], a fragment of β-LPH isolated earlier on the basis of its chemical characteristics (Bradbury *et al.*, 1976; Li and Chung, 1976) was shown later to have opiatelike activity (Lazarus *et al.*, 1976; Cox *et al.*, 1976) and has been named β-endorphin (Li and Chung, 1976). Recently we isolated, from the same starting material of hypothalamus–neurohypophysis origin from which we originally isolated α- and γ-endorphin, two peptides characterized by amino acid composition as *β-endorphin* (β-LPH[61–91]) and *δ-endorphin* (β-LPH[61–87]). No effort was made to obtain the amino acid sequences of these two samples. The synthetic replicates of these two polypeptides have identical chromatographic behavior in several systems as the native materials.

II. Biological Activities of the Hypothalamic Peptides. Experimental and Clinical Studies

As soon as they were obtained in large quantity from total synthesis, TRF and LRF were extensively studied for their biological activities, both in the laboratory and in clinical medicine. Indeed, the observation was rapidly made that TRF, and later LRF, both characterized only from tissues of ovine and porcine origin, were biologically fully active in all species of vertebrates studied, including man.

For early clinical studies with TRF, see Fleischer *et al.* (1970) and, more recently, Fleischer and Guillemin (1976); for early clinical studies with LRF, see Yen *et al.* (1972) and Rebar *et al.* (1973).

Both in the case of TRF and of LRF, chemists prepared large numbers of synthetic analogs of the primary (native) structure, for studies of correlation between molecular structure and biological activity. Also, biologists carefully screened these analogs in the hope that some of them would prove to be antagonists of the native (agonist) releasing factor. This was of particular interest in the case of the gonadotropin releasing factor; a powerful antagonist of LRF would be of considerable interest as a chemical mean of controlling or regulating fertility, thus introducing a totally new type of substance for contraception. In 1972, our laboratory reported the first partial agonist/antagonist analogs of LRF (Vale *et al.*, 1972d). They all had a deletion or a substitution of His[2] or Trp[3] in the (otherwise identical) amino acid sequence of LRF. These were extremely impotent antagonists of no possible practical value as clinically significant inhibitors of LRF. They showed, however, that analog-antagonists to the decapeptide LRF could be prepared. To this day, the most potent antagonist analogs of LRF still have the early deletion or substitution of His[2] or Trp[3] of the amino acid sequence of LRF.

Also, analogs of TRF and LRF with increased potency (over that of the native compound) were expected, searched for, and obtained.

A. Biological Activity of Thyrotropin Releasing Factor (TRF) and Luteinizing Hormone Releasing Factor (LRF)

Somewhat to the surprise of researchers in the field, of the many analogs of TRF that have been synthesized and studied biologically, only one has a significantly increased specific activity over that of the native compound. Synthesized and described by our group (Rivier *et al.*, 1971), it is the analog [3*N*-Methyl-His]-TRF. Its specific activity is approximately 10 times that of the native molecule, on the secretion of TSH as well as of prolactin. Of the several hundreds of TRF analogs synthesized, none has been found so far to be even a partial antagonist. They are all agonists with full intrinsic activity but variable specific activity; no true antagonist of TRF has been reported.

In contradistinction to the statement above regarding analogs of TRF, antagonist as well as extremely potent agonist analogs of LRF have been prepared by a number of laboratories. There are now available preparations of a series of what we may accurately call "super-LRFs," analogs that have as much as 150 times the specific activity of the native compound. In fact, in certain assays, such as ovulation, they may have 1000 times the specific activity of the native peptide. All the agonist analogs of super-LRFs possess structural variations around two major modifications of the amino acid sequence of native LRF: They all have a modification of the C-terminal glycine, as originally reported for a series of analogs by Fujino et al. (1974). The Fujino modification consists of deletion of Gly^{10}-NH_2 and replacement by primary or secondary amide on the (now C-terminal) Pro^9. In addition to the Fujino modification, they have an additional modification at the Gly^6 position by substitution of one of several D-amino acids as originally discovered by Monahan and Vale in our laboratories (Monahan *et al.*, 1973). The most potent of the LRF-analogs agonist prepared are [D-Trp^6]-LRF; (des-Gly^{10}-[D-Trp^6-Pro^9-N-Et]-LRF, [D-Leu^6, Pro^9-N-Et]-LRF (review in Vale *et al.*, 1976).

In an *in vitro* assay in which the peptides stimulate release of LH and FSH by surviving adenohypophysial cells in monolayer cultures, these analogs of LRF have a specific activity 50–100 times greater than that of the synthetic replicate of native LRF. There is no evidence of dissociation of the specific activity for the release of LH from that of FSH. All agonist analogs release LH and FSH in the same ratio (in that particular assay system) as does native LRF. Probably because of their much greater specific activity, when given in doses identical in weight to the reference doses of LRF, the super-LRFs are remarkably long acting. While the elevated secretion of LH (or FSH) induced by LRF is returned to normal in 60 minutes, identical amounts in weight, of [D-Trp^6-des-Gly^{10}]-N-Et-LRF leads to statistically elevated levels of LH up to 24 hours in several *in vivo* preparations, including man. These analogs are ideal agents to stimulate ovulation (Vilchez-Martinez *et al.*, 1975). Marks and Stern (1975) have reported that these analogs are considerably more resistant than the native structures to degradation by tissue enzymes.

Catherine Rivier and Wylie Vale in our laboratories have recently observed that the injection of 1–10 μg of the analogs [D-Trp^6-des-Gly^{10}]-N-ethylamide-LRF decreases testicular weight and, in pregnant rats, either once or on consecutive days, over the early days of gestation can cause resorption of the fetuses and prevent normal pregnancy. Johnson *et al.* (1976) have reported similar observations. The mechanism involved in these observations is not clear at the moment.

All the antagonist LRF-analogs as originally found by our group (Vale *et al.*, 1972d) or as later reported by others have deletion, or a D-amino acid substitution, of His[2]. For reasons not clearly understood, addition of the Fujino modification on the C-terminus (Fujino *et al.*, 1974) does not increase the specific activity (as antagonists) of the antagonist analogs. Administered simultaneously with LRF, the antagonist analogs inhibit LRF in weight ratios ranging from 5:1 to 15:1. The most potent of these antagonists inhibit activity of LRF not only *in vitro,* but also in various tests *in vivo.* They inhibit the release of LH and FSH induced by an acute dose of LRF; they also inhibit endogenous release of LH–FSH and thus prevent ovulation in laboratory animals. The clinical testing of some of these LRF-antagonists prepared in our laboratory has recently started in collaboration with Yen at the University of California in San Diego.

B. Biological Activity of Somatostatin

It is now recognized that somatostatin has many biological effects other than the one on the basis of which we isolated it in extracts of the hypothalamus, i.e., as an inhibitor of the secretion of growth hormone (Brazeau *et al.,* 1973). Somatostatin inhibits the secretion of thyrotropin, but not prolactin, normally stimulated by TRF (Vale *et al.,* 1974); it also inhibits the secretion of glucagon, insulin (Koerker *et al.,* 1974), gastrin, and secretin, by acting directly on the secretory elements of these peptides. I have recently shown (Guillemin, 1976) that somatostatin also inhibits the secretion of acetylcholine from the (electrically stimulated) myenteric plexus of the guinea pig ileum probably at a presynaptic locus. This may explain in part the reportedly inhibitory effects of somatostatin on gut contraction *in vivo* and *in vitro.*

It is also now well recognized that somatostatin is to be found in many locations other than the hypothalamus, from which we originally isolated it. Somatostatin has been found in neuronal elements and axonal fibers in multiple locations in the central nervous system, including the spinal cord. It has been found also in discrete secretory cells of classical epithelial appearance in all the parts of the stomach, gut, and pancreas, in which it had been first recognized to have an inhibitory effect (Guillemin and Gerich, 1976; Vale *et al.*, 1975).

Somatostatin does not inhibit indiscriminately the secretion of everything or anything. For instance, as already stated, somatostatin does not inhibit the secretion of prolactin concomitant to that of thyrotropin when stimulated by a dose of TRF; this is true *in vivo* with normal animals or *in vitro* with normal pituitary tissue. Somatostatin does not inhibit the secretion of either gonadotropin LH or FSH, the secretion of calcitonin, the secretion of ACTH in normal animals or from normal pituitary tissues *in vitro;* it does not inhibit the secretion of steroids from adrenal cortex or gonads under any known circumstances. Regarding the secretion of polypeptides or proteins from abnormal tissues of experimental or clinical sources, such as pituitary adenomas, gastrinomas, insulinomas, somatostatin has been shown to be inhibitory according to its normal pattern of activity or being now nondiscriminative. The latter must reflect one of the differences between normal and neoplastic tissue. This is in keeping with observation that TRF, or LRF can stimulate release of growth hormone from the pituitaries of acromegalic pituitaries, though that does not happen with normal tissues.

Clinical studies have confirmed, in man, all observations obtained in the laboratory. The powerful inhibitory effects of somatostatin on the secretion not only of growth hormone, but also of insulin and glucagon, have led to extensive studies over the last three years of a possible role of somatostatin in the management or treatment of juvenile diabetes. First of all, the ability of somatostatin to inhibit insulin and glucagon secretion has provided a useful tool for studying the physiological and pathological effects of these hormones on human metabolism. Infusion of somatostatin lowers plasma glucose levels in normal man despite concomitant lowering of both plasma insulin and glucagon levels (Alford *et al.*, 1974; Gerich *et al.*, 1975; Mortimer *et al.*, 1974). These observations provided the first clear-cut evidence that glucagon has an important physiological role in human carbohydrate homeostasis. Somatostatin itself has no direct effect on either hepatic glucose production or peripheral glucose utilization, since the fall in plasma glucose levels could be prevented by exogenous glucagon (Gerich *et al.*, 1974).

In juvenile-type diabetics, somatostatin diminishes fasting hyperglycemia by as much as 50% in the complete absence of circulating insulin (Gerich *et al.*, 1974). Although somatostatin impairs carbohydrate tolerance after oral or intravenous glucose challenges in normal man by inhibiting insulin secretion, carbohydrate tolerance after ingestion of balanced meals is improved in patients with insulin-dependent diabetes mellitus through the suppression of excessive glucagon responses (Gerich *et al.*, 1974). The combination of somatostatin and a suboptimal amount of exogenous insulin (which by itself had prevented neither excessive hyperglycemia nor hyperglucagonemia in response to meals) completely prevents plasma glucose levels from rising after meal ingestion in insulin-dependent diabetics (Gerich *et al.*, 1974). Through its suppression of glucagon and growth hormone secretion, somatostatin has also been shown to moderate or prevent completely the development of diabetic ketoacidosis after the acute withdrawal of insulin from patients with insulin-dependent diabetes mellitus (Gerich *et al.*, 1975).

At the moment, clinical studies with somatostatin as provided by our group at the Salk Institute are proceeding in several clinical centers in the United States.

From the foregoing description of the ability of somatostatin to inhibit the secretion of various hormones, it would appear that it may be of therapeutic use in certain clinical conditions, such as acromegaly, pancreatic islet cell tumors, and diabetes mellitus. With regard to endocrine tumors, it must be emphasized that while somatostatin will inhibit hormone secretion by these tissues, it would not be expected to diminish tumor growth. Thus, in these conditions it is unlikely that somatostatin will find use other than as a symptomatic or temporizing measure.

In diabetes mellitus, however, somatostatin might be of considerable clinical value. First, it has already been demonstrated that it can acutely improve fasting as well as postprandial hyperglycemia in insulin-requiring diabetics by inhibiting glucagon secretion. Second, since growth hormone has been implicated in the development of diabetic retinopathy, the inhibition of growth hormone secretion by somatostatin may lessen this complication of diabetes. Finally, through suppression of both growth hormone and glucagon secretion, somatostatin may prevent or diminish the severity of diabetic ketoacidosis and find application in "brittle diabetes." These optimistic expectations must be considered with the facts that the multiple effects of somatostatin on hormone secretions and its short duration of action make its clinical use impractical at the present time and that its long-term effectiveness and safety have not been established as yet. Regarding the clinical use of somatostatin, see the recent review by Guillemin and Gerich (1976).

With the considerable interest in somatostatin as a part of the treatment of diabetics, "improved" analogs of somatostatin have been in the mind of clinicians and investigators. Analogs of somatostatin have been prepared in attempts to obtain substances of longer duration of activity than the native form of somatostatin; this has not been very successful so far. Other analogs have been sought that would have dissociated biological activity on one or more of the multiple recognized targets of somatostatin. Remarkable results have recently been obtained. The first such analog so recognized by the group of the Wyeth Research Laboratories was [des-Asn^5]-somatostatin, an analog with approximately 4%, 10%, and 1% the activity of somatostatin to inhibit, respectively, secretion of growth hormone, insulin, and glucagon (Sarantakis *et al.*, 1976). Although such an analog is not of clinical interest, it shows that dissociation of the biological activities of the native somatostatin on three of its receptors could be achieved. The most interesting analogs with dissociated activities reported so far, all prepared and studied by J. Rivier, M. Brown, and W. Vale in our laboratories are [D-Ser^{13}]-somatostatin, [D-Cys^{14}]-somatostatin, and [D-Trp^8, D-Cys^{14}] somatostatin. When compared to somatostatin, this latest compound has ratios of activity such as 300%, 10%, 100% to inhibit the secretions, respectively, of growth hormone, insulin, and glucagon (Brown *et al.*, 1976). These and other analogs are obviously of much clinical interest, and are being so investigated at the moment, in several laboratories.

C. Biological Studies with the Endorphins

1. Immunocytochemical Localization of Endorphins

Cells of pars intermedia of the rat pituitary gland stain brightly and uniformly with antisera to α-endorphin or β-endorphin. Cells of the pars intermedia show reactivity within small granules, evenly distributed throughout the cytoplasm. In the pars distalis (adenohypophysis), discrete cells give bright fluorescence with either antiserum; the fluorescence observed is associated with granules somewhat larger than those of pars intermedia cells and located only at the periphery of the cells. The endorphin-reactive adenohypophysial cells appear often to be adjacent to blood vessels. The pars nervosa (neurohypophysis, posterior lobe) and the interlobular stroma of pars intermedia are completely unstained. The results are consistent in all animals (rats) so prepared, also using one cat and with pituitary glands from several cows. The fluorescence of all cells disappears entirely when the antisera are incubated with the respective peptide antigens. Discrete nerve fibers in the hypothalamus stain also by this technique, with either antiserum to α-endorphin or β-endorphin. The immunofluorescence staining of nerve fibers in the hypothalamus and other rat brain areas such as the hippocampus have been observed as late as 7 weeks after total hypophysectomy with no obvious difference from what was seen in normal animals (Bloom *et al.*, 1977). These results strongly support the suggestion that some cellular elements in the brain have the ability to synthesize β-lipotropin as the precursor of the endorphins; alternatively, they may possess enzymes that would cleave β-lipotropin as a prohormone of the endorphins, available either from its pituitary origin or from some other site in the brain. The only source of β-lipotropin reported so far has been the pituitary gland.

The results presented here raise the possibility that α- and β-endorphins may exist simultaneously with β-lipotropin in the same pituitary cells of either intermediate or anterior lobe. They could exist in the same or in different compartments. Moreover these same cells are known also to contain ACTH (1–39) as well as several fragments of ACTH, such as CLIP (i.e., ACTH 18–39).

In view of the novel information relating the presence of α- and β-endorphin to cells of the pars intermedia but not of the neurohypophysis, presence of the endorphins in the crude extract "Pitressin Intermediate" used earlier to isolate α-, β-, and γ-endorphins (Guillemin *et al.*, 1976a; Ling *et al.*, 1976b) is explained by realizing that tissues of the intermediate lobe always remain attached to the posterior lobe as it is dissected away from the whole pituitary gland. In this respect, Ling *et al.* (1976b) had reported that the extract used to isolate the endorphins had indeed melanophoretic activity—ca. one-tenth of the specific activity of pure α-MSH, which in retrospect, should be realized to be nonnegligible; it is further evidence for the presence of pars intermedia tissues in that starting material.

2. Relation of Endorphins to β-Lipotropin

So far, all morphinomimetic peptides isolated from natural sources on the basis of a bioassay or displacement assay for ^{3}H-labeled opiates on synaptosomal preparations, and chemically characterized, have been related to a fragment of the C-terminus of the molecule of β-lipotropin, starting at Tyr^{61}. In the case of Leu^5-enkephalin, the relationship still holds for the sequence Tyr-Gly-Gly-Phe; no β-lipotropin with a Leu residue in position 65 has been observed.

β-LPH has no opioid activity in any of the tests above. Incubation of β-LPH at 37°C with the 10^5g supernatant of a neutral sucrose extract of rat brain generates opioid activity suggesting that the presence of peptidase in rat brain generates opioid activity. Thus, β-LPH may be a prohormone for the opiatelike peptides (Lazarus et al., 1976). This would imply that the biogenesis of endorphins may be similar to that of angiotensin with cleaving enzymes available in the central nervous system. β-LPH[61–63] has no opioid activity at 10^{-4} M; β-LPH[61–64], β-LPH[61–65]-NH_2, (Met(O)^{65})-β-LPH[61–65]; β-LPH[61–69], β-LPH[61–76], β-LPH[61–91] all have opioid activity. β-LPH[61–65]-NH_2, LPH[61–65]-NEt, and all peptides larger than β-LPH[61–65] have longer duration of biological activity than Met-enkephalin in the myenteric plexus bioassay. All these peptides were prepared by solid-phase synthesis (see Ling and Guillemin, 1976). β-Endorphin is by far the longest-acting peptide when compared at equimolar ratios with all other fragments of the 61–91 COOH-fragment of β-LPH. In quantitative assays using the myenteric plexus, β-endorphin is approximately 5 times more potent than Met^5-enkephalin; the two analogs of Met^5-enkephalin amidated on the C-terminal residue have also 2–3 times greater specific activity than the free-acid form of the peptide, with 95% fiducial limits of the assays overlapping those of β-endorphin.

When tested in the myenteric plexus–ileum bioassay, β-LPH[61–64], Phe^1-Met^5-enkephalin, O-Me-Tyr^1 enkephalin, though of low specific activity when compared to Met^5-enkephalin, all have full intrinsic activity. [Arg-Tyr]^1-Met^5-enkephalin, i.e., β-LPH[60–65] is equipotent to Met^5-enkephalin. Thus an intact Tyr NH_2-terminal is not a requisite for full intrinsic activity. Acetyl-Tyr^1-Met^5-enkephalin has very low specific activity, which, however, cannot be further quantitated as the log-dose response function is totally divergent from that of

α-endorphin or Met[5]-enkephalin as reference standard (Ling and Guillemin, 1976).

A series of analogs of the endorphins was synthesized by N. Ling and further purified to high purity. All these peptides have parallel competition curves when studied at 5–6 dose levels in an opiate-displacement assay from rat-brain synaptosomes (Lazarus *et al.*, 1976) with the exception of β-LPH[62–91], which is definitely divergent from the other curves. Comparing the values obtained in the bioassay (myenteric plexus–longitudinal muscle) and the synaptosomal displacement assay, it is obvious that the two assay systems do not give necessarily identical values.

Of considerable interest are some results observed with the analogs of α-, β-, γ-, δ-endorphins in which residue of leucine has been substituted for methionine in position 5 from the NH[2]-terminus. [Leu[5]]-β-endorphin and [Leu[5]]-γ-endorphin are considerably more potent than their native congenors in the brain synaptosome assays, though not in the guinea pig ileum assay. It is tempting to speculate that the brain variety of endorphins might contain a residue of leucine in position 5. Proof of such a hypothesis would require isolation and characterization of such molecules. To this date, no [Leu[65]]-β-lipotropin has been recognized and characterized. On the other hand, Hughes and collaborators (Hughes *et al.*, 1975) and later Simantov and Snyder (1976) have isolated from brain extracts not only Met[5]-enkephalin, but also Leu[5]-enkephalin. Leu[5]-enkephalin might come from an allele of β-lipotropin of brain origin.

3. Release of Pituitary Hormones by Endorphins

One of our original interests in engaging in the isolation and characterization of the endorphins was that the opiatelike peptides might be involved in the secretion of pituitary hormones, particularly growth hormone and prolactin, long known to be acutely released following injection of morphine.

We showed with Rivier *et al.* (1977) that β-endorphin is a potent releaser of growth hormone and prolactin when administered to rats by intracisternal injection. Plasma levels of growth hormone or prolactin were measured by radioimmunoassays. These effects were prevented by prior administration of naloxone. The endorphins are not active directly at the level of the pituitary cells: they show no effect, even in large doses, when added directly to monolayer cultures of (rat) pituitary cells. Thus, the hypophysiotropic effects of the endorphins, like those of the opiate alkaloids, are mediated by some structure in the central nervous system and are not directly at the level of the adenohypophysis.

4. Neuronal Actions of Endorphins and Enkephalins among Brain Regions

The existence of endogenous peptides with opiatelike actions suggests that these substances may function as neuromodulators or neurotransmitters in the central nervous system (CNS). Indeed, recent iontophoretic studies have shown that the enkephalins can modify the excitability of a variety of neurons in the CNS. Most neurons tested were inhibited by these peptides (Frederickson and Norris, 1976; Hill et al., 1976; Moon et al., 1973; Zieglgansberger et al., 1976), although Renshaw cells responded with an excitation (Davis and Dray, 1976). Studies have recently appeared exploring systematically the sensitivity of neurons to the endorphins or reporting a systematic regional survey of neurons responsive to the peptides (Nicoll et al., 1977).

A surprising finding was the potent excitatory effects of the peptides and normorphine on hippocampal pyramidal cells (Fig. 5, Table I). The regional specificity of this excitatory action could be clearly demonstrated with the same electrode by recording from cells in the overlying cerebral cortex and the underlying thalamus during a single penetration. Thus as the electrode was advanced through the cortex, cells responded with inhibition to the peptides. As soon as the electrode entered the pyramidal cell layer, only marked excitatory responses were observed. Further advancement of the electrode into the thalamus again revealed exclusively inhibitory responses.

No tachyphylaxis were observed either to the excitatory or inhibitory action of the peptides in any of the regions examined, even though the peptides were often applied repeatedly to the same cell for periods in excess of 1 hour.

To determine whether the responses observed with the peptides were related to the activation of opiate receptors, the specific opiate antagonist, *naloxone,* was administered both by iontophoresis from an adjacent barrel of the microelectrode and by subcutaneous injections. Administered by either route, naloxone antagonized both the excitations and the inhibitions (Fig. 6a,b).

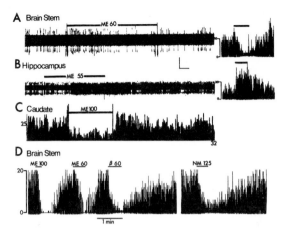

FIG. 5. The effect of opioid substances on the spontaneous activity of the central nervous system neurons. (A) Oscilloscope record of the discharge of a brainstem neuron that is inhibited by 60 nA Met⁵-enkephalin (ME). The rate meter record (1 second rate integration) of the same response is shown to the right. (B) An excitatory response from a hippocampal neuron to Met⁵-enkephalin. The calibration in A is 150 μV and 4.7 seconds and in B is 500 μV and 5.7 seconds. (C) Computer-generated drug histogram of the inhibition of a caudate neuron to Met⁵-enkephalin. This histogram sums the spikes of six sweeps, each with a duration of 66 seconds. The number on the ordinate refers to counts per bin. (D) Comparison of the action of Met⁵-enkephalin, β-endorphin (β), and normorphine (NM) on the activity of a brainstem neuron. (From Nicoll *et al.*, 1977.)

All these effects of opiatelike peptides on neuronal activity, taken with biochemical and histochemical evidence for their existence in brain, are consistent with the hypothesis that these peptides are neuro-transmitters in the CNS. When the cells of origin of these peptide-containing fibers have been determined, it may then be possible to proceed with studies into the effects on cellular activity and the secretion of the peptides in order to satisfy more completely the criteria for a neurotransmitter. Crucial points in such future analyses will be the questions of whether the endorphin- and enkephalin-containing fibers are mutually inclusive systems, whether the length of the peptide released by neuronal activity is subject to modulation, and whether peptides of intermediate length (such as the α-, γ-, and δ-endorphins) may participate in such modulatory changes. Although the endorphins and β-LPH may be prohormones for Met-enkephalin, there are at present no

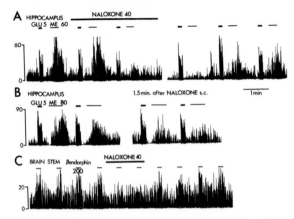

FIG. 6a. Naloxone antagonism of excitatory responses to the opioid peptides. (A) Iontophoresis of naloxone reversibly and selectively blocks the excitatory action of Met[5]-enkephalin on a hippocampal neuron. The break in the record is 8.5 minutes. (B) A subcutaneous injection of naloxone (10 mg/kg) also selectively antagonizes the Met[5]-enkephalin excitation of another hippocampal neuron. (C) The excitation of a brainstem neuron by β-endorphin is also reversibly blocked by iontophoretically applied naloxone. (From Nicoll et al., 1977.)

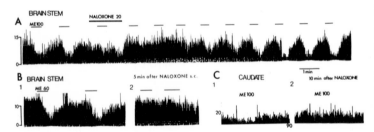

FIG. 6b. Antagonism of Met[5]-enkephalin inhibition by naloxone. (A) A short iontophoretic application of naloxone reversibly blocks the inhibitory response of a brainstem neuron. (B) A subcutaneous injection of naloxone (8 mg/kg) blocks the inhibitory response of another brainstem neuron. (C) A similar action of naloxone (8 mg/kg subcutaneously) in a caudate neuron, as documented by computer-generated drug histograms immediately before and 3 minutes after naloxone. Each histogram is composed of six sweeps of 66-second duration. (From Nicoll et al., 1977.)

such candidates for Leu-enkephalin. The results presented here indicate to us that the cellular roles of endorphin and enkephalin peptides cannot now be generalized across all brain regions where they are found, and that no simple cellular action of any peptide will yield an integrative picture of the way in which opiate alkaloids produce complex analgesic, euphoric, and addictive responses. Involvement of the endorphins in the control of adenohypophysial functions is much for further studies, at the time of writing this review. So far, no direct hypophysiotropic activities of the endorphin peptides have been clearly demonstrated.

5. Behavioral Effects of Endorphins

The pharmacological properties of endorphins have so far been screened through application of tests *in vitro* or *in vivo* previously used to characterize opiate agonists and antagonists.

When injected into the cerebrospinal fluid, endorphins affect several behavioral and physiological measures in addition to responses to noxious agents, and each of the peptides exhibits different dose-effect profiles on these measures: β-endorphin induces a marked catatonic state (Freedman *et al.*, 1975) lasting for hours (Bloom *et al.*, 1976) at molar doses 1/100 those at which Met^5-enkephalin transiently inhibits responses to noxious agents (Belluzzi *et al.*, 1976; Buscher *et al.*, 1976; Loh *et al.*, 1976). This potent effect of a naturally occurring substance suggests that its regulation could have etiological significance in mental illness.

In terms of molar dose-effectiveness on the various parameters examined, β-endorphin is clearly the most potent substance tested. Within 5–10 minutes after injection, corneal reflexes disappeared, and general locomotor activity became depressed; transient episodes of nystagmus could be seen in this period. Within 15 minutes, at doses as low as 3×10^{-10} mol (administered intracisternally) animals showed a total lack of responsiveness to pinprick or tail-pinch stimuli. After 15–30 minutes, animals injected with 7.4×10^{-9} mol of β-endorphin began to exhibit a profound catatonic state characterized by extreme generalized muscular rigidity, loss of the righting reflex, and total absence of spontaneous movement (Bloom *et al.*, 1976). As a result of these effects, animals could be placed in, and would retain, abnormal body positions (Fig. 7) for indefinite periods. Respiratory movements shifted

TABLE I

Summary of Neuronal Effects of Opioid Peptides[a]

Region (cell type)	MET-Enkephalin		β-Endorphin		Normorphine	
	%Exc.	%Inh.	%Exc.	%Inh.	%Exc.	%Inh.
Cerebellum (Purkinje)	18	21	23	23	20	60
	$N = 34$		$N = 13$		$N = 5$	
Cerebral cortex (unidentified)	1	79	25	48	26	52
	$N = 58$		$N = 44$		$N = 27$	
Brainstem (Lat. Ret. Nuc. +)	3	47	23	45	10	75
	$N = 113$		$N = 35$		$N = 20$	
Caudate nucleus (unidentified)	0	83	10	86	9	73
	$N = 18$		$N = 35$		$N = 20$	
Thalamus (unidentified)	0	100	0	100	0	100
	$N = 15$		$N = 5$		$N = 4$	
Hippocampus (pyramidal)	90	5	86	7	92	0
	$N = 19$		$M = 14$		$N = 12$	

[a] In each category the total number of cells tested and the percentage of this total that were inhibited or excited as shown. (After Nicoll et al., 1977.)

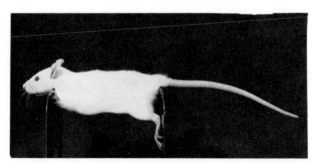

Fig. 7. Thirty minutes after the intracisternal injection of β-endorphin (14.9×10^{-9} mol) this rat exhibited sufficient rigid immobility to remain totally self-supporting when placed across metal bookends, which are in contact only at the upper neck and base of the tail. Such postures were maintained for prolonged periods. Note the erect ears and tail, widely opened eyelids, and extended lower limbs. (From Bloom et al., 1976.)

to the abdomen, and rectal temperature decreased. While in this state, the animals' eyes remained widely open (Fig. 7), with no spontaneous blinking, and showed loss of corneal and lid reflexes and often exophthalmos. With doses of 7.4×10^{-9} mol, rats remained in this state for approximately 2.5 hours. Full spontaneous recovery then occurred rapidly, with no detectable aftereffects. All these actions of β-endorphin were reversed within seconds after intravenous injection of naloxone (1.0 mg/kg); after naloxone-induced recovery, rats frequently showed several episodes of "wet-dog" shakes even though they had no prior exposure to endorphins, to exogenous opiates, or to opiate antagonists. Rats given seven daily intracisternal injections of 14.9×10^{-9} mol of β-endorphin continued to show the full set of responses and duration of action. However, 8–24 hours after as few as five daily injections such animals also showed spontaneous wet-dog shakes.

The catatonic state induced by β-endorphin was not observed with the other endorphin peptides, even at considerably higher doses. Doses of morphine or normorphine (8×10^{-9} to 132×10^{-9} mol) that suppressed responses to noxious stimuli did produce marked sedation with fixed open eyes and loss of corneal reflexes; but such animals retained considerable spontaneous locomotion (until doses of 1.3×10^{-7} mol) and showed no muscular rigidity similar to that produced by β-endorphin and only a moderate decrease in rectal temperature (0.8–$1.2°C$). At very high doses of α-endorphin, γ-endorphin, or Met[5]-enkephalin, transient losses of corneal reflexes were also observed, and α-endorphin seemed more potent in this regard than either γ-endorphin or Met[5]-enkephalin. No significant depressions of responsiveness to tail-pinch or pinprick stimuli were observed with Met[5]-enkephalin, α-endorphin, or γ-endorphin, but such effects (Bradbury et al., 1976; Buscher et al., 1976; Ross et al., 1976) could have been missed by the 5-minute interval after injection and before testing began. In contrast to the syndrome induced by β-endorphin, rats given γ-endorphin showed consistent elevations in rectal temperature (about $2.0°C \pm 0.2°C$ at 30 minutes after 281×10^{-9} mol), and sometimes exhibited some degree of hyperresponsivity to sensory testing and handling, although there were individual variations in this response.

Thus, β-endorphin in relatively small amounts induces in rats a naloxone-versible catatonia-like (Freedman et al., 1975) state reminiscent of some aspects of schizophrenia. Depending on the dose level, α-and γ-endorphins and Met^5-enkephalin also exhibited some of the other behavioral and physiological effects of α-endorphin, in which morphinelike effects (e.g., loss of response to noxious stimuli) appeared to be only a portion of a larger neuropsychopharmacological picture. As with the separate nicotinic and muscarinic actions of acetylcholine, all endorphin-mediated actions may not necessarily be explicable in terms of the alkaloid agonist morphine. Extremely puzzling in this regard is the finding that, when injected in the lateral ventricle, all three endorphin peptides and Met^5-enkephalin can elicit in *drug-naive* rats the wet-dog shaking behavior ordinarily attributable to opiate withdrawal; this effect is counteracted by naloxone (Kaymakcalan and Wood, 1956; Wei *et al.*, 1973a,b; Wei and Loh, 1976).

All our observations suggest that normal variations—either qualitative or quantitative—in the homeostatic mechanisms regulating the postulated (Lazarus *et al.*, 1976) conversion of β-LPH as a prohormone to its several endorphin cleavage products could constitute a system fundamentally involved in maintaining "normal" behavior; alterations of the mechanisms normally regulating β-lipotropin-endorphins homeostasis could lead to signs and symptoms of mental illness. Such a potential psychophysiological role of endorphins could logically be testable through the therapeutic administration of available opiate antagonists. In fact, at a recent presentation of these results and concepts (Guillemin *et al.*, 1976b), Terenius reported that administration of naloxone to two chronic schizophrenics had halted their auditory hallucinations within minutes. Recently, in collaboration with Janowsky at the Veterans Administration Hospital in San Diego, naloxone was administered in a double-blind design to ten patients with recognized active schizophrenia. So far, results observed show no improvement of the clinical picture of these patients. The ultimate identification of endorphin-sensitive behavioral events and specific treatment of their dysfunctional states may require the development of more specific "anti-endorphins" than those now available, and other naturally occurring brain peptides (Guillemin *et al.*, 1976b) have already been reported to be endorphin antagonists. Moreover, the matter of doses of the opiate antagonist remains to be more fully investigated. While their endogenous levels in physiological circumstances have not been measured as yet, there are reasons to believe that the endorphins are physiologically meaningful substances: they have already been observed by immunocytochemical methods in neurons of the CNS, both in cell bodies and in axons; they may well act as neurotransmitters, or neuromodulators at the level of multiple CNS loci. Moreover, the striking behavioral effects observed upon their injection in the CNS suggest that endorphins and their likely precursor (prohormone), β-lipotropin, may be of significance in the etiology of some neurologic and psychiatric illnesses in man. The possible participation in these profound CNS effects of a molecule of adenohypophysial origin (β-LPH) and its subunits (the endorphins) is a very unexpected observation. Relationships between brain peptides and adenohypophysial functions are far more complex and intimate at the writing of this review than they were originally expected to be.

III. LOOKING TO THE FUTURE: TWO HYPOTHESES

After this review of some of the newer developments in the expanding field of neuroendocrinology, I would like to conclude with a look to the future. This will take the form of two rather novel concepts. One of these is the concept of *low-voltage processing of information by brain cells,* as already named by Schmitt and his collaborators (1976). The other, I will call the *neural origin of endocrine glands,* or *Is endocrinology a branch of neuroendocrinology?* Both concepts have remarkable implications and point to areas of research that I think will be of importance in the next few years. What we will see also is that these two concepts lead to recognition of a remarkable unity of the mechanisms involved in physiological phenomena as widely separate as the stimulation of the secretion of ACTH or growth hormone by pituitary cells and the inhibition by β-endorphin of the firing pattern of a neuron in the cerebral cortex.

A. Low-Voltage Processing of Information by Brain Cells

Until recently the neuron has been seen primarily as a one-way communication system with a central processor for proximally received inputs and a one-way cable for output, the axon. The axon is characterized by its self-regenerating ability to conduct waves of high-voltage depolarization for rapid transmission of an essentially binary type of information, expressed at the axon terminal. The axon is usually of considerable length, many times the average diameter of the cell body. While the dendritic surface has long been recognized morphologically, and its vastness well observed, it was not granted much of an active role in the performance of the neuron, principally because experimental evidence of such activity was simply lacking. Any integrative ability or capability of the system was located at the axon hillock. One of the major characteristics of this view of the *projection neuron,* well studied for over 50 years, is the high-voltage action potential, from a few millivolts to as much as 100 mV. Classically, such a neuron will deliver its ultimate message at the limited address of its axon terminal(s) in the form of packets of a discrete neurotransmitter. For most projection neurons, we still do not know whether norepinephrine, acetylcholine, dopamine, or, in a few instances, serotonin are involved. No consensus exists as to the ultimate significance of neuropharmacologically active substances like certain amino acids, γ-aminobutyric acid, substance P, and, lately, the small peptides, such as somatostatin, the hypothalamic releasing factors, and the endorphins, traced by immunoassays or immunocytochemistry to increasing numbers of neuronal fibers and neuronal bodies far removed from the ventral hypothalamus and the pituitary.

While this simplified picture of the projection neuron is still correct, the majority appears to welcome this multiplicity of effectors; integration of these multiple effectors, with specific functional processes of individual neurons as members of a neuronal network is at the moment, an appealing hypothesis. This new view of the neuron is based on new morphology as seen by the electron microscope. Much of the discussion that follows is based on a recent review by Schmitt, Dev, and Smith (1976) and on the text of the proceedings of a Meeting of the Neurosciences Research Program devoted to local circuits (Rakic, 1975). The dendrite is seen no more as a "passive receptor surface," but rather as a locus for transmitting as well as receiving information, in traffic with dendrites of other neurons. Such communications are seen in the release or uptake of diverse small or large molecules. The electric phenomena involved are those of pinpoint depolarizations and are measured in a few microvolts. Such electrotonic currents spread only over distances measured in micrometers, not millimeters or centimeters. This type of extremely low-voltage communication constitutes the so-called local circuits. The local-circuit neuron can also modify the ultimate behavior of one or more projection neurons, which can send responses to a remote contact by a high-voltage, long axon-pathway. Such systems have been well studied in the retina, the olfactory bulb, and the lateral geniculate body. There is increasing evidence that such local circuitry is actually present in all parts of the CNS. It actually represents the structure of the greatest mass or volume of the CNS, with the projection neurons in their classical anatomical arrangements, probably a minority in number as well as in occupied space.

Such multiple dendritic connections have been observed in the electron microscope. Figure 8 is a diagram of possible connections [redrawn from the recent review by Schmitt *et al.* (1976)], between one axon terminal and two dendrites, one of which also is in contact with three other dendrites at about ten other locations. The diagram conveys the observation that dendrites may be both presynaptic and postsynaptic to each other, as in reciprocal synapses. There is also electron microscope evidence of *gap junctions* between dendrites. Such electrotonic coupling has been demonstrated in the CNS. Several neurons so coupled will respond synchronously, with extremely low activating voltages required. Oscillatory behavior has been observed in populations of neurons in some invertebrates (Gettings and Willows, 1974) when elec-

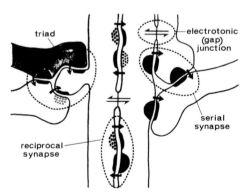

FIG. 8. Diagram illustrating the proposal that dendrites in their reciprocal interactions can be presynoptic and postsynaptic to one another. One axon only is shown in the diagram; all other connections are between dendrites. The hypothesis is that several neurochemicals may be involved at the several junction points (peptides, enzymes, catecholamines, etc.), with either inhibitory or excitatory activity. Redrawn from Fig. 1 of Schmitt *et al.* (1976).

trically coupled. Such electronic junctions are frequently observed in immediate proximity to chemical synapses (Schmitt *et al.*, 1976). None of these phenomena require, and none of these structures produce, high-voltage spikes. Information transfer by such mechanisms is relatively slow, in seconds or longer, not milliseconds.

1. Peptidergic Neurons and Peptidergic Endocrine Cells

What are the relationships between this new view of neurons and the peptides of neuroendocrinology? They become apparent when one asks about the nature of the chemicals involved in these dendro-dendritic contacts? The fragmentary emerging picture is most interesting. It has long been considered that dendrites are involved in uptake of necessary metabolites, such as sugars, free amino acids, adenosine. Such uptake can proceed from extracellular fluid and also from capillary vessels, through endothelial cells. Molecules of much larger size appear similarly to be taken up by dendrites. For instance, an enzyme like acetylcholinesterase, after being released in extracellular compartments, has been reported (Kreutzberg *et al.*, 1975) to be first bound to the outer surface of the dendritic membrane and later taken up by dendrites.

Thus an interesting *hypothesis* would be the release at dendritic points of (still to be characterized) enzymes of neuronal origin that would specifically cleave a biologically active peptide, such as one of the endorphins, from a biologically inactive precursor, such as β-lipotropin, available in extracellular compartments or perhaps to be found in the axoplasm.

Classical transmitters appear to be released and taken up by the dendrites. Similar release and reciprocal uptake of the small peptides, such as substance P, neurotensin, somatostatin, TRF, endorphins, have not been demonstrated as yet. That this is possible and actually happens is a working hypothesis worth investigating. It would go a long way to explain the multiplicity of effects of the polypeptides on the CNS. See, for instance (Table II), the multiplicity of effects of the tripeptide TRF on biological events that have nothing to do with the release of pituitary thyrotropin, the well known hypophysiotropic activity of TRF, for which it was originally named and recognized. The possibility of an enormous number of such dendritic transfer sites might also explain the psychotropic effects of some of these peptides. Cajal as early as 1899 had made the comment that local-circuit neurons may well play an

TABLE II

CENTRAL NERVOUS SYSTEM-MEDIATED ACTIONS OF THYROTROPIN RELEASING FACTOR (TRF)[a]

Increases spontaneous motor activity

Alters sleep patterns

Produces anorexia

Inhibition of condition avoidance behavior

Head-to-tail rotation

Opposes actions of barbiturates on sleeping time, hypothermia, lethality

Opposes actions of ethanol, chloral hydrate, chlorpromazine, and diazepam on sleeping time and hypothermia

Enhances convulsion time and lethality of strychnine

Increases motor activity in morphine-treated animals

Potentiates DOPA-pargyline effects

Amelioration of human behavioral disorders?

Central inhibition of morphine-mediated secretion of growth hormone and prolactin

Alteration of brain cell membrane electrical activity

Increases norepinephrine turnover

Releases norepinephrine and dopamine from synaptosomal preparations

Enhances disappearance of norepinephrine from nerve terminals

Potentiates excitory actions of acetylcholine on cerebral cortical neurons

[a]From W. Vale, C. Rivier, and M. Brown, *Annu. Rev. Physiol.* **39,** 473–527 (1977).

important role as the substrate of complex behavior because of their "prodigious abundance and unaccustomed wealth of forms." Considering such enormous dendritic trees, with each dendrite ending possibly involved in multiple synaptic junctions (see Fig. 8), the number of contacts and control points for a single neuron defies the imagination. Such cellular anatomy, when considered with the hypotheses mentioned above for chemical inputs and outputs, shows the considerable possible functional significance of an expanded dendritic connection network.

The hypothesis of networks with multiple terminals capable of releasing and/or utilizing biologically active peptides, may also be involved in another way in explaining some current data. It has been recognized that the total amounts, as well as the concentrations, of TRF, or LRF, or somatostatin in the extrahypothalamic CNS as measured by bioassays or radioimmunoassays are considerably higher than can be accounted for by the number of cell bodies shown to contain such peptides by immunocytochemistry. A hypothesis to consider is that there would be relatively few neurons manufacturing, say, TRF or LRF (primarily) located in the hypophysiotropic area of the hypothalamus with perhaps a few more cells in the amygdala, and that these neurons have long axons with *multiple axon collaterals,* all with peptide-containing and -secreting boutons terminals (Martin *et al.,* 1975).

There is already evidence that the dendritic traffic of chemicals works both ways with release and uptake. Thus, in a reciprocally functioning system, if the endorphins and enkephalins are enzymically cleaved extracellularly from β-lipotropin as a circulating extracellular precursor in a manner reminiscent of the biogenesis of angiotensin, they could then be picked up by the multiple dendritic endings and carried by retrograde axoplasmic flow whatever distance is necessary for their physiological function.

In summary, we see the small peptides as substances released locally, and perhaps produced locally, at innumerable possible source points. The specific functions each would subserve, would thus be dependent on the effector cell each would be affecting (homonymic information). The same peptide could have vastly different ultimate effects depending on the target cell it would be acting upon. This is now well recognized, for instance, for somatostatin. In other words, the same message could have multiple meanings depending on which receptor–effector receives it. (''Go'' received–effected by the conductor of a train has an entirely different result than when received–effected by a swimmer ready to dive.) They could also be either transmitters or modulators, depending on their locus of release. If the effect of the small peptides is then the activation of the adenylcyclase–cAMP system of their effector neurons, as they may well do in other target tissues, such as the adenohypophysis, their effects in neuronal networks could be amplified, long-lasting as well as possibly expanding from their exact source point. Such a system involving neuronal cAMP has already been demonstrated by Siggins *et al.* (1973) for neurons of the locus coeruleus.

2. *Endocrinology vs Paracrinology*

This concept of a *local* release and *local* immediate effect of the peptides from multiple sources in the CNS is a point to remember for future discussion. It does not belong to substances classically defined as hormones. This is true even if each local event may lead to ultimately widespread effects, which is the usual result of hormonal actions. Needless to say that the technology involved in exploring such secretory functions of the dendrites or of the boutons of axon collaterals will be particularly challenging.

TRF activity, LRF activity, somatostatin activity were demonstrated by bioassays and radioimmunoassays in the extrahypothalamic CNS. Later reports appeared showing effects of somatostatin in inhibiting secretion of glucagon and insulin by direct action at the level of the endocrine pancreas. Because somatostatin has a short biological half-life upon injection in peripheral blood it was unlikely that any physiological effect of endogenous somatostatin on the endocrine pancreas would be due to somatostatin of hypothalamic origin. Looking originally for somatostatin in pancreatic nerve endings, somatostatin was found by immunofluorescence in discrete endocrine *cells,* of the pancreas, now well characterized as the D cells (Dubois, 1975; Luft *et al.,* 1974). The same studies showed somatostatin in discrete cells in the jejunum, the colon, the duodenum, and the gastric mucosa. Other observations indicated also that somatostatin can inhibit the secretion of gastrin, secretin, gastric HC1, and acetylcholine from the myenteric plexus. TRF and LRF, though found in extrahypothalamic CNS, have not been found, as yet, to my knowledge in extra-CNS tissues. This is certainly worth investigating. As early as 1957 I had observed CRF activity in extracts of gut tissues also containing substance P (Guillemin, 1957). Brodish has also described extrahypothalamic CRF. Besides somatostatin, other peptides are now known to be present and most likely synthesized by cellular elements, in *both* the central and peripheral nervous system and also in glandular elements of the gastrointestinal tract. The first peptide so observed was substance P in the remarkable experiments of Ulf von Euler and Gaddum as early as 1931 (von Euler and Gaddum, 1931). There is now evidence that neurotensin, gastrin, VIP, GIP, the endorphins, enkephalin(s) are found in the brain as well as in the gastrointestinal tract and the pancreas. This is also true for several of the small peptides, such as bombesin, caerulein, physalaemin, isolated years ago from extracts of the skin of frogs. Furthermore there are remarkable analogies and homologies between the amino acid sequences of several of these peptides of CNS origin and gastrointestinal origin as well as those isolated from the frog skin. These peptides have been found by immunocytochemistry essentially in two types of cells: (1) they are seen in cell bodies and nerve fibers, i.e., neural and dendritic processes of *neurons* in brain, in spinal cord, in spinal ganglia, and in the myenteric plexus; (2) they are seen also in typical *endocrine* cells, for instance, in the pancreatic islets of Langerhans, in the enterochromaffin cells of the gut, and in the adrenal medulla. Neuroblastomas have been reported to contain high levels of the vasointestinal peptide (VIP) (Said and Rosenberg, 1976). An undifferentiated mediastinoma has been found to contain somatostatin, calcitonin, ACTH, prolactin (private communication from Iain MacIntyre).

All these results are based on radioimmunoassays, immunocytochemistry, in some instances also bioassays, in most cases with evidence of parallelism of the responses to the known peptide-reference standard and the crude tissue extracts. In cases involving immunological methods there is modest evidence for specificity of the antibodies utilized. More significant, reports are beginning to appear that demonstrate identity of the primary structure of the gastrointestinal variety of a peptide when compared to its CNS variety; for instance, neurotensin (Carraway *et al.*, 1976) and substance P. Our laboratory has already reported the complete sequencing of hypothalamic α-MSH and found it to be identical to that of pituitary α-MSH (Burgus *et al.*, 1976). Thus there is every reason to believe that we are dealing with the same peptides regardless of their tissue origin.

What is the message to be read in these observations of startling commonalities between the CNS and endocrine tissues, and what does it imply for future research?

B. *The Neural Origin of Peptidergic Endocrine Cells*

There is already an interesting unifying concept: Much credit must go to A. G. E. Pearse (1968) for his visionary concept, formulated some 10 years ago, of the APUD cells: Pearse observed that neurons and some endocrine cells producing polypeptide hormones shared a set of common cytochemical features and ultrastructural characteristics. APUD is an acronym referring to *A*mine content and/or amine *P*recursor *U*ptake and *D*ecarboxylation, as common qualities of these cells (Pearse, 1968). The APUD concept postulated that these endocrine cells were derived from a common neuroectodermal ancestor, the transient *neural crest*.

Pearse postulated further that a still larger number of endocrine cells, would be eventually found sharing these common properties if one were to explore further in the adult, endocrine tissues derived from the neural crest. Recent observations with refined techniques, particularly the work of Le Douarin on topical chimeras with chromosomal markers have led Pearse to modify the original APUD concept, but, as we will see, in a remarkable manner. The new evidence regarding the multiple sources of the several peptides mentioned above, showed that tissues were involved that were not of neural crest origin; this is particularly true for the peptide-secreting cells of the gut. All these cells have been shown to arise from specialized neuroectoderm (Pearse and Takor, 1976), that is, not only the neural crest but also the neural tube, the neural ridges, and the placodes.

The expanded concept now postulates that all peptide hormone-producing cells are derived from the neural ectoderm, as are all neurons. For instance recently Takor and Pearse have reexamined the early stages of development of both the hypophysis and the hypothalamus (Pearse and Takor, 1976). They confirmed and expanded earlier conclusions of Ballard, who as early as 1964 had recognized that Rathke's pouch does not come from the stomodeum (the pharyngeal origin) as is classically written, but it originates from the ventral neural ridge (from studies in the chick embryo) (Ballard, 1964).

Thus, the hypophysis would share with the hypothalamus the same ventral neural ridge of the neuroectoderm for its origin. Recent work by Ferrand and Hraoui (1973) using the chromosomal markers in topical chimeras has also indicated an exclusively neuroectodermal origin of the adenohypophysis. Thus Pearse and Takor (1976) have recently concluded: "It is therefore necessary to postulate a neuroectodermal derivation for *all* the endocrine cells of the adenohypophysis and to regard the whole hypothalamo-hypophysial complex as a neuroendocrine derivative of the ventral neural ridge."

I mentioned earlier that we have recently observed with well characterized antisera to α-endorphin and β-endorphin that these peptides can be seen by immunocytochemistry in discrete nerve fibers in the hypothalamus and in all cells of the intermediate lobe plus some cells of the adenohypophysis (Bloom *et al.*, 1977). These same cells in the pars intermedia have long been known from the work of several groups of investigators also to contain ACTH[1–39], CLIP, i.e. ACTH[18–39],

α-MSH, i.e. ACTH[1–13], β-LPH[1–91], γ-LPH[1–48]. Cells of the pars intermedia have also been considered to belong to the APUD series.

The conclusion from all this is that the peptide-secreting cells and tissues appear to be as much part of the nervous system as is the adrenal medulla, or what has been called traditionally the neurohypophysis. The word *neuroendocrinology* is now taking a fuller meaning than ever. Pearse has gone so far as to propose that the nervous system should be recognized as composed of three divisions: somatic, autonomic, and endocrine.

Perhaps the time has come to redefine the word *hormone*. The hypothalamic hypophysiotropic peptides, TRF, LRF, somatostatin, are really not hormones according to the current definition, which is still that proposed by Starling in 1905. The definition implies a single source of secretion and, fundamentally, the direct ingress of the secretory product into blood vessels for distribution to a distant receptor tissue, itself thus triggered to respond by its own secretion, change in metabolism, etc. At the level of the dendritic network discussed above, between median eminence and adenohypophysial cells, in the endocrine pancreas or in the gastric mucosa, TRF, LRF, somatostatin appear to have remarkably localized ranges of extracellular movements ranging from angstroms, to micrometers, at most a few millimeters through the hypothalamohypophysial portal capillaries. There is no incontrovertible evidence so far that these peptides circulate in peripheral blood in physiologically significant concentrations. They have multiple sources, possibly, as hypothesized above, innumerable. They would thus not be hormones in the classical sense. The concept of *paracrine* secretion first proposed by Feyrter in 1938 seems much more appropriate to describe products from cells that act on immediate neighbors. The distinction with *neurotransmitters* is not obvious. I proposed earlier the name *cybernin* for these substances, the etymology of the word implying "local information" or "local control." I have not pushed that new terminology too boldly as it is still another word, and an entirely new root (in biology). As we discussed above, there is good evidence that the small peptides can act as *modulators* of the function of neuronal system. They are not necessarily neurotransmitters in the classical sense and, so far, have not been demonstrated as such. We may want to redefine a *hormone* to be any substance released by a cell and which acts on another cell near or far, regardless of the singularity or ubiquity of the source and regardless of the means of conveyance—blood stream, axoplasmic flow, immediate extracellular space. If we do not do so, because of the old definition and to be consistent, hormones would be the steroids, the products of the adenohypophysis, of the thyroid, insulin, glucagon, etc.—that is, those messengers that really circulate wide and far in peripheral blood. The neuroendocrine peptides would have to be something else. I think that it is becoming of heuristic significance to reconsider that terminology. The choice of words or of definitions that will be proposed should take into consideration the remarkable developments I have summarized briefly here.

IV. CONCLUSIONS

The remarkable picture that emerges is not only that more and more neurophysiologists and endocrinologists are dealing with similar concepts, but that they are, and have been all along, talking about various forms or embodiments of a single anatomical structure fundamentally devoted to the centrifugal dispatch of information. This structure comes as the classical neuron or as the classical endocrine cell and as several overlapping forms.

From the increasing number of studies using specific radioimmunoassays as well as methods of immunocytochemistry, more and more neurons are being recognized as containing specific peptides. Immunoreactive gastrin—or a closely related peptide—is found in cells of the cerebral cortex; substance P, angiotensin, somatostatin, vasoactive-intestinal peptide, peptide sequences corresponding to fragments of ACTH and to fragments of β-LPH are located in neurons, their axons and dendrites. When one realizes that all our current classical neurophysiology as well as all current classical thinking in neurology and neuropsychiatry simply ignores this increasing, overwhelming morphological and biochemical information, one wonders what will be the significance of these peptides in the physiology of the brain. This has to be the beginning of a new era in our knowledge, and prospective of the central nervous system, both normal and diseased.

ACKNOWLEDGMENTS

Research of the Laboratories for Neuroendocrinology at the Salk Institute is currently supported by research grants from the NIH (HD-09690-03 and AM-18811-03), National Foundation (1-411), and the William Randolph Hearst Foundation.

REFERENCES

Alford, F. P., *et al.*, (1974), *Lancet* **2**, 947.

Amoss, M., Burgus, R., Ward, D. N., Fellows, R., and Guillemin, R. (1970). *Endocrinology* **87**, A61.

Amoss, M., Burgus, R., Blackwell, R., Vale, W., Fellows, R., and Guillemin, R., *Biochem. Biophys. Res. Commun.* (1971), **44**, 205–210.

Ballard, W. W. (1964). *In* "Comparative Anatomy and Embryology," Ronald Press, New York, 1964.

Belluzzi, J. D., Grant, N., Garsky, V., Sarantakis, D., Wise, C. C., and Stein, L. (1976), *Nature (London)* **260**, 625.

Bloom, F., Segal, D., Ling, N., and Guillemin, R. (1976). *Science* **194**, 630–632.

Bloom, F., Battenberg, E., Rossier, J., Ling, N., Leppaluoto, J., Vargo, T., Guillemin, R. (1977). *Life Sci.* **20**, 43–48.

Bøler, J., Enzmann, F., Folkers, K., Bowers, C. Y., and Schally, A. V. (1969). *Biochem. Biophys. Res. Commun.* **37**, 705.

Bowers, C. Y., Schally, A. V., Enzmann, F., Bøler, J., and Folkers, K. (1969). *Proc. 45th Meet. Am. Thyroid Assoc.,* p. 15.

Bowers, C. Y., Schally, A. V., Enzmann, F., Bøler, J., and Folkers, K. (1970). *Endocrinology* **86**, 1143–1153.

Bradbury, A. F., Smyth, D. G., and Snell, C. R. (1975). *In* "Proceedings of the Fourth American Peptide Symposium" (R. Walter and G. Meienhofer, eds.), pp. 609–615. Ann Arbor Sci. Publ., Ann Arbor, Michigan.

Bradbury, A. F., Smyth, D. G., Snell, C. R., Birdsall, N. J. M., and Hulme, E. C. (1976). *Nature (London)* **260**, 793–795.

Brazeau, P., Vale, W., Burgus, R., Ling, N., Butcher, M., Rivier, J., and Guillemin, R. (1973). *Science* **179**, 77–79.

Brazeau, P., Rivier, J., Vale, W., and Guillemin, R. (1974). *Endocrinology* **94**, 184–186.

Brown, M., Rivier, J., and Vale, W. (1976). *Metabolism* **25**, 1501–1503.

Burgus, R., and Guillemin, R. (1967). *Fed. Proc., Fed. Am. Soc. Exp. Biol.* **26**, 255.

Burgus, R., and Guillemin, R. (1970). *In* "Hypophysiotropic Hormones of the Hypothalamus" (J. Meites, ed.), p. 227. Williams & Wilkins, Baltimore, Maryland.

Burgus, R., Stillwell, R. N., McCloskey, J. A., Ward, D. N., Sakiz, E., and Guillemin, R. (1966a). *Physiologist* **9**, 149.

Burgus, R., Ward, D. N., Sakiz, E., and Guillemin, R., (1966b). *C. R. Acad. Sci.* **262**, 2643.

Burgus, R., Dunn, T. F., Desiderio, D., Vale, W., and Guillemin, R. (1969a). *C. R. H. Acad. Sci. Ser. D* **269**, 226. 1969a.

Burgus, R., Dunn, T. F., Ward, D. N., Vale, W., Amoss, M., and Guillemin, R. (1969b). *C. R. H. Acad. Sci. Ser. D* **268**, 2116.

Burgus, R., Dunn, T. F., Desiderio, D., and Guillemin, R. (1969c). *C. R. H. Acad. Sci. Ser. D* **269**, 1870.

Burgus, R., Dunn, T. F., Desiderio, D., Ward, D. N., Vale, W., and Guillemin, R. (1970a). *Nature (London)* **226**, 321.

Burgus, R., Dunn, T. F., Desiderio, D., Ward, D. N., Vale, W., Guillemin, R., Felix, A. M., Gillessen, D., and Studer, R. O. (1970b). *Endocrinology* **86**, 573.

Burgus, R., Butcher, M., Ling, N., Monahan, M., Rivier, J., Fellows, R., Amoss, M., Blackwell, R., Vale, W., and Guillemin, R. (1971). *C. R. H. Acad. Sci. Ser. D* **273**, 1611–1613.

Burgus, R., Butcher, M., Amoss, M., Ling, N., Monahan, M., Rivier, J., Fellows, R., Blackwell, R., Vale, W., and Guillemin, R. (1972). *Proc. Natl. Acad. Sci. U.S.A.* **69**, 278–282.

Burgus, R., Ling, N., Butcher, M., and Guillemin, R. (1973). *Proc. Natl. Acad. Sci. U.S.A.* **70**, 684–688.

Burgus, R., Amoss, M., Brazeau, P., Brown, M., Ling, N., Rivier, C., Rivier, J., Vale, W., and Villarreal, J. (1976). *In* "Hypothalamus and Endocrine Functions" (F. Labrie, *et al.*), p. 355. Plenum, New York, 1976.

Buscher, H. H., Hill, R. C., Romer, D., Cardinaux, F., Closse, A., Hauser, D., Pless, J., (1976). *Nature (London)* **261**, 423–425.

Campbell, H. T., Feuer, G., Garcia, J., and Harris, G. W. (1961). *J. Physiol. (London)* **157**, 30.

Carraway, R. E., Kitabgi, P., and Leeman, S. (1976). *Int. Congr. Endocrinol., Hamburg 6th* (Abstract), p. 178, A435.

Courrier, R., Guillemin, R., Jutisz, M., Sakiz, E., and Aschheim, P. (1961). *C. R. H. Acad. Sci.* **253**, 922.

Cox, B. M., Goldstein, A., and Li, C. H. (1976). *Proc. Natl. Acad. Sci. U.S.A.* **73**, 1821–1823.

Davies, J., and Dray, A. (1976). *Nature (London)* **262**, 603–604.

Dhariwal, A. P. S., Watanabe, S., Antunes-Rodrigues, J., and McCann, S. (1967). *Neuroendocrinology* **2**, 294–303.

Dubois, M. (1972). *Lille Med.* **17**, 1391–1394.

Dubois, M. (1975). *Proc. Natl. Acad. Sci. U.S.A.* **72**, 1340–1343.

Fales, H. M., Nagai, Y., Milne, G. W. A., Brewer, H. B., Bronzert, R. J., and Pisano, J. J. (1971). *Anal. Biochem.* **43**, 288–299.

Fellows, R. E., and Mudge, A. (1970). *Fed. Proc., Fed. Am. Soc. Exp. Biol.* **30**, 1078.

Ferrand, R., and Hraoui, S. (1973). C. R. *Soc. Biol.* **167**, 740.

Feyrter, F. (1938). "Uber diffuse Endokrine Epitheliale Organ," p. 259. Barth, Leipzig.

Fleischer, N., and Guillemin, R. (1976). *In* "Peptide Hormones" (J. A. Parsons, ed.), pp. 317–335. Macmillan, New York.

Fleischer, N., Burgus, R., Vale, W., Dunn, T., and Guillemin, R. (1970). *J. Clin. Endocrinol.* **31**, 109–112.

Folkers, K., Enzmann, F., Bøler, J., Bowers, C. Y., and Schally, A. F. (1969). *Biochem. Biophys. Res. Commun.* **37**, 123.

Freedman, A. M., Kaplan, H. I., and Saddock, B. J. (eds.) (1975). "Comprehensive Textbook of Psychiatry," p. 2578. William & Wilkins, Baltimore, Maryland.

Frederickson, R. C. A., and Norris, F. H. (1976). *Science* **194**, 440–442.

Fujino, M., Yamazaki, I., Kobayashi, S., Fukuda, T., Shinagawa, S., Nakayama, R. (1974). *Biochem. Biophys. Res. Commun.* **57**, 1248–1256.

Gerich, J. E., Lorenzi, M., Schneider, V., Karam, J., Rivier, J., and Guillemin, R. (1974). *N. Engl. J. Med.* **291**, 544–547.

Gerich, J. E., Lorenzi, M., Gustafson, G., Guillemin, R., and Forsham, P. (1975). *Metabolism* **24**, 175.

Gettings, P. A., and Willows, A. O. D. (1974). *J. Neurophysiol.* **37**, 358-361.

Gillessen, D., Felix, A. M., Lergier, W., and Studer, R. O. (1970). *Helv. Chim. Acta* **53**, 63.

Guillemin, R. (1957). *Rev. Suisse Zool.* **64**, 37.

Guillemin, R. (1964). *Rec. Prog. Horm. Res.* **20**, 89.

Guillemin, R. (1967). *Annu. Rev. Physiol.* **29**, 313.

Guillemin, R. (1968). *In* "Pharmacology of Hormonal Polypeptides and Proteins" (N. Back *et al.*, eds.), p. 148. Plenum, New York.

Guillemin, R. (1973). *In* "Advances in Human Growth Hormone Research" (S. Raiti, ed.), Vol. 1, p. 139-143. U.S. Gov't. Printing Office, Pub. No (NIH)74-612.

Guillemin, R. (1976). *Endocrinology* **99**, 1653.

Guillemin, R., and Gerich, J. (1976). *Annu. Rev. Med.* **27**, 379-388.

Guillemin, R., and Rosenberg, B. (1955). *Endocrinology* **57**, 599-697.

Guillemin, R., and Sakiz, E. (1965). *Nature (London)* **207**, 297.

Guillemin, R., and Vale, W. (1970). *In* "Hypophysiotropic Hormones of the Hypothalamus" (J. Meites, ed.), p. 21. Williams & Wilkins, Baltimore, Maryland.

Guillemin, R., Yamazaki, E., Jutisz, M., and Sakiz (1962). E., *C. R. Acad. Sci.* **255**, 1018-1020.

Guillemin, R., Yamazaki, E., Gard, D. A., Jutisz, M., and Sakiz, E. (1963). *Endocrinology* **73**, 564.

Guillemin, R., Sakiz, E., and Ward, D. N. (1965). *Proc. Soc. Exp. Biol. Med.* **118**, 1132.

Guillemin, R., Burgus, R., Sakiz, E., and Ward, D. N. (1968). *C. R. H. Acad. Sci. Ser. D* **262**, 2278.

Guillemin, R., Ling, N., and Burgus, R. (1976a). *C. R. H. Acad. Sci. Ser. D* **282**, 783-785.

Guillemin, R., Ling, N., Burgus, R., Lazarus, L. (1976b). *Psychoneuroendocrinology* **2**, 59-62.

Gunne, L. M., Lindstrom, L., and Terenius, L. (1977). *J. Neural Transmission* **40**.

Hagenmaier, H., Ebbighausen, W., Nicholson, G., and Votsch, W. (1970). *Z. Naturforsch.* **25B**, 681-689.

Hill, R. G., Pepper, C. M., and Mitchell, F. J. (1976). *Nature (London).* **262**, 604-606.

Hughes, J. (1975). *Brain Res.* **88**, 295-308.

Hughes, J., Smith, T. W., Kosterlitz, H. W., Fothergill, L. A., Morgan, B. A., and Morris, H. R. (1975). *Nature (London)* **258**, 577-579.

Igarashi, M., and McCann, S. M. (1964) *Endocrinology* **74**, 440-445.

Johnson, E. S., Gendrich, R. L., and White, W. F. (1976). *Fertil. Steril.* **27**, 853-860.

Jutisz, M., de la Llosa, P., Sakiz, E., Yamazaki, E., and Guillemin, R. (1963a). *C. R. Soc. Biol.* **157**, 235.

Jutisz, M., Yamazaki, E., Berault, A., Sakiz, E., and Guillemin, R. (1963b). *C. R. H. Acad. Sci.* **256**, 2925.

Kamm, O., Aldrich, T. B., Grote, I. W., Rowe, L. W., and Bugbee, E. P. (1928). *J. Am. Chem. Soc.* **50**, 573.

Kaymakcalan, S., and Wood, L. A. (1956). *J. Pharmacol. Exp. Ther.* **117**, 112.

Koerker, D. J., *et al.* (1974). *Science* **184**, 482-484.

Kreutzberg, G. W., Schubert, P., and Lux, H. D. (1975). "Neuroplasmic Transport in Axons and Dendrites" (M. Santini, ed.), p. 161-166. Raven, New York.

Krulich, L., Dhariwal, A. P. S., and McCann, S. M. (1968). *Endocrinology* **83**, 783.

Lazarus, L. H., Ling, N., and Guillemin, R. (1976). *Proc. Natl. Acad. Sci. U.S.A.* **73**, 2156–2159.

Li, C. H., and Chung, D. (1976). *Proc. Natl. Acad. Sci. U.S.A.* **73**, 1145–1148.

Ling, N., and Guillemin, R. (1976a). *Proc. Natl. Acad. Sci. U.S.A.* **73**, 3308–3310.

Ling, N., Rivier, J., Burgus, R., and Guillemin, R. (1973). *Biochemistry* **12**, 5305–5310.

Ling, N., Burgus, R., and Guillemin, R. (1976b). *Proc. Natl. Acad. Sci. U.S.A.* **73**, 3942–3946.

Loh, H. H., Tseng, L. F., Wei, E., and Li, C. H. (1976). *Proc. Natl. Acad. Sci.* **73**, 2895–2896.

Luft, R., Efendic, S., Hökfelt, T., Johansson, O., and Arimura, A. (1974). *Med. Biol.* **52**, 428–430.

McCann, S. M., and Porter, J. C. (1969). *Phsyiol. Rev.* **49**, 249.

McCann, S. M., Taleisnick, S., and Friedman, H. M. (1960). *Proc. Soc. Exp. Biol. Med.* **104**, 432.

Marks, N., and Stern, F. (1975). *FEBS Lett.* **55**, 220–224.

Martin, J. B., Renaud, L. P., and Brazeau, P. (1975). *Lancet* **8**, 393–395.

Matsuo, H., Nair, R. M., Arimura, A., and Schally, A. V. (1971a). *Biochem. Biophys. Res. Commun.* **43**, 1334.

Matsuo, H., Arimura, A., Nair, R. M. G., and Schally, A. V. (1971b). *Biochem. Biophys. Res. Commun.* **45**, 822–827.

Monahan, M., Rivier, J., Burgus, R., Amoss, M., Blackwell, R., Vale, W., and Guillemin, R., *C. R. H. Acad. Sci. Ser. D* **273**, 205.

Monahan, M., Amoss, M., Anderson, H., and Vale, W. (1973). *Biochemistry* **12**, 4616–4620.

Moon, H. D., Li, C. H., and Jennings, B. M. (1973). *Anat. Rec.* **175**, 529–538.

Mortimer, C. H., *et al.* (1974). *Lancet* **1**, 697.

Nair, R. M. G., Barrett, F. J., Bowers, C. Y., and Schally, A. V. (1970). *Biochemistry* **9**, 1103.

Nicoll, R., Siggins, G., Ling, N., Bloom, F., and Guillemin, R. (1977). *Proc. Natl. Acad. Sci. U.S.A.* **74**, 2584–2588.

Pasternak, G., Goodman, R., and Snyder, S. H. (1975). *Life Sci.* **16**, 1765–1770.

Pearse, A. G. E. (1968). *Proc. R. Soc. London Ser. B* **170**, 71.

Pearse, A. G. E., and Takor, T. (1976). *Clin. Endocrinol.,* Suppl., 229s–244s.

Rakic, P. (1975). *Neurosci. Res. Program Bull.* **13**, 291.

Rebar *et al.* (1973). *J. Clin. Endocrinol. Metab.* **36**, 10–16.

Redding, T. W., Bowers, C. Y., and Schally, A. V. (1966). *Endocrinology* **79**, 229.

Rivier, C., Vale, W., Ling, N., Brown, M., and Guillemin, R. (1977). *Endocrinology* **100**, 238–241.

Rivier, J. (1974). *J. Am. Chem. Soc.,* **96**, 2986–2992.

Rivier, J., Burgus, R., and Vale, W. (1971). *Endocrinology* **88**, A86.

Ross, M., Su, T.-P., Cox, B. M., and Goldstein, A. (1976). *In* "Opiates and Endogenous Opioid Peptides." H. Kosterlitz, ed.), pp. 35–40. Elsevier, Amsterdam.

Said, S. I., and Rosenberg, R. N. (1976). *Science* **192**, 907.

Sarantakis, D., McKinley, W. A., Jannakais, I., Clark, D., and Grant, N. (1976). *Clin. Endocrinol.* **5** Suppl., 275s–278s.

Schally, A. V., Bowers, C. Y., and Redding, T. W. (1966a). *Endocrinology* **78**, 726.

Schally, A. V., Bowers, C. Y., Redding, T. W., and Barrett, J. F. (1966b). *Biochem. Biophys. Res. Commun.* **25**, 165.

Schally, A. V., Redding, T. W., Barrett, F. J., and Bowers, C. Y. (1966c). *Fed. Proc., Fed. Am. Soc. Exp. Biol.* **25**, 348.

Schally, A. V., Saito, T., Arimura, A., Muller, E. E., and Bowers, C. Y. (1966d). *Endocrinology* **79**, 1087-1094.

Schally, A. V., Arimura, A., Bowers, C. Y., Kastin, A. J., Sawano, S., and Redding, T. W. (1968). *Rec. Prog. Horm. Res.* **24**, 497.

Schally, A. V., Redding, T. W., Bowers, C. Y., and Barrett, F. J. (1969). *J. Biol. Chem.* **244**, 4077.

Schally, A. V., Arimura, A., Baba, Y., Nair, R. M. G., Matsuo, H., Redding, T. W., Debeljuk, L., and White, W. F. (1971a). *Biochem. Biophys. Res. Commun.* **43**, 393-399.

Schally, A. V., Nair, R. M. G., Redding, T. W., and Arimura (1971b). A., *J. Biol. Chem.* **246**, 7230-7236.

Schmitt, F. O., Dev. P., and Smith, B. H. (1976). *Science* **193**, 114.

Schroder, E., and Lübke, K. (1965). "The Peptides," Vol. 2. Academic Press, New York.

Siggins, G. R., Battenberg, E. F., Hoffer, B. J., and Bloom, F. E. (1973). *Science* **179**, 585.

Simantov, R., and Snyder, S. H. (1976). *Life Sci.* **18**, 781-788.

Terenius, L., and Wahlstrom, A. (1975). *Life Sci.* **16**, 1759-1764.

Teschemacher, H., Opheim, K. E., Cox, B. M., and Goldstein, A. (1975). *Life Sci.* 1771-1776.

Tsuji, S., Sakoda, M., and Asami, M. (1968). *In* "Integrative Mechanisms of Neuroendocrine System" (S. Itoh, ed.), p. 63. Hokkaido Univ. School of Med., Houston, Texas (Publ).

Vale, W., Burgus, R., Dunn, T. F., and Guillemin, R. (1970). *J. Clin. Endocrinol. Metab.* **30**, 148.

Vale, W., Rivier, J., and Burgus, R. (1971). *Endocrinology* **89**, 1485-1488.

Vale, W., Brazeau, P., Grant, G., Nussey, A., Burgus, R., Rivier, J., Ling, N., and Guillemin, R. (1972a). *C. R. H. Acad. Sci.* **275**, 2913-2915.

Vale, W., Grant, G., Amoss, M., Blackwell, R., and Guillemin, R. (1972b) *Endocrinology* **91**, 562-572.

Vale, W., Grant, G., Amoss, M., Blackwell, R., and Guillemin, R. (1972). *Endocrinology* **91**, 562-572.

Vale, W., Grant, G., Rivier, J., Monahan, M., Amoss, M., Blackwell, R., Burgus, R., and Guillemin, R. (1972d). *Science* **176**, 933-934.

Vale, W., Rivier, C., Brazeau, P., and Guillemin, R. (1974). *Endocrinology* **95**, 968-977.

Vale, W., Brazeau, P., Rivier, C., Brown, M., Boss, B., Rivier, J., Burgus, R., Ling, N., and Guillemin, R. (1975). *Rec. Prog. Horm. Res.* **31**, 365-397.

Vale, W., Rivier, C., Brown, M., Leppaluoto, J., Monahan, M., Rivier, J., (1976). *Clin. Endocrinol.* **5**, Suppl., 261-273.

Vilchez-Martinez, J., Coy, D., Coy, E., De la Cruz, A., Nishi, N., and Schally, A. V. (1975). *Endocrinology* **96**, 354A.

von Euler, U. S., and Gaddum, J. H. (1931). *J. Physiol. (London)* **72,** 74.

Wei, E., and Loh, H. (1976). *Science* **193,** 1262–1263.

Wei, E., Loh, H. H., and Way, E. L. (1973a). *Life Sci.* **12,** 489.

Wei, E., Loh, H. H., and Way, E. L. (1973b). *J. Pharmacol. Exp. Ther.* **185,** 108–115.

Yamazaki, E., Sakiz, E., and Guillemin, R. (1963a). *Experientia* **19,** 480–483.

Yamazaki, E., Sakiz, E., and Guillemin, R. (1963b). *Ann. Endocrinol.* **24,** 795.

Yen *et al.* (1972). *J. Clin. Endocrinol. Metab.* **35,** 931–934.

Zieglgansberger, W., Fry, J. P., Herz, A., Moroder, L., and Wunsch, E. (1976). *Brain Res.* **115,** 160–164.

THE SENSORY PHYSIOLOGY OF ANIMAL ORIENTATION*

DONALD R. GRIFFIN

The Rockefeller University, New York, New York

I. INTRODUCTION

A number of animals maintain orientation with respect to their surroundings under conditions where it has been difficult to understand what sort of information from the animals' environment is employed, or what sensory "window" conveys such information into the
central nervous system. In some cases we remain ignorant about both
aspects of the matter. Because of the surprises that have resulted from
discoveries about animal orientation, this field has become a significant
area of comparative neurobiology. Again and again it has turned out that
the previous thinking of scientists had been constrained by what might
figuratively be called "simplicity filters." Puzzling phenomena have
tended to be neglected in efforts to restrict scientific consideration to
relatively simple explanations. When certain of these have eventually
been studied with adequate methods, the animals have turned out to be
doing things that had scarcely been thinkable. The theoretical
framework previously taken for granted has then required modification.
Simplicity filters are an important part of scientific thinking, inasmuch
as it is impracticable to bear constantly in mind all conceivable complexities. But their use involves the danger that they will cause us to rule
out in advance hypotheses that may in fact be correct.

Another limitation of perspective results from an understandable concentration on problems and phenomena of importance in our own
bodies, or those of a few convenient animal surrogates such as cats or
rats. But when an experimental biologist limits his thinking in this way
he misses a great deal of significant interest. Furthermore, as stressed by
many physiologists from August Krogh to T. H. Bullock, important
advances have come from the strategic use of species in which a particu-

---

*Lecture delivered February 19, 1975.

lar function is especially well developed or for other reasons especially accessible for investigation (Krebs, 1975).

This paper will concentrate on five examples of orientation behavior the investigation of which has revealed unexpected sensory processes. They have been chosen largely because enough is known to permit a fairly complete discussion in physiological terms. Many other examples could serve the same purpose, and full explanations are by no means complete in these five cases. It is encouraging to realize that so much has been learned since I prepared a comparable review in the early 1950s (Griffin, 1953).

II. NEW SENSORY WINDOWS

Not many years ago it was generally believed that fish do not hear, and that aquatic animals are silent. Today it is difficult to understand how such an ill-informed belief could have lingered well into the 1950s. For example, in the 1920s and early 1930s von Frisch and his students had conducted a meticulous series of experiments demonstrating excellent hearing in several species of fish (reviewed by von Frisch, 1936). By modern standards, the transducers available at this time were crude and uncalibrated, but the experiments were so thorough that sensitivity to a broad frequency range could scarcely be doubted. Furthermore, comparative anatomists had described in detail the elaborate morphological specializations of the Weberian apparatus that mechanically links the inner ear labyrinth to the swim bladder in fishes of the order Ostariophysi (including catfish, carp, and the common goldfish). This reluctance to recognize a well documented fact of comparative physiology exemplifies the effectiveness of simplicity filters, especially when they are combined with an "anthropocentric" bias that tends to underrate the scientific significance of any structure or function not clearly related to human physiology (Griffin, 1955; Popper and Fay, 1973; Fay and Popper, 1975; Tavolga, 1976).

Not only fishes but marine mammals have excellent hearing, and their cochleas are efficiently coupled to water rather than to air. Both dominant groups of aquatic vertebrates are also well equipped with apparatus for generating sounds, and these are sometimes used for communication over long distances. Underwater hearing is also an essential component of a highly specialized type of orientation behavior discussed below in Section V.

In a somewhat parallel fashion comparative sensory physiologists have found that insects and certain other animals can see the plane of polarization of light, although for a long time this capability was not recognized or considered to be a serious possibility (von Frisch, 1967). It is thus important to keep an open mind concerning the sensory channels available to animals, without of course jumping to the conclusion that all forms of energy are detectable by animals even though we can think of uses that they might make of such information if they could perceive it.

III. Infrared Detection by Snakes

Behavioral studies of the detection of prey by two groups of snakes, the pit vipers (Crotalidae) and the boas (Boidae), indicated that thermal radiation from a warmblooded animal such as a mouse was at least one source of information guiding the striking motion of the snake (Noble and Schmidt, 1937). Snakes can aim accurately at warm targets under conditions where vision is impossible, but not at those having the same temperature as the surroundings. Experimental impairment of the facial pits of the pit vipers and smaller depressions above the lips of the boas suggested that the heat receptors were located in these structures, even though only simple undifferentiated nerve endings were present.

Careful experiments by Bullock and Diecke (1956) showed that long-wavelength infrared radiation would indeed excite these nerve endings in pit vipers, and further anatomical and physiological studies by Bullock and Fox (1957), Bullock and Barrett (1968), and others have added substantially to our understanding of a specialized radiation detecting system. The whole subject has been recently reviewed by Barrett et al. (1970) and Hartline (1974). Hartline's experiments have shown that directional localization is possible with an accuracy on the order of $10°$ even though the pit itself is only crudely directional and admits radiation over a cone of approximately $75°–90°$. Thus even so simple a structure as this biological radiometer involves integration of sensory information in the central nervous system to improve significantly upon the directional capabilities of the peripheral sense organs.

IV. ELECTRORECEPTION

Charles Darwin remained seriously perplexed by a few attributes of animals that seemed to defy a reasonable explanation in evolutionary terms. Among these were the electric organs of fish, such as the electric eel, which as far as was then known served only as weapons. Large electric organs can administer severe shocks to predators or prey, but Darwin was at a loss to understand how such an elaborate organ could have evolved through intermediate stages, because it seemed that a weak electric organ would have no survival value at all. Nor were weak electric organs merely hypothetical stages postulated in the evolutionary history of electric eels. Several species of fish were discovered with small electric organs capable of producing only feeble discharges. Modern measurements have shown that many of these fishes produce only a few millivolts when their electric organs discharge maximally. Even the inspired imagination of Charles Darwin could not find a plausible function for such trivial discharges.

This paradox was solved by Hans Lissmann (1958), who demonstrated that weakly electric fish could detect objects in their immediate vicinity by sensing changes in the electric fields produced by their own electric organs. Most of these fish are nocturnal and many live in turbid waters where vision is of limited usefulness, but electroreception suffices for finding their way about and for avoiding obstacles. It probably also helps them to locate appropriate cavities for shelter during the day. Receptors of the lateral-line system allow these fish to detect voltage gradients at least as small as $0.1~\mu V/cm$. The sensory and neurophysiology of electroreception have been intensively studied since Lissmann's original discovery, and the resulting knowledge of this unanticipated sensory window has been thoroughly reviewed by Bennett (1971), Bullock (1973), Fessard (1974), and Heiligenberg (1975, 1976).

Not only can sensory neurons of the lateral-line system respond to artificially applied electric fields, their activity is coordinated with the nervous control of electric organ discharges and the patterns of afferent impulses show clear changes when objects of varying dielectric constant are moved in the vicinity of the fish. A greatly enlarged cerebellum is active in analyzing the patterns of afferent electrosensory input.

Further studies by Black-Cleworth (1970), Bell *et al.* (1974), Hopkins (1974), Russell *et al.* (1974), and Westby (1974a,b) have shown that weakly electric fish also use their electric organs for social communication. Relatively simple patterns of change in the electric organ discharge serve to signal aggressiveness, submission, and probably courtship. In certain species the frequency of electric organ discharge varies inversely with body length, so that frequency is an indication of the size of a conspecific individual. Females tend to have higher frequencies for a given size than males. Hopkins reported the intriguing observation, limited unfortunately to two cases, that mated pairs may have frequencies an octave apart.

Another unexpected development in the electrosensory world of fish was the discovery by Dijkgraaf (1968), Kalmijn (1971), and Peters and van Wijland (1974) that many fishes not equipped with electric organs of any kind nevertheless have electrical sensitivities equalling or even exceeding those of species specialized for electrical orientation. Sharks and rays, catfish, and other species have low enough electrical thresholds to detect electrical potentials from other aquatic animals, and certain sharks find their prey by this means. A smaller fish buried in the mud is located and seized even when it is invisible and not detectable by the chemical senses. This remarkable discovery was supported in part by experiments in which electrodes replaced the buried prey, and potentials simulating those of a live fish of appropriate size would consistently elicit attack behavior from a hungry shark. Many species of fish can also detect a variety of naturally occurring electric fields of both animate and inanimate origin (Peters and Bretschneider, 1972; Kalmijn, 1974, and Akoev *et al.*, 1976).

One important physiological feature of electroreceptor systems in many fishes are elongated canals having walls with high electrical resistance and interior lumens filled with jellylike material of low resistance. Such structures serve to concentrate the environmental gradient of electrical potential across relatively thin membranes where electrosensitive cells are located. This anatomical device produces local potential gradients that greatly exceed the overall environmental gradient, and this seems to account in large measure for the remarkably low thresholds measured from some species (in extreme cases as low as 0.01 μV/cm).

The information available to Darwin thus involved only the tip of the proverbial iceberg. In the final section of this paper I will return briefly to the subject of electrical sensitivity in fishes because it throws significant light on another unsolved problem of animal navigation.

V. ECHOLOCATION

The ability of bats to orient their flight in darkness by emitting specialized sounds and locating objects through echoes of these orientation sounds has been one of the more thoroughly analyzed examples of animal orientation behavior that falls into the general "eye-opening" category selected for discussion in this paper. The history of this problem has been reviewed by Griffin (1958), and it is merely appropriate to point out that in the 1790s Cuvier appealed to a sort of simplicity filter when he argued that bats must simply *feel* the proximity of obstacles, and on this basis dismissed the experiments of Jurine and Spallanzani in which bats were drastically disoriented when their ears were blocked.

The fact that most bats use orientation sounds lying above the frequency range of human hearing delayed the discovery of echolocation until twentieth century electronic apparatus became available. Even now many scientists feel that there is something suspect about experiments with sounds above roughly 20 kHz (see, for example, the discussion following Suga, 1973). Yet echolocation is not a behavior pattern limited to the bats or to ultrasonic frequencies. One of the two suborders of the Chiroptera, the Old World fruit bats, have large eyes and lack echolocation altogether, except for one genus (*Rousettus*), which has secondarily acquired this mode of perception. On the other hand, two genera of cave-dwelling birds (*Steatornis* and *Collocalia*) use echolocation to guide their flight into dark caves. *Rousettus, Steatornis,* and *Collocalia* all use clicks that are clearly audible to human ears. Aside from the bats of the suborder Microchiroptera, the most advanced development of echolocation occurs in the marine mammals, which of course use underwater sounds. While both orientation sounds and communication signals overlap with the frequency range of human hearing, many of them also have strong ultrasonic components extending to well above 100 kHz. Certain terrestrial mammals, especially the shrews, employ a limited form of echolocation (Buchler, 1976). Furthermore, as will be discussed in more detail below, it also occurs in our own species.

The orientation sounds of echolocating bats and cetaceans appear to be well adapted for this purpose, although the relative advantages of the different types are only beginning to be worked out. The marine mammals use very brief clicks containing only a few individual waves, which, as transients, generate a very broad band of frequencies approximating the entire range audible to the animals involved. Echolocating bats, on the other hand, usually employ signals that contain many sound waves with well defined frequency structure. By far the commonest pattern is a rapid downward frequency sweep, usually an octave or more within a single brief pulse containing roughly 10 to several hundred waves. In many cases there are two or more harmonically related components that sweep together. The recent experiments of Simmons and his colleagues (reviewed by Simmons *et al.,* 1975, and Simmons, 1977) have shown that these FM pulses are well adapted for determining the distance of a target through the time interval between its emission and its return to the bat's ears. Range discrimination capabilities and detection of faint signals in noise approach very close to the limits set by the mathematical theory of signal detection (Griffin *et al.,* 1963; Simmons, 1977).

The FM pulses also provide information about the nature of the echoing target through spectral differences in the echoes. Within the octave or more of frequency sweep a given target may return a varying fraction of the incident acoustic energy, and this pattern of echo spectrum seems to provide the bat with qualitative information about the nature of the target (Griffin *et al.,* 1965). Recent experiments by Simmons and others (1974) have confirmed, under more precisely controlled conditions, that bats are capable of distinguishing between echoes having very nearly the same overall intensity but different frequency spectra.

When bats are faced with difficult orientational problems, such as avoiding small obstacles, drinking by skimming a water surface, landing, or catching flying insects, the duration of the orientation sounds and the rate of frequency sweep vary widely. In extreme cases the frequency may remain almost constant for a substantial fraction of the pulse duration. Constant frequency components are apparently used for two general purposes: (1) to concentrate most of the emitted energy into a narrow frequency band and thus detect faint echoes with improved signal-to-noise ratio, including those from small or distant targets; (2) to detect relative motion of the target through Doppler shifts in the echo frequency. The first type of echolocation is being found more and more frequently as detailed studies of the orientation sounds are carried out under a variety of natural conditions. The same species of bat may employ a wide range of signal patterns under different conditions. These may include very brief purely FM sweeps, such sweeping frequencies followed by a relatively long period of nearly constant frequency, or a number of intermediate patterns. The nearly constant frequencies tend to be used when flying relatively high above the ground and searching for insect prey.

Certain groups of bats have become highly specialized for echolocation that relies on precisely controlled constant-frequency signals, and these are often called for convenience the CF bats. The highly specialized CF bats include one large family found in warmer regions of Africa, Eurasia, and Australia (the Rhinolophidae) and a single species from one genus of neotropical bats (*Pteronotus parnellii*). The CF signals always contain at least a brief terminal portion with a downward frequency sweep, and the constant-frequency portion seems to be employed primarily when searching for insects. When active pursuit and interception are underway, the constant frequencies are reduced in duration and the FM sweep becomes more prominent. Simmons and his colleagues have recently demonstrated that the same bat may adjust the duration and other properties of its orientation sounds according to the specific problem presented by a given experimental situation, for example, range discrimination or detection of faint echoes partially masked by interfering noise (Simmons, 1977).

A. Neurophysiological Adaptations for Echolocation in Bats

For a considerable period after the convincing demonstration that echolocation was used by bats, the only available information concerning their hearing was the demonstration by Galambos (1942) that cochlear microphonics were measurable at frequencies up to about 100 kHz. The fact that orientation sounds well above the human range were emitted and utilized by bats provided strong general evidence that they could be heard. As might be expected from their heavy reliance on echolocation, the brains of insectivorous bats have a strong emphasis on the auditory system at the expense of other sensory systems. Grinnell

(1963) opened up the neurophysiological analysis of the auditory areas of bat brains, and his experiments have been followed by the substantial and increasingly detailed investigations of Suga, Henson, Neuweiler, Schnitzler, and others. Since most of these have been reviewed by Suga (1973) and by Simmons *et al.* (1975), no general summary of this extensive work is appropriate here. But it is important to consider the degree to which these experiments have disclosed auditory mechanisms that differ from those of other mammals in ways that adapt the nervous systems of bats for extracting useful information from echoes.

Initially it seemed that one important element in such specialization was a simple matter of frequency. Bats were the first animals definitely demonstrated to use frequencies well above the range of human hearing. But later investigations have clearly established that all small mammals share with bats the ability to hear at ultrasonic frequencies. While only a few of the many groups of mammals have been adequately studied, the available data support the rough generalization that the smaller the mammal, the higher the frequencies it can hear (von Bekesy, 1960; Sales and Pye, 1974). This approximate scaling of auditory frequency range to body size should not be taken as a rigid formula, at least until a wider range of species have been adequately studied. But it is clear that the smaller rodents have excellent sensitivity up to roughly 80 kHz and useful hearing extending above 100 kHz. The shrews and other small members of the order Insectivora are logical candidates for high-frequency sensitivity. Although they have not yet been studied with adequate methods, they may well prove to have ultrasonic sensitivity matching or even exceeding that of the smaller bats.

The simple question of frequency range of auditory sensitivity can be studied in two general ways, by behavioral experiments in which the animal is induced to give consistent responses to sounds of various frequencies and its auditory threshold determined at enough frequencies to plot the type of curve generally called an audiogram. Such experiments are tedious, and variability is often great. Spontaneous responses such as the Preyer pinna reflex suffer from rapid habituation, and such spontaneous behavioral responses usually begin only at levels well above the absolute threshold. Electrophysiological methods are appealing in that conditions can be controlled and much more reproducible results obtained. Cochlear microphonic potentials have been measured in great detail by E. G. Wever and his colleagues from a number of

animals including bats (Wever and Vernon, 1961). While these potentials arise at, or very close to, the hair cells of the basilar membrane, and
hence appear to monitor the earliest processes in auditory response, they
are ordinarily discernible only at levels considerably above the absolute
threshold determined by behavioral experiments.

Since the orientation sounds and their echoes are brief stimuli lasting
at most for several milliseconds, they excite nearly simultaneously large
numbers of afferent neurons of the bat's VIIIth nerve. Grinnell (1963)
found that even gross electrodes on the dorsal surface of the inferior
colliculus pick up a series of positive potentials, the earliest of which
have a latency of 1 msec or slightly less and hence must be the primary
afferent input to the medullary nuclei of the auditory system. A bat,
such as *Myotis lucifugus* under barbituate anesthesia, yields prominent
evoked potentials whenever the orientation sounds of other bats, or
indeed almost any impulsive sound, impinges on the animal's ears. The
dorsal surface of the inferior colliculus typically yields the lowest
thresholds for such evoked potentials. Subsequent experiments by Suga
have shown that the most prominent component is the synchronized
firing of axons of the lateral lemniscus, so that this wave is now called
LL. It is the fourth wave evident after arrival of a brief pulse of sound
and is therefore also designated as N_4. Comparable recordings from
small rodents give similar results and have provided a major portion of
the evidence that they too can hear well at a broad range of ultrasonic
frequencies.

Neurophysiologists are seldom satisfied with field potentials recorded
by large electrodes, since they comprise an unknown mixture of axonal
or synaptic responses. Microelectrodes recording from single cells are
far preferable in providing specific information about the responses of
one neuron at a time. Such recordings were first made by Grinnell
(1963) and, later, more extensively, by Suga and his colleagues (reviewed by Suga, 1973). A relatively recent development, fraught with
many difficulties but nevertheless yielding important results, has been
the use of implanted electrodes capable of monitoring neurophysiological potentials in unanesthetized bats (Suga *et al.*, 1974).

An unexpected result of the measurement of many audiograms from
bats and other small mammals has been the common, but not universal,
tendency for the higher ultrasonic frequencies (above roughly 50 kHz)
to show a second minimum. That is, the threshold in the vicinity of
55–60 kHz is often lower than at 20–40 kHz. Other evidence suggests

that this higher ultrasonic frequency range is differentially more sensitive to physiological factors that depress sensitivity in general, such as reduced body temperature or lowered oxygen tension (Harrison, 1965). This hints at a specialized mechanism more vulnerable than the responses to lower frequencies, but definitive evidence is not yet available.

Because downward FM sweeps are so prominent in the orientation sounds of bats, Suga has made a special effort to search for "feature detectors" in bat brains that might show selective sensitivity to signals of this type. FM-sensitive neurons have indeed been found, and Suga has explained the mechanism by which they operate. As in most other mammalian auditory systems, sounds over a certain range of frequencies and intensities have an excitatory effect on particular central neurons. When these data are plotted on a graph of auditory threshold versus frequency, these stimuli with excitatory properties fall into what can conveniently be described as an excitatory area. This is of course the area above the conventional threshold curve for the cell in question. By presenting stimuli in pairs, however, it can also be demonstrated an inhibitory effect of sounds falling in other areas on this graph of intensity versus frequency. Individual neurons in the midbrain and more anterior auditory areas show a wide variety of such excitatory and inhibitory response areas. In the inferior colliculus and auditory cortex of bats Suga found numerous units whose inhibitory areas were asymmetrical, with a larger inhibitory area lying at either higher or lower frequency than the minimum of the excitatory area. Such units are differentially responsive to sweeping frequencies. A stimulus is quite effective if it begins at a frequency that lies in the excitatory area, and only later enters an inhibitory area. But the reverse situation produces sufficient inhibition to eliminate any response to a similar stimulus sweeping in the opposite direction. Units with similar behavior have been recorded from cats and other nonecholocating mammals, and it is not clear whether their abundance in bats as described by Suga has resulted from a special effort to search for them or whether, on the other hand, an adaptation for echolocation is to have a relatively large proportion of central auditory neurons selectively sensitive to sweeping frequencies.

All the CF bats so far studied have a narrow frequency band of auditory sensitivity close, but not absolutely equal to, the constant frequency in the orientation sounds (Schnitzler, 1968, 1970; Pollak *et al.*,

1972). A large part (but probably not all) of their central auditory system seems to be concerned with this sharply tuned "window" (Suga and Jen, 1976). Under many conditions these bats control the emitted frequency with a precision on the order of 0.1%. When their attention is directed at a particular target, they adjust this emitted frequency so that its echo, which may be Doppler shifted owing to relative motion, falls in this narrow frequency band where their auditory sensitivity is maximum (Schuller and Suga, 1976a,b; Suga *et al.*, 1976; Schnitzler *et al.*, 1976; Bruns, 1976a,b).

Another type of auditory mechanism that appears to be at least quantitatively specialized as an adaptation for echolocation is what might be called transmit–receive switching. The auditory system of an echolocating animal, like a radar or sonar system, faces the problem of protecting its sensitive receiver from severe overloading during the emission of an intense probing signal. All mammals have small muscles attached to the middle ear ossicles which have a protective function in that their contraction reduces auditory sensitivity—at least to certain frequencies. These muscles are greatly hypertrophied in echolocating bats, being enormously larger relative to the size of the animal than in nonecholocating mammals. It was therefore reasonable to speculate that these muscles might serve as a transmit–receive switching system; but before direct evidence was available, this speculation faced the difficulty that very rapid recovery of sensitivity would be necessary so that echoes returning within a few milliseconds could be heard.

Henson (1965) provided such evidence by showing that in certain echolocating bats the middle ear muscles do reduce the sensitivity of hearing by an appreciable amount (on the order of 20–30 dB) and furthermore that they can also relax very rapidly, so that within a very few milliseconds full auditory sensitivity has been restored. Suga and Jen (1975) have recently shown that these muscles contract in approximate synchrony with the emission of orientation sounds, and there is little doubt that they function as transmit–receive switches. Contraction of the laryngeal muscles is appropriately coordinated (Jen and Suga, 1976).

Suga and Jen (1975) also analyzed an additional, central, mechanism which augments the transmit–receive switching function of the middle ear muscles. They found that the orientation sounds of FM bats are less effective in stimulating the auditory system central to the lateral lemniscus if they are emitted by the bat itself than if they are played back from an appropriate tape recorder. Control stimuli consisting of tape-recorded orientation sounds from the same bat were adjusted to elicit approximately equal response as the bat's own vocalizations at the VIIIth nerve and the medullary auditory nuclei. But the tape-recorded signal produced a considerably larger response at the lateral lemniscus and more anterior auditory areas. If the intensity of the tape-recorded signal was adjusted to produce equal amplitude of response, or equal thresholds, at the lateral lemniscus, the tape-recorded signal had to be roughly 12 dB lower than the bat's emitted sound. These experiments demonstrate that some process of neural attenuation occurs in approximate synchrony with the emission of orientation sounds and that this renders the more anterior portions of the auditory system less sensitive to the emitted signal than otherwise would be the case. Suga and Jen concluded that the combined action of this process of neural attenuation and the middle ear muscles together achieve something on the order of 30–35 dB of reduction in auditory sensitivity at the time the orientation sounds are being generated.

While these transmit–receive switching mechanisms may well be especially prominent in echolocating animals, somewhat similar processes are apparently at work in other mammals including men. The human and feline middle ear muscles are also known to contract in at least approximate synchrony with vocalization, but no experimental evidence is yet available to indicate how closely their action resembles the situation in echolocating bats.

B. Human Echolocation

Echolocation may appear at this point to be an esoteric zoological specialization found only in animals remote from practical or human concerns. But in fact it has a direct relevance to one of the most distressing of human afflictions. It has long been known that blind persons have some residual ability to detect obstacles before colliding with them. Subjective, introspective reports from even the most skillful blind people strongly suggest that some tactile mechanism is involved. The blind say simply that they feel something is there before bumping into it, and hence the customary term for such obstacle detection is "facial vision." The history of investigation of nonvisual orientation by the blind and by bats has followed a curiously parallel course, although the published record suggests very slight interaction between the scientists studying these two questions. But at about the same time when Pierce, Galambos, and I were able to demonstrate the existence of echolocation in bats, Supa, Cotzin, and Dallenbach (1944) carried out the first clearly definitive experiments showing that blind people also rely heavily on echolocation. Blind subjects or sighted subjects wearing tight blindfolds lost most of the ability to detect objects when their ears were tightly plugged. Furthermore the entire process could be carried out by means of a loudspeaker and microphone carried by one subject while a second person listened from a remote room to the sounds picked up by the microphone. Rice (1967) has shown that under favorable conditions the most proficient subjects can detect objects as small as quarter inch rods at a distance of roughly two meters, and can discriminate between objects located in different directions or having different acoustic reflectivities. Differential judgments of acoustic size or target strength are also possible with practice.

Despite the surprising capabilities of experienced subjects in laboratory experiments, human echolocation has obviously not been perfected to a level remotely approaching that achieved by bats. Since the brain of a typical insectivorous bat weighs approximately 1 g, and since 1500 g of human brain are proficient at analyzing complex such sounds as speech and music, it is appropriate to ask what explains this enormous gap in ability to obtain pertinent information from echoes. Since bats catch flying insects on the wing, it is not altogether outrageous to inquire why a blind man could not fly an airplane and catch birds.

There are several possibilities to explain this unfortunate performance gap. The use of ultrasonic frequencies by bats does not appear to be the crucial factor. A few species of bats and the two species of cave-dwelling birds achieve reasonably proficient echolocation using sounds that overlap the human frequency range (roughly from 6 to 15 kHz). Furthermore the most specialized echolocating bats can detect such small obstacles as fruit flies or wires 0.2 mm in diameter. If a simple scaling of wavelengths were all that separated the capabilities of bats and blind people, one might suppose that what a bat can do with 80 kHz a blind man should be able to do with a 10-fold larger object returning echoes of 8 kHz. Another less obvious advantage of ultrasonic frequencies will be mentioned below.

A potential limitation to human echolocation is suggested by many experiments on human hearing which demonstrate a temporary loss of sensitivity for a substantial fraction of a second after a loud sound impinges on the ear. This is usually called the temporary threshold shift (TTS), and can be quite large for many tens of milliseconds after the end of a moderately intense sound. This of course is the time period within which echoes important to a blind man return. (A convenient constant to bear in mind in this connection is that sound travels 34.4 cm/msec. Hence most objects close enough to a blind man to be of crucial importance for him to detect will return echoes within roughly 10–30 msec.)

The importance of this phenomenon of temporary threshold shift is easily demonstrated when a sharp click lasting only a few milliseconds is tape-recorded both in a typical indoor room and also out-of-doors or in an anechoic chamber where only weak echoes return to the microphone after the end of the click itself. If such tape recordings are played back in the normal fashion, they do not sound very different under the two conditions, except that the "indoor" click will sound louder. If the amplitudes are adjusted so that the perceived loudness is approximately equal, there are only very slight qualitative differences in the sound of the two recordings. If another simple experiment is now performed by reversing the direction of motion of the tape over the playback heads, a striking qualitative difference is immediately apparent. The click recorded out-of-doors is relatively little changed, but the indoor click now sounds like "shhhiCK." Part of this difference is probably due to the gradual onset of the reversed signal. But the hissing component preceding the major portion of the click consists of the complex of echoes which return to the original microphone after reflection from the walls, floor, and other objects in the room. It is this complex of echoes which contains information that would be extremely helpful to a blind man if his auditory system could put it to use.

One way to get around the difficulty of the temporary threshold shift would be to protect the ear of a person attempting to echolocate objects in his environment from the outgoing signals. This might be done by simple mechanical baffles, or conceivably in other ways. In some preliminary experiments I have used electronic switching to "dissect" the echo complex from the original signal. Since in a typical room the echo complex may last for 50 msec or more after an emitted signal of 10 msec duration, the isolated echoes sound more or less like the original, combined sound. Much more extensive additional investigations will be necessary to examine whether, with practice, a human listener could extract helpful information from these echo complexes even when they are experimentally separated from the original, outgoing signals.

It seems quite likely that a major limitation to human echolocation is not so much that the echoes are inaudible as that they are masked by what students of sonar and radar call clutter. If a blind man is looking for a chair, he needs to obtain information about its location and to separate such information from that provided by echoes from the floor, ceiling, or other furniture not directly in his line or approach to the chair. The optimal conditions under which human echolocation has been analyzed involve test targets isolated from other echoing surfaces by 2 or 3 meters. This is of course a highly unnatural situation, far removed from the real world faced by the blind. Bats too face severe problems of clutter, especially those that catch insects in the midst of relatively dense forests. Much louder echoes must return from the vegetation, the ground, and all sorts of clutter other than the minute moving insect prey. The superiority of bat brains may lie in the realm of neurophysiological clutter rejection.

The atmosphere becomes increasingly murky or absorptive as frequencies increase through the higher parts of the human range and into the ultrasonic frequencies employed by bats. The reduction in sound due to its absorption and conversion to heat is completely negligible over a few meters at all but the highest frequencies audible to our ears. But under certain conditions of humidity, the higher frequencies used by some bats may suffer absorption at rates up to 10 dB per meter. Bats using such high frequencies can almost certainly detect nothing at all by echolocation at more than a few meters. Indeed even their emitted orientation sounds are often undetectable by the best available equipment when they are flying 10 meters overhead, although they become readily apparent if the same apparatus is carried to the treetops where the bats are flying. It may be that this acoustic murkiness of the air is a distinct advantage in overcoming the clutter problem, and that one serious limitation to human echolocation is that we are forced to use frequencies so well transmitted by the air that innumerable multiple echoes from all objects within many meters contribute to a hopeless clutter. Yet in typical indoor situations the recognition of speech, including individual identification of the speaker, involves an impressive discrimination between important and unimportant components of a chaotic mixture of direct signal coming straight from the speaker and a complex of overlapping echoes from other surfaces nearby. It may be that our auditory system has become specialized for this type of fine analysis and that such specialization interferes with the discriminatory responses required for understanding what can be called, figuratively, the language of echoes.

Pursuing this speculative approach a little further, let us suppose tentatively that speech recognition and echo recognition are to some degree competing processes. It would then become relevant to inquire whether the neural mechanisms for such pattern recognition are inherently different in bat and human brains. Or are such patterns largely learned in childhood, as we learn to recognize speech? In this case appropriate experiments might disclose significant differences between young children and adults. Furthermore if such patterns are the result of individual experience and learning, it is not unthinkable that they could be modified in the case of blind persons to help them understand the language of echoes. Persons who are totally blind but otherwise in good health differ widely in their abilities at echolocation. But no one has succeeded in correlating these differences with other factors such as age at which vision was lost, type of subsequent experience, auditory skills of other sorts, such as musical ability or linguistic competence. Perhaps in this area of obvious human concern our progress has also been held back by simplicity filters that have hindered us from thinking adequately about the questions that most deserve to be asked.

VI. BIRD NAVIGATION

The challenging problems posed by the long-distance migrations and homing flights of birds are well known in a general way, almost too well known in some respects for balanced scientific appraisal. Many observations and experiments provide tantalizing but inconclusive evidence which has very recently been reviewed in detail in the proceedings of a symposium edited by Schmidt-Koenig (1977). Not only are major questions still unanswered, in certain important areas we do not even know what are the important questions to ask. The available evidence can conveniently be classified into two interrelated categories, directional orientation and goal-directed homing.

A. Directional Orientation

1. Sun-Compass Orientation

For a long time it seemed unrealistic, and even foolishly speculative, to postulate that birds might compensate for the apparent motion of the sun across the skies and maintain a constant direction of flight by heading at a gradually changing angle to the sun's azimuth. But in the early 1950s Matthews and Kramer demonstrated experimentally that birds are quite capable of doing just this. These developments have been well reviewed by Matthews (1968), Schmidt-Koenig (1965), and Emlen (1975).

Kramer (1959) developed a type of apparatus that, with minor modifications, has been widely used for many significant experiments on the orientation of birds. This "orientation cage" is a cylindrical enclosure roughly 1 meter in diameter, screened by an opaque barrier to conceal local landmarks but allow the bird inside a clear view of the sky. The direction in which a small bird orients itself is recorded by visual observation, or by one of several types of automatic devices. Under suitably controlled conditions Kramer showed that when birds were in the physiological state appropriate for migration they would flutter back and forth as though attempting to go roughly north in spring or south in fall.

Having, so to speak, brought bird navigation under experimental control, Kramer was able to show that the sun was one important cue. If the bird's view of the sky was manipulated appropriately with plane mirrors, the direction of its attempted migratory flights was deflected more or less as would be expected. In order to obtain more extensive data under better-controlled conditions, Kramer soon turned from spontaneous migration to directional choices motivated by hunger. Starlings, homing pigeons, and other species of birds learned to seek food in a symmetrically constructed, cylindrical orientation cage by going to one of several identical feeders located at the periphery. The food could not be seen until the bird pushed its bill into the feeder, and for critical tests all the feeders were empty. By making everything as uniform as possible, and by randomly rotating the cage at frequent intervals, all cues except compass direction were eliminated. Provided the sun was visible the birds chose the correct direction with an accuracy of roughly ±30°, regardless of the time of day and the resulting azimuth direction of the sun. In certain experiments the sun was replaced by an artificial light which remained in one position throughout the day, and the birds then changed their directional choices in a pattern that would have compensated for the normal motion of the sun across the sky. McDonald (1973, 1975) has shown that reactions to shadows may complicate such experiments.

Experiments of this type were then extended by resetting the endogenous biological clocks of the birds by keeping them for several days on a shifted light–dark cycle. The orientation of such clock-shifted birds was deflected in approximately the predicted fashion (Schmidt-Koenig, 1965).

2. Star-Compass Orientation

Most species of birds migrate at night, for reasons that we can only guess. Thus the sun is directly available only to diurnal migrants, which tend in general to be waterfowl and other relatively large birds. Although Kramer performed a few preliminary experiments under the night sky, it was Franz Sauer who perfected the technique of using orientation cages to study the reactions of migratory birds to the stars. He found, like Kramer, that seasonally appropriate orientation occurred under the natural sky, and he was able to demonstrate comparable orientation under the artificial light patterns of a planetarium. Similar experiments were later perfected by Emlen (1967) with the addition of important improvements and controls not feasible with the planetarium originally available to Sauer. The net result of these experiments has been to show that directional orientation by means of the stars is quite within the capabilities of migratory birds. In the northern hemisphere the area of sky within roughly 30° of Polaris seems to be of primary importance, although the limited data available suggest that no one star, including Polaris itself, is essential.

Emlen has also carried out ingenious developmental experiments indicating that, while young birds can orient to the stars with very limited prior experience, the genetic information with which they come to this problem is not a detailed star map. Instead, Emlen's birds paid attention to the apparent rotation of the stars, and in fall they tended to orient in a direction roughly opposite from that part of the sky that did not rotate (Emlen, 1970, 1975).

3. The Problem of Overcast Skies

For a few years after the discovery of time-compensated sun-and star-compass orientation, it seemed that the problem of directional orientation was largely solved, and it was easy to overlook the fact that much migration occurs under cloudy skies. But radar observations disposed of this simplicity filter. Some of the earliest observations of extensive migration, with the airport surveillance radar at Zurich, suggested that birds were disoriented when flying below clouds and yet on the same night were migrating in appropriate directions above the overcast. But most later observations with many types of radar in several parts of the world showed that there was little correlation between the accuracy of migratory orientation and the presence or absence of opaque clouds (reviewed by Eastwood, 1967; Griffin, 1969; Emlen, 1975). By concentrating on nights with low clouds, I have observed that some migrants maintain accurate orientation even when flying in or between layers of opaque cloud (Griffin, 1973).

It is important to point out that the volume of nocturnal migration is strongly influenced by weather conditions. The majority of migrants fly on nights when the temperature has changed in the characteristic direction for the season, that is, has turned warmer in spring and colder in fall than the previous day or so. In many areas there is also a strong tendency for the more abundant and smaller birds to fly primarily downwind. In those areas where the most extensive radar data are available these two meteorological patterns tend to coincide, and as a result a considerable proportion of the smaller migrants are able to take advantage of tail winds. Nights with low cloud do not, in general, produce nearly as abundant migration, and usually there are many more birds above or below the clouds than in or between them.

When migrants fly below opaque layers of cloud they can probably see something of the surface of the earth even on moonless nights. But many migrants fly above clouds, over relatively homogeneous terrain, or over the open ocean, where it seems unlikely that sight of the ground or water would provide useful information concerning the direction appropriate for migratory flight.

4. Other Potential Sources of Directional Information

It is appropriate at this point to digress briefly to certain other sources of information that might be important to migratory birds even though none of them seems likely to provide as generally helpful guidance as the sun or stars.

Wind direction, while highly changeable over long periods of time or large distances, does tend to remain roughly constant at the altitudes where birds migrate during considerable fractions of any one day or night through the distances covered by most migrants. It has been suggested that a migration initiated on the basis of other information, such as the position of the sun, might be continued for several hours by orientation with respect to the wind. There is, however, a troublesome problem for the majority of migrants that fly at night and at altitudes of many hundreds of meters. If the entire air mass is moving uniformly, as is approximately the case under most conditions, no direct effect of the wind would be felt by a flying bird. Only with the aid of information from some outside source can a pilot, or presumably a migrating bird, determine whether he is flying upwind, crosswind, or downwind in a homogeneously moving air mass (Able, 1977).

There are, however, some second-order possibilities that might help a bird determine wind direction even when the ground provides no visible patterns that could be used to estimate wind drift. Sounds reaching a migrant from the surface might substitute for visible landmarks and provide indication of wind drift (D'Arms and Griffin, 1972; Griffin, 1976). The air itself may not in fact always move as a homogeneous mass. Especially near the surface, turbulence is known to involve a wide range of changing velocities which locally differ from, although in aggregate they add up to, the net motion of the wind. It used to be generally believed that atmospheric turbulence is isotropic and hence lacking any consistent patterns that might enable a flying bird to determine the net direction of the wind. But recent studies of micrometeorology have weakened this particular simplicity filter, and it now seems possible that under many conditions patterns of small-scale atmospheric flow might convey to a flying bird information about the net wind through which it is flying (Griffin, 1969; Lenschow, 1970; Hines, 1972; Hooke et al., 1972).

A final possibility, which remains almost entirely at the level of attractive speculation, is that a group of birds might greatly improve the accuracy of their orientation by communicating with one another and pooling whatever information they may have individually concerning the appropriate direction of flight. Some, but as far as we know not all, migrating birds emit characteristic flight calls. Radar observations strongly indicate that nocturnal migrants are aggregated, but not into tight flocks. Spacings of a few tens of meters between individuals seem to be the rule, with these groups separated by relatively large distances. Some reports suggest that flight calls are more abundant on nights with low clouds, but it remains to be ascertained whether this is because birds fly lower, and hence are more easily heard by observers on the ground, or whether those that are present emit more calls. My colleague Dr. Ronald Larkin has demonstrated through computer simulations that a hypothetical group of migrants individually provided only with very crude means of orientation could greatly reduce their errors and deviations from the appropriate direction by relatively simple communication strategies. But at present we lack the necessary data to judge whether migrants actually employ such strategies.

B. Goal-Directed Homing

Many birds return to an area where they have been captured even after artificial transportation to distances of hundreds of kilometers. While such homing behavior has been demonstrated in several species of wild birds, in only a few of these, and in the most proficient homing pigeons, do the percentage and speed of returns suffice to demonstrate approximately direct flights from release point to the home. Simple homing experiments of this type often fail to provide data adequate to distinquish between two possibilities: (1) relatively slow progress in approximately the correct homeward direction, with long pauses for rest or feeding, and (2) rapid and prolonged flights that deviate from the correct direction but eventually reach the home area by a process of random wandering or systematic exploration. The appeal of parsimony and related simplicity filters made the second explanation appealing at one time (Griffin, 1952). But improved experiments by Matthews (1968) and Kramer (1959) demonstrated that homing pigeons and at least one species of wild bird (the Manx shearwater) may head roughly toward home within the first few minutes after release. The best homing pigeons do this so consistently as to rule out any explanation based on wandering or exploration (reviewed by Keeton, 1974).

Thus a very challenging problem is posed by the ability of pigeons to select approximately the homeward direction when transported to an arbitrarily selected release point. In the best of such experiments there is adequate evidence that the release point is in unfamiliar territory, far from any point the bird has ever visited previously. The birds are transported in opaque containers providing no visual information concerning the route of transportation, and a variety of methods ranging from simple visual observation through binoculars, to following from aircraft, or tracking by means of miniature radio transmitters carried by the birds, have all shown that by one or a few minutes after release the best strains of homing pigeons select the homeward direction within $\pm$ 30°– 45°.

For several years after consistent homeward initial headings had been demonstrated it seemed that clear skies were necessary, because in most (but not quite all) homing experiments when the sky was overcast the initial headings were randomly oriented. More recently, however, Keeton (1974) found that pigeons accustomed to fly on cloudy days also showed accurate homeward headings when the sky was completely overcast. Doubts concerning the possibility that the birds could detect the sun's position through the clouds were dispelled by experiments in which endogenous biological clocks of the pigeons were reset. Schmidt-Koenig (1965) had previously reported that birds with a 6-hour clock shift deviated approximately 90° in the expected direction. Keeton's pigeons showed this same result when released under clear skies after a 6-hour clock shift. But if the skies were overcast, clock-shifted birds did not differ significantly from untreated controls; both headed toward home with reasonable accuracy. This elegant experiment demonstrated at one stroke that goal-directed homing involved some other source of information than the position of the sun.

It is of course evident that no simple directional system of orientation, whether based on the sun or any other source of environmental information, can by itself account for homeward orientation after displacement in an arbitrarily chosen direction into unfamiliar territory. Gustav Kramer expressed this problem in terms of the need for the equivalent of a map as well as the equivalent of a compass. What has thus come to be called the "map component" of homeward orientation remains the central mystery of animal navigation.

One approach to the problem of goal-directed homing is to inquire whether birds capable of this impressive type of orientation acquire the information on which it is based during transportation to the release point or only after release. A variety of experiments appear to provide an unequivocal answer in favor of the latter alternative by Walcott and Schmidt-Koenig (1973). But more recently, some experiments, though not all, have indicated that information obtained on the way to the release point may, after all, play a role in goal-directed homing (Schmidt-Koenig, 1977). Birds transported under deep anesthesia, or in containers subjected to irregular and complex mechanical oscillations, show just as accurate initial headings and as rapid homing flights as controls subjected to identical procedures before or after the actual outbound journey. Most of the information on which goal-directed homeward orientation seems to be based is obtained between the moment a bird is released from its opaque cage and the time when it has made its directional choice. In most experiments with the best homing pigeons this is on the order of a minute, or in some experiments as little as 10 or 15 seconds. In almost all cases a better than random homeward orientation is demonstrated within 5 minutes at the very most.

It would obviously be a large step forward if goal-directed homing could be elicited in some type of cage or under any other circumstances that would permit experimental control of the situation and the environmental cues available to the bird. But numerous attempts by almost every student of the problem to discover such a procedure have so far failed. No one has yet accomplished for goal-directed homing what Kramer achieved when he perfected his orientation cage.

C. The Question of Magnetic Sensitivity

It has been repeatedly suggested that birds and other animals that migrate over long distances might have some physiological equivalent of a magnetic compass. The earth's magnetic field is universally available over the surface of the earth, and it would obviously be of great advantage to animals if they could utilize its horizontal component as a basis for directional orientation.

Until the last few years the evidence in favor of sensitivity to the earth's magnetic field was limited to experiments that were difficult to replicate. The situation has now changed, and a considerable amount of positive evidence has been presented. Yet none of those who are convinced by this evidence would consider the present situation a satisfactory one, for several gaps and difficulties are evident. We are thus faced with a perplexing situation in which a new sensory channel may be in process of being adequately demonstrated. I shall therefore attempt to present both the strong and weak points of the available evidence.

Frank Brown has reported many experiments which he interprets as evidence that a variety of animals can respond to a variety of geophysical energy fluxes that are not ordinarily considered within the range of sensitivity of physiological receptors. These include cosmic rays, atmospheric tides, and the earth's magnetic field. In reviewing this work, Brown (1971) emphasized experiments in which the directional choices made by planarians and marine snails showed *average* deviations of about 1° to 5° in their direction of locomotion correlated with experimental changes in the earth's magnetic field. As pointed out in the published discussion of this paper, the raw data consisted of estimates of the directions that were ordinarily recorded in units of about 5° or 10°. Since these effects are so small and require such massive application of statistical averaging, they have not been widely accepted as adequate to demonstrate that animals can actually orient with respect to the earth's magnetic field.

Somewhat larger effects have been reported by Southern (1971, 1975) with ring-billed gulls. In most of Southern's experiments young gulls are released in relatively large circular cages, and their directional choices and recorded in terms of the portion of the cage periphery to which they move. While there is considerable variability, the data show a consistent tendency to orient in an approximately southeasterly direction. This statistical tendency weakened during some but not all periods when the earth's magnetic field fluctuated by an unusual amount, that is, during magnetic storms, (Schmidt-Koenig, 1977). Similar variations in directional orientation were reported when gulls were transported to the vicinity of a very large low-frequency radio antenna which generated alternating electromagnetic fields approximating, at the location of the orientation cage, the magnitude of the earth's field but fluctuating at about 70 Hz. Radar tracking of migrating birds flying within a few hundred meters of this antenna also showed a tendency to turn more often when the antenna was turned on or was changing its level of emission than when it was turned off (Larkin and Sutherland, 1977).

Wiltschko (1968) and Wiltschko and Wiltschko (1975, 1976) have reported in a series of papers growing out of earlier reports by Merkel and others at Frankfurt that, even without any opportunity to see the sun or stars, migratory birds in cages similar to the orientation cage originally developed by Kramer show approximately correct seasonal orientation when in the physiological state appropriate for migration. The orientation is much weaker, however, with very much more variability than in the experiments described by Sauer and Emlen, which have convincingly demonstrated star-compass orientations. In typical experiments of the type described by the Wiltschkos, the number of directional choices registered in each of eight radially symmetrical directions differs by only about 1 or 2% from the proportion expected by change. Nevertheless, statistically significant trends emerge from the averaging of hundreds or thousands of responses, and these are biologically appropriate in the sense that migrants tend to orient toward the north in the spring and toward the south in the fall. Furthermore the Wiltschkos have reported that these average directional tendencies can be experimentally shifted by means of artificially applied magnetic fields in a manner consistent with a compasslike sensitivity to the earth's magnetic field.

The results of these experiments appear quite sensitive to minor details of the experimental arrangements. The cage that the Wiltschkos have found to be most effective is actually a doughnut-shaped enclosure approximately 1 meter in diameter with a central cylinder blocked off to form a ring-shaped cage in which the birds can move freely. Eight radial bars provide resting places, and touching or landing on these bars is electrically recorded by microswitches. On nights when the birds are in the physiological state that produces migration restlessness, they tend to hop or fly round and round this enclosure activating the radial perches to a varying degree, but commonly at rates of several hundred times during an 8-hour night. Wiltschko (1968) described these procedures in full detail and presented the raw data in tabular form. Summing the perch activations shows slightly more landings or touches in certain sectors than others, but the variability in number of perch activations by a given bird during a particular night is very great. Only occasionally are the data from one bird averaged over one night significantly different from random. But when data from several bird nights are combined, statistically significant departures from randomness do emerge, and they appear consistently different according to the season, roughly north in the spring and south in the autumn.

The Wiltschkos ordinarily present their data in terms or radial graphs in which each point represents the weighted average direction from a single bird night. While many of these individual points do not in themselves represent statistically significant departures from a random circular distribution, a significant trend emerges when a number of such points are plotted for a given set of conditions. Such trends show appropriate seasonal differences and appear to be altered by artificially applied magnetic fields. It should be emphasized that large numbers of experiments of this general type have been reported by the Wiltschkos and that similar results have been obtained by other investigators (Wallraff, 1972; Emlen, 1975).

Procedural details of these experiments have caused some concern. The doughnut-shaped cages are constructed with their parts as uniform as practicable, but it is known that birds are sensitive to small local differences in such cages. The cage is therefore rotated from time to time, and in the most recent replications reviewed by Emlen *et al.* (1976) great care was taken to randomize these rotations and to avoid statistical biases that might result from unequal numbers of bird nights under different experimental conditions. Nevertheless it is puzzling to find that if the cage is rotated at frequent intervals the birds become disturbed, and the results are reported to deteriorate. As a result the cages are ordinarily rotated only once each night. Another puzzling aspect of the behavior recorded in these cages is that the birds spend most of their time flying around the doughnut-shaped enclosure, and when activating the northern radial perch they are actually heading either east or west. In one unsuccessful attempt to replicate these experiments, tangential perches were used so that a bird whose body was actually pointing north would activate the north, rather than the east or west perch (Perdeck, 1963). It is also perplexing that even after many years of work with these doughnut-shaped orientation cages the directional preferences remain so very small, barely significant even when hundreds of perch activations are summed.

Keeton's extensive experiments with homing pigeons have included tests on the possibility that magnetic sensitivity plays a significant role in the orientation of these highly trained and selected birds. In the most clear-cut of these experiments, small bar magnets were cemented to the backs of pigeons just before they were released. While homing success (speed and percentage of return) were not significantly affected, there was a clear tendency for birds fitted with magnets to show less well oriented initial headings than control birds carrying brass bars of the same size. These differences were more pronounced under overcast skies, and magnets had a somewhat greater effect on relatively inexperienced young pigeons. These results are consistent with the hypothesis that sensitivity to the earth's magnetic field provides an alternate source of directional information that is called in play under overcast skies. It is important to bear in mind that the effects of magnets were evident within a minute or two after release, but that the birds which initially headed away from home returned as soon as those which started in the homeward direction. In other words the effects of the magnets were relatively brief and did not prevent normally rapid homing.

In other experiments Keeton and his colleagues have reported that when pigeons are repeatedly released at the same place, so that the vicinity of the release point and the route home presumably become very familiar, nevertheless their initial headings show a slight statistical tendency to deviate from the actual home direction. Furthermore these deviations show statistically significant correlations with the fluctuations of the earth's magnetic field (Keeton, 1974; Larkin and Keeton, 1976).

Walcott and Green (1974) and Walcott (1977) reported tests with homing pigeons similar to Keeton's but employing miniature coils above and below the bird's head to generate a small local magnetic field. The initial headings of these pigeons released under overcast skies, while showing the usual amount of variation (roughly $\pm 30°$), were significantly different when the coils were connected so that the current flowed in opposite directions. When the artificial magnetic field had its local magnetic north pole pointed upward the initial headings were less well oriented toward home, and indeed there was a tendency to fly in roughly the opposite direction. With the current reversed, however, there was no significant difference from the headings of control birds carrying identical apparatus but with the battery disconnected. These results add an important element to the others described above in that there appeared to be a change in the direction chosen by the birds during the first minute or two after release rather than a simple deterioration of orientation.

These experiments have been interpreted by the Wiltschkos and by Walcott and Green to be consistent with the hypothesis that pigeons detect the dip of the earth's magnetic field, which is more than 45° downward in the north temperate regions where these experiments have been carried out. For instance, the inclination of the earth's field where Walcott and Green's experiments were conducted is about 70°. If birds can do this, they can presumably also detect the direction of the horizontal component, which is equivalent to having a conventional magnetic compass. In experiments where bar magnets or coils are carried by the birds, the resultant field at any point on the bird's body varies according to the bird's vertical and horizontal orientation with respect to the earth's field. Since pigeons do a great deal of turning shortly after release, it is difficult to evaluate all the complicated interactions between the earth's field and that carried by the bird. Nevertheless, the Walcott and Green experiments do indicate that a short-term effect on directional orientation can be produced experimentally by relatively small changes in the earth's magnetic field.

Very recently Bookman (1977) has reported that three pairs of homing pigeons showed a clear and consistent difference in behavior correlated with the presence or absence of a magnetic field having approximately the intensity of the normal earth's field. The apparatus employed was a wooden tunnel about 1 meter square and 4 meters long, closed at one end. The pigeons were placed by hand into the open end and trained to move along the length of the tunnel to the closed end, where two doors, symmetrically placed in the side walls, led to chambers, of which only one contained food located in a bin not visible from the main chamber. The tunnel was located in a room shielded with mu-metal, which reduced the earth's magnetic field to $0.02 \pm 0.01\ g$ or roughly 1/25th of its normal value. Three "Helmholtz coils" about 1 meter in diameter were located above and below the wooden tunnel, and when a direct current was turned on they produced a vertical magnetic field estimated at $0.5\ g$—or approximately the field near one of the earth's magnetic poles. One door led to food when a current of 0.1 amp flowed through these coils, the other when they were turned off. The vertical field produced by the three coils could not have been uniform along the length of the tunnel, especially since the diagram of the apparatus indicates that the coils were separated by approximately their diameters rather than by their radii, as in true Helmholtz coils.

Only the choice of the first member of the pair to enter one of the feeding chambers was recorded. Performance was above the chance level only if two conditions were met: (1) The two pigeons had to be a mated pair; single birds or a pair of nonmated birds were reported to be less active in the tunnel and apparently did not achieve any significant discrimination. (2) At least 3 seconds of "fluttering" had to occur before the bird entered a feeding chamber (Schmidt-Koenig, 1977).

When these two conditions were satisfied, correct choices were made in 68 out of 89 trials with one pair, 50 out of 61 with another, and 13 out of 16 with the third. The two-tailed binomial probability of these results occurring by chance is less than 0.0001 for the first two pairs and less than 0.025 for the third. It is not clear whether the fluttering birds jumped into the air and hovered in place or flew along the length of the tunnel. Since the experiments were apparently not conducted "blind," inadvertent cues could have been provided by the experimenter who placed the bird in the open end of the tunnel at the beginning of each trial.

Bookman's experiments may nevertheless have supplied the first clear-cut experimental demonstration of sensitivity to magnetic fields comparable in intensity to the normal earth's field. Since the experiment indicates only that the birds can distinguish between a field roughly equal to the normal earth's field and a field of very greatly reduced intensity, it could be argued that an ability to distinguish between the presence and the virtual absence of an environmental signal is not sufficient to demonstrate that it is used for directional orientation. But if Bookman's experiments can be confirmed, they will prove to be an exciting new development. They may even mark the beginning of a new stage in the experimental analysis of magnetic sensitivity, in which clear-cut and repeatable responses of individual organisms can be analyzed in detail.

When all this recent evidence in favor of sensitivity to the earth's magnetic field is reviewed, one may wonder why any doubt remains. Indeed almost all investigators of bird navigation seem convinced that the earth's magnetic field has some influence on bird orientation. Two significant uncertainties, however, must be seriously considered. The first is the fact that numerous attempts have been made to elicit unequivocal responses from pigeons or other birds to magnetic fields comparable in strength to the earth's, and in every case the results have been overwhelmingly negative. Negative results are viewed by scientists with justifiable suspicion, but in this case such a diversity of experiments have been attempted that their uniform failure cannot easily be overlooked. The most thorough of these experiments, and the only ones for which complete details have been published, are those of Kreithen and Keeton (1974) and Beaugrand (1976). A very effective method was developed for classical conditioning of pigeons to show a distinct change in heart rate when a stimulus that they could sense was followed after a few seconds by an electric shock. This method worked well not only for stimuli known to be easily detected, such as lights and sounds, but also for two other classes of stimuli to which pigeons had not previously been shown to be sensitive. These were the plane of polarization of light, and relatively small fluctuations in atmospheric pressure down to roughly 1 millibar (equivalent to about 10 meters change in altitude). Thus the method was demonstrated to be effective not only for grossly obvious stimuli, but for relatively subtle ones. A determined experimental effort using the same individual pigeons which had showed inaccurate initial headings when carrying magnets yielded completely negative results.

A second problem is the very small magnitude of all the effects reported from these experiments to date except for those of Bookman discussed above. After many years of experimental work, the methods employed by the Wiltschkos achieve marginal statistical significance only by pooling the data recorded by several birds over several hours in the apparatus. Yet in the real world of a homing or migrating bird orientational choices must be made over short periods of time by individual birds. To be sure, under some conditions migrants might pool information by communicating, but individual homing pigeons released one at a time show as accurate initial headings as those flying in groups (Keeton, 1974). It has been suggested that sensitivity to the earth's magnetic field is such a marginal matter for birds that only by averaging information received over many hours can even an approximate orientation be achieved. The Wiltschkos have indeed postulated (Wiltschko and Wiltschko, 1975) that while magnetic orientation is in a sense primary, birds learn to "calibrate" other sources of information such as the stars, or possibly wind direction, and then base their immediate orientational responses on these nonmagnetic cues. These explanations postulate that the magnetic sense has a very long time constant. But this does not suffice to explain the effects on the initial headings of homing pigeons reported by Keeton and by Walcott and Green to occur within a few minutes after application of the bar magnet or activation of the coils, and within a minute or two after the bird begins to fly. Bookman's pigeons appear to have required only a few seconds to detect the presence or absence of a 0.5 g field.

Another possibility that has been discussed by Keeton (1974) and others is that the earth's magnetic field can be detected only by a bird in rapid motion through the earth's field. The physical basis for detecting the earth's field might be the detection of induced voltage gradients or currents flowing through the bird's body as a result of its motion through the earth's field. But in many of the experiments in which responses to weak magnetic fields have been sought, including those of Kreithen and Keeton, changing magnetic field strengths have been employed. These should induce voltage gradients similar to those resulting from motion through the earth's field.

On balance then the whole question of avian sensitivity to the earth's magnetic field stands in a puzzling state. The positive evidence for a weak effect is far from trivial (Schmidt-Koenig, 1977), and yet the negative evidence is also relatively strong. It thus seems that the case might best be described as suggestive but not proved. It may be best to reserve judgment until more definitive evidence becomes available.

Evidence of Magnetic Sensitivity in Animals Other Than Birds

The experiments deriving from Lissmann's original demonstration that weakly electric fish orient themselves by sensing electric fields have led to the recent demonstration by Kalmijn and others that many fishes have sufficient electrical sensitivity that they should be able to detect the voltage gradients resulting from motion through the earth's magnetic field. Indeed Lissmann originally showed responses to moving magnets, and in recent experiments reviewed by Kalmijn (1974) fish have responded to weak magnetic fields, comparable to the earth's. Akoev *et al.* (1976) have reported thresholds for rate of change of a magnetic field in electrosensitive skates and found thresholds of about $0.8\,g$ per second. Since the earth's field is about $0.5\,g$, these fish would have to execute very rapid turns or other maneuvers to reach this threshold level by swimming through the natural earth's field. One can therefore argue: If fish can do this, why not birds? But a serious physical difficulty remains to be explained away, and this is the fact that electrosensitive fish concentrate voltage gradients across their bodies so that local potential differences across receptor cells are much greater than the average gradient. An important part of the physical mechanism by which this is accomplished is the flow of current not only through the fish but through the surrounding water, which provides an electrical return path. A much more difficult problem is faced by a bird surrounded by air, which has an enormously lower electrical conductivity than even the purest fresh water. While the same voltage gradient would be established, or perhaps a greater one owing to higher speeds of motion, the estimated difference in current flow remains very large.

Experiments by Lindauer and Martin (1972) on a wholly different kind of terrestrial animal, the honeybee, provide important support for the general conclusion that the earth's magnetic field can be sensed by animal nervous systems. As is well known from the pioneering experiments of von Frisch (1967), under conditions where the colony is in great need of food returning foragers execute a figure eight-shaped waggle dance, the straight portion of which indicates directions relative to the azimuth position of the sun. When bees are executing these dances with reference to a source of food at a fixed location, the actual angle of the dance relative to the vertical changes progressively during the day as the sun moves through the sky. Yet, as von Frisch noted many years ago, the dances do not precisely follow the change in the sun's azimuth, but rather show slight deviations of up to 10°–15° from time to time during the day. Lindauer and Martin (1972) showed that these minor deviations disappeared in an artificial magnetic field of the appropriate strength and orientation to cancel the natural earth's field to within less than 5%. Under these conditions the dances shifted smoothly with the sun's azimuth and underwent only random variations of about 2° or 3°. Another important finding described in preliminary fashion by Lindauer and Martin (1972) is that when bees are induced to occupy a new cavity, the plane of the parallel layers of honeycomb which they build can be altered by suitable Helmholtz coils. In other experiments Lindauer (1976) reported effects on honeybee dances of daily fluctuations in the earth's field. Martin and Lindauer (in press) describe experiments on gravity orientation of bees that appear to provide additional evidence that honeybees can react consistently to the earth's magnetic field or to small changes in it. Thus a stronger line of argument than comparing birds to electrically sensitive fish would be: If bees can orient to the earth's magnetic field, why not birds?

Finally it is important to add to this long series of experiments on magnetic sensitivity the recent report by Blakemore (1975) that bacteria of a type living in marine sediments move toward the north magnetic pole under laboratory conditions. These magnetotactic bacteria are provided with cellular inclusions containing considerable amounts of iron. All a bird would seem to need is an appropriate infection of its inner ear with such bacteria!

From all this evidence it is clear that living cells have the capability of responding to the earth's magnetic field, but it still remains to be demonstrated in any satisfactory fashion that birds actually use the earth's magnetic field for their orientation. The evidence reviewed above has certainly stimulated many investigators to search by a variety of methods for clear physiological or behavioral evidence of the sort so conspicuously lacking to date; thus we may anticipate that unequivocal evidence will be forthcoming in the reasonably near future. Otherwise we may be forced to remain in the uncomfortable situation where animals that have less pressing need than birds for the equivalent of a magnetic compass are nevertheless the only ones in which this new sensory capability is unequivocally demonstrable.

D. The Problem of Kramer's Map Component

It is important to reiterate that the goal-directed homing after arbitrary displacement into unfamiliar territory requires more than directional orientation. Neither magnetic nor sun compass, nor both together, seem capable of furnishing the map component, as it was termed by Kramer. We are in the embarrassing position of lacking even a plausible hypothesis to account for goal-directed homing, and this, to put it mildly, hinders the design of adequate experiments. One natural reaction is simply to ignore the problem, to take refuge behind yet another simplicity filter, and hope the disturbing business will simply go away. But the history of this field provides little comfort for this attitude. Real animals persist in doing things with which our scientific Zeitgeist is not yet prepared to cope. This situation clearly presents a challenge and the opportunity for creative investigators to open new chapters in the history of this field which has already yielded so many significant surprises.

VII. SUMMARY

Investigations of comparative sensory physiology have disclosed several previously unsuspected "windows" by which information from an animal's environment reaches its central nervous system. The excellent underwater hearing of certain fishes and of marine mammals is one outstanding example. Another is the ability of insects and other animals to utilize the plane of polarization of light. In certain snakes (pit vipers and boas) undifferentiated nerve endings located in specialized sense organs serve as effective radiometers. These are used to detect warmblooded prey, such as mice, with surface temperatures that differ from the background by a few degrees.

Many groups of fishes have lateral-line systems which are remarkably sensitive to small voltage gradients—down to well below 1 μV/cm. By a previously unsuspected mode of perception, weakly electric fishes detect changes in the electric fields set up by their own relatively feeble electric organs. Further investigations of this electrical "window" showed that electric signals are also used for communication. Aggressive interactions and probably also courtship are mediated, at least in large part, by weak electric signals.

Still further investigations of electrosensitive fishes disclosed that many groups, such as the sharks and rays, that have no electric organs nevertheless have sufficiently sensitive electroreceptors that they can detect other fish, especially prey, by sensing direct current and low-frequency electric potentials of biological origin. Some fish can also detect naturally occurring electric fields originating from physical or chemical processes in the aquatic environment. Even the earth's magnetic field can be sensed through induced voltage gradients as fish swim or are carried by currents.

One of the best known examples of animal orientation based on an extension of previously appreciated sensory spectra is the echolocation of bats and marine mammals. Specialized orientation sounds yield echoes that convey important information via the auditory system. Although clicks audible to human ears are used by a few species of bats and two genera of cave-dwelling birds, the existence of echolocation was unsuspected until the late 1930s because the orientation sounds of most bats are above the frequency range of human hearing.

The underwater orientation sounds of marine mammals are very brief clicks with extremely broad frequency spectra, whereas echolocating bats usually employ orientation sounds with a definite frequency structure. Commonly this consists of a very rapid downward frequency sweep, typically an octave in roughly 50–100 waves. Usually each orientation sound is of short enough duration to avoid overlap between the emitted probing signal and returning echoes. Repetition rates almost always increase sharply when the animal is faced with a difficult problem of orientation, such as a bat pursuing flying insects.

Echolocating animals have developed auditory nervous systems exquisitely specialized for extracting pertinent information from echoes, including identification of targets and discrimination between them on the basis of frequency spectra of echoes. Discrimination between targets at slightly different distances and detection of faint echoes masked by interfering noise are both accomplished with a proficiency very close to the theoretical limits set by signal detection theory.

The auditory system of echolocating animals is basically similar to that of other mammals, but certain features are at least quantitatively accentuated. These include neural networks that achieve selective sensitivity to sweeping frequencies and "transmit–receive switches" of two sorts. The best known are the relatively hypertrophied middle ear muscles which contract synchronously with the emission of orientation sounds and yet relax within a very few milliseconds so that full auditory sensitivity is restored before echoes return. A second mechanism of this type, only recently discovered, is "neural attenuation" somewhere between the VIIIth nerve and lateral lemniscus also synchronized with the emission of orientation sounds. In the bats, where they have been best studied, these two mechanisms together reduce auditory sensitivity by about 30 decibels at the time when intense orientation sounds are being emitted.

Echolocation is not limited to specialized animals. In the human blind a simple sort of obstacle detection based on hearing echoes is well known. Unfortunately the proficiency achieved by bats and dolphins has not been matched even by the most skillful and experienced blind people. Since the physiological reasons underlying this regrettable performance gap are not known, it is unclear whether appreciable improvement in human echolocation is possible.

Major scientific challenges still confront us concerning the well known ability of birds to maintain correct orientation during migrations and homing flights. Birds and many other animals are capable of time-compensated sun- or star-compass orientation in which they head at an angle to the sun or to particular groups of stars which shifts progressively with time. But many migrants, and some of the most proficient homing pigeons, can orient almost as well under completely opaque clouds as when the sun or stars are visible.

A sensitivity to the earth's magnetic field is a possible alternate sensory window used by birds for directional orientation when the sky is not visible. In several types of experiments, deterioration in orientation or a shift in the average direction of flight has been observed when the natural magnetic field is distorted. But most laboratory experiments designed to test unequivocally for sensitivity to the earth's magnetic field have yielded negative results. It therefore seems best to reserve judgment as to whether or not a new sensory window is in the process of being discovered. Yet investigations of animal orientation have led to so many extensions of our conceptual horizons that a continuation of this process would not be altogether surprising.

REFERENCES

Able, K. P. 1977. *Anim. Behav.* **25**, 924–925.
Akoev, G. N., Ilyinsky, O. B., and Zadan, P. M. (1976). *J. Comp. Physiol.* **A 106**, 127–136.
Barrett, R., Madison, P. F. A., and Meszler, R. M. (1970). *In* "The Biology of the Reptilia" (C. Gans and T. S. Parsons, eds.), Vol. 2, pp. 277–304. Academic Press, New York.
Beaugrand, J. P. (1976). *J. Comp. Physiol.* **A110**, 343–355.
Bell, C. C., Myers, J. P., and Russell, C. J. (1974). *J. Comp. Physiol.* **92**, 201–228.
Bennett, M. V. L. (1971). *In* "Fish Physiology" (W. S. Hoar and D. J. Randall, eds.), Vol. 5, pp. 493–574. Academic Press, New York.
Black-Cleworth, P. (1970). *Anim. Behav. Monograph* **31**, 1–77.
Blakemore, R. (1975). *Science* **190**, 377–380.
Bookman, M. A. (1977). *Nature (London)* **267**, 340–342.
Brown, F. A., Jr. (1971). *Ann. N. Y. Acad. Sci.* **188**, 224–241.
Bruns, V. (1976a) *J. Comp. Physiol.* **A106**, 77–86.
Bruns, V. (1976b). *J. Comp. Physiol.* **A106**, 87–97.
Buchler, E. R. (1976). *Anim. Behav.* **24**, 858–873.
Bullock, T. H. (1973). *Am. Sci.* **61**, 316–325.
Bullock, T. H., and Barrett, R. (1968). *Commun. Behav. Biol.* **A.1**, 19–29.
Bullock, T. H., and Diecke, P. J. (1956). *J. Physiol.* (London) **134**, 47–87.
Bullock, T. H., and Fox, W. (1957). *Quart. J. Microsc. Sci.* **98**, 219–234.
D'Arms, E., and Griffin, D. R. (1972). *Auk* **89**, 269–279.
Dijkgraaf, S. (1968). *Experientia* **24**, 187–188.
Eastwood, E. (1967). "Radar Ornithology." Methuen, London.
Emlen, S. T. (1967). *Auk* **84**, 309–342, 463–489.
Emlen, S. T. (1970). *Science* **170**, 1198–1201.
Emlen, S. T. (1975). *In* "Avian Biology" (D. S. Farner and J. R. King, eds.), Vol. 5, pp. 129–219. Academic Press, New York.
Emlen, S. T., Wiltschko, W., Demong, N., Wiltschko, R., and Bergman, S. (1976). *Science* **193**, 505–508.
Fay, R. R., and Popper, A. N. (1975). *J. Exp. Biol.* **62**, 379–387.
Fessard, A. (ed.) (1974). "Electroreceptors and Other Specialized Receptors in Lower Vertebrates," Vol. III of "Handbook of Sensory Physiology." Springer Publ., New

York. (Detailed reviews by A. Fessard, T. Szabo, R. W. Murray, A. Kalmijn, H. Schleich, and T. H. Bullock.)

Galambos, R. (1942). *J. Acoust. Soc. Am.* **14,** 41–49.

Griffin, D. R. (1952). *Biol. Rev. Cambridge Philos. Soc.* **27,** 359–400.

Griffin, D. R. (1953). *Am. Sci.* **41,** 209–244, 281.

Griffin, D. R. (1955). *Deep Sea Res.* **3,** Suppl., 406–417.

Griffin, D. R. (1958). "Listening in the Dark." Yale Univ. Press, New Haven, Connecticut (reprinted by Dover, New York, 1974).

Griffin, D. R. (1969). *Quart. Rev. Biol.* **44,** 255–276.

Griffin, D. R. (1973). *Proc. Am. Philos. Soc.* **117,** 117–141.

Griffin, D. R. (1976). *Anim. Behav.* **24,** 421–427.

Griffin, D. R., McCue, J. J. G., and Grinnell, A. D. (1963). *J. Exp. Zool.* **152,** 229–250.

Griffin, D. R., Friend, J. H., and Webster, F. (1965). *J. Exp. Zool.* **158,** 155–168.

Grinnell, A. D. (1963). *J. Physiol. (London)* **167,** 38–127.

Harrison, J. B. (1965). *Physiol. Zool.* **38,** 34–48.

Hartline, P. H. (1974). *In* "Electroreceptors and Other Specialized Receptors in Lower Vertebrates," Vol. III/3 of "Handbook of Sensory Physiology" (A. Fessard, ed.), Springer Publ., New York.

Heiligenberg, W. (1975). *J. Comp. Physiol.* **103,** 247–272.

Heiligenberg, W. (1976). *J. Comp. Physiol.* **A109,** 357–372.

Henson, O. W., Jr. (1965). *J. Physiol. (London)* **180,** 871–887.

Hines, C. O. (1972). *Nature (London)* **239,** 73–78.

Hooke, W. H., Young, J. M., and Beran, D. W. (1972). *Boundary-layer Meteorology* **2,** 371–380.

Hopkins, C. D. (1974). *Am. Sci.* **62,** 426–437.

Jen, P. H.-S., and Suga, N. (1976). *Science* **191,** 950–952.

Kalmijn, A. J. (1971). *J. Exp. Biol.* **55,** 371–383.

Kalmijn, A. J. (1974). *In* "Electroreceptors and Other Specialized Receptors in Lower Vertebrates," Vol. III/3 of "Handbook of Sensory Physiology" (A. Fessard, ed.). Springer Publ., New York.

Keeton, W. T. (1974). *In* "Advances in the Study of Behavior" (D. S. Lehrman, R. A. Hinde, and E. Shaw, eds.), Vol. X, pp. 47–132. Academic Press, New York.

Kramer, G. (1959). *Ibis* **101,** 399–416.

Krebs, H. A. (1975). *J. Exp. Zool.* **194,** 221–226.

Kreithen, M. L., and Keeton, W. T. (1974). *J. Comp. Physiol.* **91,** 355–362.

Larkin, R. P., and Sutherland, P. J. (1977). *Science* **195,** 777–779.

Larkin, T. S., and Keeton, W. T. (1976). *J. Comp. Physiol.* **A110,** 227–231.

Lenschow, D. H. (1970). *J. Appl. Meterol.* **9,** 874–884.

Lindauer, M. (1976). *Verh. Dtsch. Zd. Ges.* pp. 156–183.

Lindauer, M., and Martin, H. (1972). *In* "Animal Orientation and Navigation" (S. R. Galler, K. Schmidt-Koenig, G. J. Jacobs, and R. E. Belleville, eds.), NASA SP-262. U.S. Govt. Printing Office, Washington, D.C.

Lissmann, H. (1958). *J. Exp. Biol.* **35,** 156–191.

McDonald, D. L. (1973). *J. Exp. Zool.* **183,** 267–278.

McDonald, D. L. (1975). *J. Exp. Zool.* **191,** 161–167.

Martin, H., and Lindauer, M. *J. Comp. Physiol.* (In press).

Matthews, G. V. T. (1968). "Bird Navigation," 2nd ed. Cambridge Univ. Press, London and New York.

Noble, G. K., and Schmidt, A. (1937). *Proc. Am. Philos. Soc.* **77,** 263–288.

Perdeck, A. C. (1963). *Ardea* **51,** 91–104.

Peters, R. C., and Bretschneider, F. (1972). *J. Comp. Physiol.* **81,** 345–362.

Peters, R. C., and van Wijland, F. (1974). *J. Comp. Physiol.* **92,** 273–280.

Pollak, G., Henson, O. W., Jr., and Novick, A. (1972). *Science* **176,** 66–68.

Popper, A. N., and Fay, R. R. (1973). *J. Acoust. Soc. Am.* **53,** 1515–1529.

Rice, C. E. (1967). *Science* **155,** 656–664.

Russell, C. J., Myers, J. P., and Bell, C. C. (1974). *J. Comp. Physiol.* **92,** 181–200.

Sales, G., and Pye, J. D. (1974). "Ultrasonic Communication in Mammals." Chapman & Hall, London.

Schmidt-Koenig, K. (1965). *In* "Advances in the Study of Behavior" (D. S. Lehrman, R. A. Hinde, and E. Shaw, eds.), Vol. 1, pp. 217–278. Academic Press, New York.

Schmidt-Koenig, K., ed. (1978). Animal Migration, Navigation and Homing. Springer, New York, in press.

Schnitzler, H.-U. (1968). *Z. Vergl. Physiol.* **57,** 376–408.

Schnitzler, H.-U. (1970). *Z. Vergl. Physiol.* **68,** 25–38.

Schnitzler, H.-U., Suga, N., and Simmons, J. A. (1976). *J. Comp. Physiol.* **A106,** 99–110.

Schuller, G., and Suga, N. (1976a). *J. Comp. Physiol.* **A105,** 9–14.

Schuller, G., and Suga, N.(1976b). *J. Comp. Physiol.* **A107,** 253–262.

Simmons, J. A. *In* "Dahlem Workshop on Complex Acoustic Signals" (T. H. Bullock, ed.). Dahlem Konferenzen, Berlin, 1977.

Simmons, J. A., Lavender, W. A., Lavender, B. A., Doroshow, C. A., Kiefer, S. W., Livingston, R., Scallet, A. C., and Crowley, D. E. (1974). *Science* **188,** 1130–1132.

Simmons, J. A., Howell, D. J., and Suga, N. (1975). *Am. Sci.* **63,** 204–215.

Southern, W. E. (1971). *Ann. N. Y. Acad. Sci.* **188,** 295–311.

Southern, W. E. (1975). *Science* **189,** 143–145.

Suga, N. (1973). *In* "Basic Mechanisms in Hearing" (A. R. Møller, ed.), pp. 675–744. Academic Press, New York.

Suga, N., and Jen, P. H.-S. (1975). *J. Exp. Biol.* **62,** 277–311.

Suga, N., and Jen, P. H.-S. (1976). *Science* **194,** 542–544.

Suga, N., Simmons, J. A., and Shimozawa, T. (1974). *J. Exp. Biol.* **61,** 379–399.

Suga, N., Neuweiler, G., and Möller, J. (1976). *J. Comp. Physio.* **A106,** 111–125.

Supa, M., Cotzin, M., and Dallenbach, K. M. (1944). *Am. J. Psychol.* **57,** 133–183.

Tavolga, W. N. (ed.) (1976). "Sound Reception in Fishes." Dowden, Hutchinson, & Ross, Stroudsburg, Pennsylvania.

von Bekesy, G. (1960). "Experiments in Hearing" (translated by E. G. Wever). McGraw-Hill, New York.

von Frisch, K. (1936). *Biol. Rev. Cambridge Philos. Soc.* **11,** 210–246.

von Frisch, K. (1967). "The Dance Language and Orientation of Bees." Harvard Univ. Press, Cambridge, Massachusetts.

Walcott, C. (1977). *J. Exp. Biol.* **70,** 105–123.

Walcott, C., and Green, R. P. (1974). *Science* **184,** 180–182.

Walcott, C., and Schmidt-Koenig, K. (1973). *Auk* **90,** 281–286.

172 DONALD R. GRIFFIN

Wallraff, H. G. (1972). *Z. Tierpsychol.* **30,** 374–382.
Westby, G. W. M. (1974a). *J. Comp. Physiol.* **92,** 327–341.
Westby, G. W. M. (1974b). *J. Comp. Physiol.* **96,** 307–341.
Wever, E. G., and Vernon, J. A. (1961). *J. Auditory Res.* **2,** 158–175.
Wiltschko, W. (1968). *Z. Tierpsychol.* **25,** 537–558.
Wiltschko, W., and Wiltschko, R. (1975). *Z. Tierpsychol.* **37,** 337–355.
Wiltschko, W., and Wiltschko, R. (1976). *J. Comp. Physiol.* **A109,** 91–99.

LEUKEMIA VIRUS GENOMES IN THE CHROMOSOMAL DNA OF THE MOUSE*

WALLACE P. ROWE

Laboratory of Viral Diseases,
National Institute of Allergy and Infectious Diseases,
National Institutes of Health,
Bethesda, Maryland

As with most disease problems, the approaches to the control of cancer fall into two general strategies. Relatively empirical approaches, such as chemotherapy, immunotherapy, and antiviral vaccines, may result in control of the disease without requiring a deep understanding of the cellular or molecular basis of malignancy. Alternatively, control may come only when basic research has provided a full, in-depth understanding of the biological and molecular processes involved. Central to both of these approaches is one biological system—the laboratory mouse. The empirical approaches in large part rely on the mouse as the test system and disease model, while basic research on mammalian genetics, oncogenic viruses, chemical carcinogenesis, cellular immunology, tissue transplantation, and vertebrate development and differentiation is focused primarily on the inbred mouse.

Surprisingly, in each of these areas, there is known or suspected involvement of the murine C-type viruses. The developmental biologist must deal with the implications of the programmed expression of C-type virus antigens during embryogenesis (Huebner *et al.,* 1970); the cellular immunologist must question whether an immunosuppressive effect of a given manipulation could be secondary to activation of a C-type virus that replicates in T lymphocytes; a new transplantation antigen must be analyzed from the point of view that it may be a virus-coded cell-surface antigen. Regardless of whether C-type viruses have this much biologic importance or just have good press agents, they presently constitute a major problem in biological research, even apart from their importance as models for the possible etiology of cancer.

*Lecture delivered March 18, 1976.

An interesting parallel to this situation dates back almost 20 years to the period when the impact of the discovery of polyoma virus was at its peak. Here was a virus of incredible oncogenic potential; it was widespread in mice, and often found in their tumors. The air was thick with the implication that the cause of mouse cancer was in hand. This hypothesis was clearly and definitively put to rest by a very simple approach. Techniques for detecting the virus and for identifying infected animals were developed, refined, and evaluated; and the ridiculously simple, but crucial, observation was made that some mouse colonies were infected, while others were not. The infection was horizontal, spreading like any classical infectious disease, and the chain of infection could be readily interrupted. From this point on, it was easy to show that positive and negative animals and colonies did not differ in their spontaneous tumor occurrence, and that the polyoma virus therefore could not be responsible. A knowledge of the natural history of the virus allowed its biological role to be put in perspective (Rowe *et al.*, 1961).

Why has this type of straightforward, epidemiological approach not cleared the air with respect to C-type viruses of the mouse? Techniques have been devloped, and an immense amount is known about the viruses. The reason: simply that one cannot make the assertion that *these* mice have the virus, and *those* do not. All mice "have the virus," in that genetic material of murine C-type viruses is carried as chromosomal DNA by all members of the species *Mus musculus*. The basis for this assertion, and for some of its implications, are the subject that I will address here.

It is essential to recognize that the mouse C-type viruses constitute a family of viruses that are related to each other but fall into several biologically distinct categories. It is useful to consider them as having group-specific and type-specific components. By group-specific I mean proteins common to all murine C-type viruses, analogous to group-specific antigens of adenoviruses. Type-specific means a component unique to a certain subgroup within the family. The major group-specific components of the C-type viruses are the gs (p30) antigen and the reverse transcriptase; these appear to be serologically identical for all such viruses. As with other enveloped viruses, the type-specific components are chiefly virion envelope components; these are the glycoproteins that play a major role in determining host range, interference specificity, and reactivity with neutralizing antibody. For this discussion, the naturally occurring C-type viruses of laboratory mice can be considered to fall into two types, of which one has two subtypes. Ecotropic, also called mouse-tropic, viruses can enter and replicate in murine cells, but not cells of other mammals. Xenotropic viruses have essentially the opposite host range; they can infect a wide variety of mammalian cells, but cannot initiate infection from without when applied onto mouse cells (Levy and Pincus, 1970; Levy, 1973; Todaro *et al.*, 1973). There is a third major class, amphotropic viruses (Hartley and Rowe, 1976; Rasheed *et al.*, 1976), which have the host range of both mouse-tropic and xenotropic viruses, but to date these have been found only in wild *Mus musculus*, not in laboratory mice. These three classes not only differ in their host ranges, but form distinct serologic and interference groups.

The ecotropic viruses fall into two important host-range subclasses, defined by their ability to replicate in different inbred mouse strains. A gene of the mouse, *Fv-1* (Lilly, 1970), determines sensitivity to the two types of ecotropic virus; $Fv-1^n$ mice are sensitive to the so-called N-tropic strains, while mice of the other type, $Fv-1^b$, are sensitive to the other viruses, called B-tropic. Heterozygotes, $Fv-1^{nb}$, are resistant to both N- and B-tropic viruses, resistance being dominant (Pincus *et al.*, 1971). There is a third allele of *Fv-1*, provisionally termed *nr*, which confers resistance to both types of virus (W. P. Rowe and J. W. Hartley, unpublished data).

It may seem strange that host range receives so much emphasis in the taxonomy of these viruses, while host range is being progressively abandoned in general virology as an outmoded taxonomic criterion. In part this results from the paucity of other markers that might be used for classification, but chiefly it is because host range is so informative in envisioning some of the biology of these viruses. Thus, if we are speaking of ecotropic virus, we must think of a virus that can spread from cell to cell within the mouse, whereas with xenotropic viruses a cell that is producing virus does not infect any others. Also, when dealing with ecotropic viruses, we can envision a more permissive host environment if the *Fv-1* type matches the virus type, or a partially restrictive environment if there is a mismatch.

It is very likely that there are additional types of murine C-type virus that have not been detected by the presently available virus assay systems, and this should always be borne in mind in considering a given system as being free of virus.

When inbred mouse strains are tested for C-type viruses, several distinct patterns emerge. With ecotropic viruses, there are three patterns. In high-virus strains, every mouse has moderate to high titers of virus, virus being first detectable early in life, even in the last few days of embryonic development (Rowe and Pincus, 1972). Low-virus strains have the capacity to produce ecotropic virus that is indistinguishable from that in high-virus mice; however, the virus is found later in life, in small amount, and in only a fraction of individuals (i.e., 5% to 60%, after a year or more of age, depending on strain). In these low-virus mice, production of virus can often be induced by experimental manipulations such as radiation and graft-vs-host reactions, and generally accompanies the induction of tumors. Finally, there are virus-negative strains of mice, from which ecotropic virus has never been isolated or induced. There is a generally good correlation between these ecotropic virus patterns and the occurrence of spontaneous lymphoid neoplasms, high-lymphoma strains in all cases being high-virus strains. With regard to xenotropic virus infection, there are also strain-specific patterns of infection. The NZB mouse is a high-xenotropic virus strain, but most other strains appear to be in the low-virus category. To date, there is no proved xenotropic virus-negative strain of mice.

To summarize these patterns, inbred mouse strains differ both as to the presence or the absence of ecotropic virus and the level of its expression in the positive strains, while with respect to xenotropic virus there is polymorphism in level of expression, but probably not in the presence or the absence of the capacity to produce the virus.

Briefly stated, the evidence that these patterns are determined by chromosomally integrated viral genomes comes from many directions and makes a compelling argument. It is most clear with the ecotropic viruses, where the virus detection techniques are most highly sensitive and reliable. There are four types of evidence for this.

1. The virus expression patterns are strain-specific and independent of the environmental conditions; even rearing of mouse embryos in the uterus of mice with different virus expression patterns does not change their phenotype in postnatal life (Fekete and Otis, 1954; T. Pincus, K. Bechtel, and W. P. Rowe, unpublished data).

2. Cell cultures derived from embryos of high- or low-ecotropic virus-positive mice can be carried as noninfectious cell lines, but every cell has the potential ability to produce virus (Rowe *et al.,* 1971; Aaronson *et al.,* 1971). In particular, iodo- and bromodeoxyuridine (IUdR and BUdR) induce rapid synthesis of viral antigens and infectious virus in a significant proportion of cells (Lowy *et al.,* 1971). With high-virus strains this can be as high as 70% of cells producing gs antigen, and 5–10% of cells producing infectious virus within 3 days of adding the drug, whereas with cultures from low-virus mice the efficiency is generally many orders of magnitude less.

3. In matings between high-virus and negative or low-virus mice, the high-virus phenotype follows classical mendelian segregation patterns (Taylor *et al.,* 1971; Rowe, 1972), and in two instances the chromosomal loci responsible for the high-virus phenotype have been mapped in the mouse genome (Rowe *et al.,* 1972; Rowe, 1973).

4. As will be shown later, viral nucleic acid sequences are present at these chromosomal loci.

Let us first examine some of the general biological characteristics of these ecotropic virus-inducing (V) loci. There are several interesting correlations, which provide some insight about these loci. As mentioned above, there is a good correlation between high spontaneous activation of virus, both *in vivo* and *in vitro,* and high activation by IUdR, suggesting that the various virus-inducing genes are under one basic type of molecular control mechanism. When genetic analysis is carried out by the standard procedure of making an F_1 hybrid between a high-virus and virus-negative mouse, and backcrossing to the negative strain, the segregation ratios show that the high-virus strains generally carry more than one locus for virus induction. Strain AKR, the prototype high-virus mouse, carries two such loci, *Akv-1* and *Akv-2;* these segregate independently of one another and give indistinguishable high-virus phenotypes in mice inheriting one or the other locus (Rowe, 1972). The high-virus subline of C3H, C3H/Fg, carries 3 such alleles (Rowe, 1973), and C58 carries 3 or possibly 4 (Stephenson and Aaronson, 1973; W. P. Rowe and J. W. Hartley, unpublished data). On the other hand, one relatively high-virus, high-leukemia strain, PL/J, appears to carry only one locus (A. Ishimoto, J. W. Hartley, and W. P. Rowe, unpublished studies). Multiple loci are certainly not necessary for the high-virus phenotype, since the various single-gene heterozygotes that we have studied in the course of isolating these loci are as high in virus titer as is AKR, which, being a double homozygote, has four times as many V-loci per cell.

Whether low-virus mice will be found to have multiple V-loci as well is not known; the one strain analyzed to date, BALB/c, appears to have only one locus for production of ecotropic virus (Aaronson and Stephenson, 1973).

A most important feature of the V-loci is that they seem to be at nonallelic sites in the different inbred mouse strains. As shown in Fig. 1, the two such loci which have been mapped are both on chromosome 7 (linkage group I), but at different sites; the AKR locus *Akv-1* is on the centromeric side of Gpi-1 (Rowe *et al.*, 1972), while one of the 3 loci in C3H/Fg is very close to the *Hbb* locus (Rowe, 1973). Further, it is quite clear that C3H/Fg does not have a V-locus at the site of *Akv-1*, nor AKR

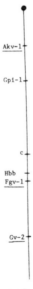

FIG. 1. Chromosome 7 (linkage group I) of the mouse. *Akv-1* and *Fgv-1* are virus-inducing loci of AKR and C3H/Fg, respectively. *Gv-2* is a murine leukemia virus-related gene described by Stockert *et al.* (1971), which is required for the expression of G_{IX} antigen on strain 129 thymocytes.

a locus where *Fgv-1* is; also, C58 does not have any of its 3 or 4 V-loci on this chromosome (W. P. Rowe and J. W. Hartley, unpublished data). It is conceivable that there is one constant V-locus site, i.e., *Akv-2*, occupied in all high-virus mice, or possibly in all high- and low-virus mice; once *Akv-2* is mapped, this hypothesis can be tested readily.

It is important to note that presence of a chromosomal V-locus does not confer any resistance to exogenous infection with ecotropic virus; there is no analog to lysogenic immunity.

Incorporation of nucleic acid hybridization techniques into the study of the virus-inducing loci has provided great insight. These studies, by Dr. Sisir Chattopadhyay in our laboratory, have been done with single-stranded, radiolabeled DNA probes prepared from ecotropic and xeno-tropic virus strains. The probes are allowed to react with a vast excess of separated strands of cellular DNA from mouse embryos, and the extent of binding of radiolabel into double-stranded DNA is measured, using hydroxyapatite columns to isolate the double-stranded DNA. Since the viral probe does not undergo self-annealing, being composed of only one strand type, any entering of probe label into double-stranded molecules has to be from its matching with complementary sequences in the cellular DNA.

These assays can give three types of information. The saturation level, meaning the proportion of the probe that reacts with an excess of cellular DNA when the reaction is carried to completion, tells what proportion of the viral genome is present in the cell DNA. Analysis of the kinetics of the reaction can show how many copies there are of the viral sequences in the cell genome; if some of the viral sequences are more abundant than others, this also can be deduced from the kinetic curves, along with an estimate of the number of copies of each of the classes. And third, the thermal stability of the cell-probe hybrid molecules (expressed as $\Delta TE50$, the difference between the midpoints of the melting curves of probe-cell hybrid molecules and cell–cell rean-nealed molecules) tells how close is the complementarity between the two, that is, whether the sequences would be considered as being essentially identical or more distantly related.

The sequence homology studies using the ecotropic, AKR virus probe with embryo cell DNA from inbred mouse strains have given completely consistent confirmation of the patterns obtained from the biological studies (Chattopadhyay *et al.,* 1974a,b, 1975). The saturation level analyses (Fig. 2) show that all strains from which ecotropic virus can be obtained, whether high- or low-virus yielders, contain the whole viral genetic information in the embryo cell DNA, while the ecotropic virus-negative strains uniformly show lower saturation levels, at a level that indicates that about one-fourth of the viral genome is lacking. The kinetic analyses show further correlations. All the virus-yielding strains show two populations of viral sequences in the cell DNA; one set is present as multiple copies, roughly between 10 and 50 per haploid genome, while the remainder are present in much smaller numbers, that is, no more than 4 per haploid genome. When we look at the number of copies of the latter sequences in relation to the virologic status (Fig. 2, right), we again have an excellent correlation between the biological and biochemical findings. The high-virus mice that carry 2–4 V-loci as shown by mendelian genetic analysis show 3 or 4 copies of this set of sequences per haploid genome, while the high-virus strain with a single such locus, PL/J, and all the low-virus mice show only 1 or 2 copies. In the DNA of the virus-negative strains there is only the one class of sequences, the multiple-copy set. By cross-absorption studies, it was shown that the multiple-copy set is the group of sequences that are present in both the virus-positive and virus-negative strains, and thus the set present in small numbers in virus-positive mice includes the

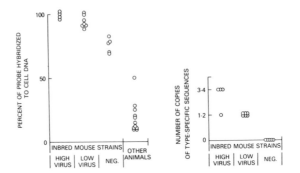

FIG. 2. Characterization of ecotropic murine leukemia virus sequences in cellular DNA of various mouse strains, in relation to the pattern of expression of ecotropic virus. The high value in the tests of cell DNA of other animals is *Microtus arvalis* (S. K. Chattopadhyay and W. P. Rowe, unpublished data).

sequences that are missing from the virus-negative mice (Chattopadhyay *et al.*, 1974a).

The comparable data obtained with the xenotropic virus probe are shown in Fig. 3. Again in full agreement with the biological studies, which indicate that all laboratory mice carry xenotropic virus, DNAs from all mouse strains show comparably high saturation levels, corresponding to the whole virus genome being present. The kinetic analysis of these data is not complete, but it is clear that some of the sequences are present in the 10–50 copies range.

In cross homology tests between probes and viral RNA, the ecotropic and xenotropic viruses have about 50% of their sequences in common.

Our interpretation of these patterns is that the C-type viral genome contains group-specific and type-specific regions, corresponding to the group- and type-specific proteins and glycoproteins mentioned earlier. The set of viral sequences that is present in multiple (10–50) copies in the cell DNA corresponds to the group sequences and is present in all mice, both laboratory and wild; thus the ecotropic virus probe detects this class of sequences in virus-negative mouse DNA, where it is part of the genome of xenotropic and perhaps other C-type viruses, and possibly as defective, incomplete genome segments as well. The sequences present in small number (0–4) include the part of the viral genome that codes for type-specific functions.

Further confirmation of the importance of these type-specific sequences comes from analyses of hybrid mice. Table I shows the eco-

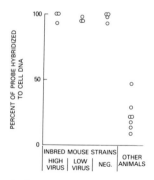

FIG. 3. Xenotropic murine leukemia virus sequences in cellular DNA of various mouse strains, in relation to pattern of expression of ecotropic virus.

TABLE I

DNA HOMOLOGY STUDIES OF HYBRIDS BETWEEN HIGH- AND LOW-VIRUS MICE,
USING ECOTROPIC MURINE LEUKEMIA VIRUS (MuLV) PROBE[a]

			Hybridization against ecotropic MuLV probe		
	Genotype			No. of copies of type-specific sequences per haploid genome	ΔTe_{50} (°C)
Mouse	Akv-1	Akv-2	Saturation level (%)		
AKR	+/+	+/+	100	3.3	1.3
NIH	−/−	−/−	78	0	7.0
(AKR × NIH)F$_1$	+/−	+/−	100	1.6	4.5
NIH congenic for Akv-1	+/+	−/−	95	1.4	3.0

[a] Cellular DNA of mouse embryos was tested with [^{3}H]DNA probe prepared from AKR virus. Saturation level is the proportion of the viral probe that is represented in the cellular DNA, and ΔTe_{50} is a measure of the relatedness between the viral and cellular sequences, the lower values corresponding to closer relatedness.

tropic virus probe analysis of two types of hybrid between AKR and NIH Swiss (a virus-negative strain): the F$_1$ hybrid, and NIH made partially congenic for *Akv-1* by 5 generations of serial backcrossing to NIH followed by inbreeding. In addition to showing that the high saturation level and low ΔTE_{50} (which indicates close matching of sequences) are seen in the virus-positive hybrids, these data are most useful for validating the analysis of the number of type-specific sequences. In full agreement with the genetic model, the F$_1$ mice show half the number seen in AKR, while the *Akv-1* congenic line, which has the same number of virus-inducing loci per cell as the F$_1$ hybrid, shows the same copy number as the F$_1$.

Furthermore, we have tested for these sequences, using saturation level and $\Delta TE50$ analyses, in individual embryos of a cross which is segregating for *Akv-1* (Chattopadhyay *et al.*, 1975). A mouse heterozygous for *Akv-1, c,* and *Gpi-1* was mated to a virus-negative NIH mouse, and 9 embryos were obtained. Each was scored for eye color, *Gpi-1* type, and for IUdR-inducibility of the cells in culture, as the marker for inheritance of *Akv-1;* the DNA was analyzed for the hybridization characteristics (Table II). The five embryos which carried *Akv-1* showed high saturation level and relatively low ΔTE_{50}s, while the 4 *Akv-1*-negative segregants were like the NIH mice. Five of the 9 mice were recombinants, either between *c* and *Gpi-1,* or between *Gpi-1* and *Akv-1,* and in all cases the sequences went with inducibility. Thus, a 4-point genetic cross confirmed that *Akv-1* contains the type-specific sequences of ecotropic virus.

I would like to turn now to a more speculative view of these studies, particularly with regard to their implications and the next level of questions needing study. The present stage of C-type virus research is a most exhilarating one—the questions and hypotheses jump out in all directions, techniques are available in abundance, paradoxes remain which must contain the germs of future surprises, and cold, hard facts have not yet caught up with us.

Where did these genes come from? Are similar genes present in man? What regulates their expression? Can a gene segment within a virus-inducing locus function as a classical gene? What is the arrangement of

TABLE II

ECOTROPIC MURINE LEUKEMIA VIRUS PROBE ANALYSIS
OF CELLULAR DNA FROM MOUSE EMBRYOS OF A
CROSS SEGREGATING FOR *Akv-1*

Akv-1 positive embryos		*Akv-1* negative embryos	
Saturation level (%)	ΔTE_{50}	Saturation level (%)	ΔTE_{50}
97	5.5	87	8.3
96	5.0	81	9.0
94	5.5	78	8.5
94	5.4	78	8.0
94	5.0		

[a] An *Akv-1* heterozygote on NIH Swiss background was bred to an NIH Swiss. The nine embryos obtained were scored for virus inducibility by IUDR, and the DNA was allowed to react with AKR virus DNA probe for determination of saturation level and ΔTE_{50}.

the multiple copies of the group-specific sequences in the mouse genome? Are they at allelic sites in different mice? How did the multiple V-loci of the high-virus mice arise? Does a high-virus locus derive from alteration or reinsertion of a low-virus locus? Is the viral genome carried in the chromosome as a complete linear genome, or does a recombination or rearrangement occur during the induction process? Does exogenous virus integrate into the viral chromosomal sequences? Does the state of differentiation of the cell affect the integration site or the ability of a given locus to be induced? The questions can go on and on. What is really remarkable is not just that we can now formulate these questions, but that they are potentially answerable. I will deal with a few of these, and give a few guesses and preliminary data which bear on them.

What is the origin of the C-type viral sequences in mouse DNA? I suspect that there are several answers to this, at least to the extent that the group-specific sequences and the ecotropic type-specific sequences may be of different origin. The group-specific, multiple-copy sequences, being uniformly present in all mice, both laboratory and wild, may well have been present in *Mus musculus* throughout most of its evolution and may be derived from a horizontally acquired C-type virus infection of an ancestor of *Mus musculus*. Attempts to detect these sequences in the phylogenetic relatives of *Mus musculus* have not given clear-cut evidence of coevolution; even with as close a relative as *Mus caroli,* the cell DNA reacts with only about 15% of the probe (S. K. Chattopadhyay, M. R. Lander, and W. P. Rowe, unpublished data). However, these studies are in a very preliminary state.

The fact that laboratory mice, and wild mice as well, are not uniformly positive for the ecotropic type-specific sequences suggests a number of interesting possibilities about their origin. It seems possible that these sequences are derived from a more recent horizontal infection by a C-type virus of some species with which *Mus musculus* has contact in nature; the ecotropic virus may represent a genetic recombinant between that C-type virus and the murine group-specific sequences already present in the cell DNA. Another possible explanation of this polymorphism is that the ecotropic virus entered the mouse genome at the time that the group sequences were acquired, but that the ecotropic virus produced enough of a negative selective pressure to maintain heterozygosis, thus allowing for subsequent segregation of virus-negative inbred strains and wild mouse populations. A variation of this hypothesis would be that the ecotropic type-specific sequences can be lost from the germ line, analogous to lysogenic curing in phage biology.

It is implicit in much of what we have been discussing that the difference in C-type virus expression between mouse strains lies not in the presence or absence of the complete viral genome, but in the mechanisms that affect or regulate its expression. It is precisely because of this that C-type viruses may have much to offer for the analysis of gene regulation in general. However, it is necessary to point out that the complexity of the systems, and the multiplicity of genomes involved make this a hazardous undertaking at present. First we must differentiate between regulation of expression by factors within the same cell, and factors which can suppress the viral expression phenotype without acting in the same cell. With regard to the latter, there are two powerful mechanisms that can suppress the expression of ecotropic virus. The $Fv-1$ gene, by preventing spread of a mismatched virus, can give a false negative phenotype. Also, some mother mice of certain strains transmit through their milk a maternal resistance factor (MacDowell and Richter, 1935; Law, 1954; W. P. Rowe and J. W. Hartley, unpublished data), presumably an antibody which cannot be detected by conventional tests, which produces a marked inhibition of ecotropic virus growth in their nurselings. These two mechanisms act by inhibiting spread of virus once induced, but do not appear to affect the induction process itself.

In studying the C-type viruses at the true gene regulation level there are two basic problems. First, if one measures virus expression by two different parameters, as for example by measuring the number of cells producing gs antigen and the number producing infectious virus following IUdR induction, the two assays could, in large part, be measuring products of different loci. Second, it would be of much interest to compare the regulation of ecotropic virus production in cells producing their endogenous virus, with the same kind of cells exogenously infected. It is a common fallacy to assume that an AKR cell culture chronically producing virus after exposure to IUdR, or even after spontaneous activation of virus, represents endogenous virus production. This is a semantic trap; in one sense it is endogenous virus, but, in the sense that is relevant to the problem, it is mostly not endogenous virus of the cells that are producing it. That is, a fraction of the cells in the culture produced virus from their endogenous viral genomes, and from them the rest of the culture became infected, by normal exogenous infection.

Being able to make this distinction would be very helpful for getting at the question of reversibility of the induced virus production. When mouse cells are infected with ecotropic virus from without, virus production is irreversible; the cell and its descendants produce virus forever, presumably by transcription of chromosomally integrated viral genomes. In contrast, the chromosomal V-loci can remain unexpressed, without producing virus, for hundreds of cell generations; once induced, either spontaneously or by IUdR, do they similarly become irreversibly committed to virus production? With induction, does the V-locus excise and reinsert at a site that is not subject to the same control mechanisms? Does the V-locus synthesize a DNA copy that inserts at such a site? Or does an irreversible loss of a control mechanism occur, without a change in the sequence or topology of the viral DNA? In the case of induction of xenotropic virus, the work of Aaronson and Stephenson makes it very likely that virus production is quite reversible; that is, following IUdR induction of BALB/c cells, there is production of virus, measured by polymerase activity in culture fluids, followed by a marked decline several days later (Aaronson, 1971). This is reminiscent of data reported by Huebner (Huebner *et al.,* 1970), showing that gs antigen appears in mouse embryos at certain stages of embryogenesis and is again undetectable several days later. It seems that these viruses may be a most useful model system for study of reversible and irreversible differentiation controls, and may even be involved in control of differentiation themselves.

Another question: Is there cooperation between genes in the induction of virus, or are both the probability of induction and the genotype of the resulting virus determined solely by the V-locus and its immediate chromosomal environment? From our work with the highly inducible loci of the high-virus AKR mouse, it would appear that the latter is true; that is, the V-loci themselves determine the virus expression phenotype, unaffected by the rest of the cellular genotype. However, several recently studied systems involving less readily inducible V-loci suggest that there may be genetic interactions, in one case affecting the level of inducibility, and in the other case, the N-B type of the induced virus. The former is work being done by Dr. Rex Risser in our laboratory; he had found that mating of two very poorly inducible strains, C56BL/6 and BALB/c, can give rise to moderately inducible mice in the F_2 generation, at a frequency of about 1 in 16. The second system is a mouse strain, Dr. Frank Lilly's subline of B10.BR, which is a relatively high-virus mouse for B-tropic virus; Dr. Bernice Moll, in our laboratory, found this mouse to be inducible for both N- and B-tropic viruses. In genetic analysis of this double inducibility, we are finding that in some mating combinations, N- and B-tropic virus inducibility segregate together, while in other combinations, only B-tropic virus can be induced. This system, which is in a very preliminary stage, suggests either that the genome of the IUdR-induced virus may contain gene segments derived from two separate sites in the cell DNA, or that one locus can induce two types of virus, and the cell genome can selectively suppress induction of one of them.

A major question about these genomes is whether they can be transcribed in part, or only can function via induction of the complete virus genome. There are a number of *in vivo* systems where there is "noninfectious" expression of viral genome or where only one viral marker is found, particularly the G_{IX} (Stockert *et al.,* 1971) and gs antigens. However, to my knowledge, there is still no tissue culture system where this pattern occurs, or where there is high level production of a viral antigen in the absence of viral particle production; until such systems are found it will be very difficult to clarify this important problem.

Up to this point I have been scrupulously avoiding the aspect of C-type virology that is generally foremost in interest—that is, the role of these viruses in causing tumors. I have done this for a purely political reason—to illustrate that, at least in our present state of knowledge, these viruses are important and interesting in and of themselves. Also, I want to express my conviction that the study of these viruses will contribute greatly to the understanding of cancer independently of whether they are eventually shown to have a significant etiologic role.

The problem of establishing an etiologic role for these chromosomally transmitted genomes is replete with semantic and logical pitfalls. A question such as: Is this DNA segment of host or viral origin? is a linguistic mine field, and can only be answered in the framework of to what use will the answer be put.

In this regard, there is a truism that is not often stated, but which lies at the heart of the experimental method. That is, we can evaluate only when there is a contrast. For example, every disease is genetic, in the sense that one can conceive of a different genotype in which the disease would not occur. But we consider a disease as being genetic only when there is polymorphism, some individuals having the trait and others not. For example, scurvy is a genetic disease, in that we lack the genes for synthesis of ascorbic acid. However, since we all have the same genetic lack, we do not bother to make a point of it. This problem must be recognized in talking about mouse cancer, and our hypotheses must be framed with this problem in mind.

The etiologic role of those viruses and viral sequences that are present in all mice may never be able to be evaluated, at least in the usual framework of our thinking about etiology. However, with the recognition that mice are polymorphous for ecotropic viruses, it is now possible to rigorously evaluate their role in murine tumorigenesis. The great majority of carcinogenesis research in mice has been done with strains that are now known to be low-ecotropic-virus producers, chiefly C57BL and BALB/c. Would the same patterns of spontaneous and physical or chemical carcinogen-induced tumorigenesis be seen if the ecotropic V-loci were bred out of these strains and they were made congenic for the absence of the ecotropic-specific sequences? This is a difficult prospect, but it is entirely feasible, and in the long-term view may be the only way to put the ecotropic viruses in a true perspective. Even comparing different strains for their response to different carcinogens on the basis of whether they are low-virus or virus-negative strains could be very rewarding. Part of this could be done just by a literature search.

That ecotropic virus can cause thymic lymphoma has been known since the classical experiments of Gross (Gross, 1951), but on the mechanism there is still very little knowledge. I would like to present very briefly two studies which can help define some of the parameters of the disease. The first is the lymphoma experience of NIH Swiss mice, normally a very low leukemia strain, made congenic for *Akv-1* or *Akv-2* from AKR (Table III). Both lines have become high-lymphoma strains, but with disease occurring significantly later in life than in AKR. In the *Akv-2* mice, the virus-negative segregants were not high leukemic. This study illustrates the key role that ecotropic virus plays in this type of leukemogenesis, and shows that the viruses from both loci are essentially equivalent in this regard.

TABLE III

Mortality (Primarily Lymphoma) in NIH Mice Congenic for *Akv-1* or *Akv-2*

Gene	Generations of inbreeding	Virus	No. of mice	Mortality (%)	
				12 months	18 months
Akv-1	5	Positive	39	13	70
Akv-2	1	Positive	65	40	74
		Negative	24	12	17
Control NIH Swiss		Negative	32	0	6

The second experiment, done with Drs. Frank Lilly and Maria Duran-Reynals (Lilly *et al.*, 1975), studied a cross from AKR in which all segregants inherited 2–4 V-loci, but in which the replication of virus was inhibited in some mice by inheritance of a restrictive *Fv-1* allele or by the maternal immune factor; the virus titer in the tail tissue at 6 weeks of age, and the incidence of leukemia at 18 months were determined (Table IV). There was a striking relationship, which we interpret as proving the need for large numbers of exogenous infections to occur

TABLE IV

Leukemia Incidence in (BALB/c × AKR) × AKR Mice in Relation to Virus Titer in Tail at 6 Weeks of Age

Ecotropic MuLV[a] titer ($\log_{10}$)	Leukemia incidence	
	No. dying of leukemia/no. in category	%
$\geqslant 3.0$	22/25	88
2–2.9	47/80	59
1–1.9	16/38	42
0.3–0.9	11/30	37
Negative	15/162	9

[a] Murine leukemia virus.

early in life for lymphoma to be induced. That is, inheritance of the V-genes and their expression within induced cells does not produce lymphoma; only spread of virus can do this. This may result simply from the greater number of infected cells at risk; or the multiple cycles of virus growth could produce viral mutants, transducing defectives, phenotypic mixes between different endogenous viruses, or pseudovirions carrying host RNA sequences, which could result in loss of regulation in cells infected with one of these abnormal particles.

While it is clear that these viruses can and do cause lymphomas in high-virus mice, it is essential to avoid the logical trap of assuming that all lymphomas are caused by them. The ecotropic virus-negative mice also develop lymphomas, spontaneously at low frequency, but in high frequency following treatment with X-irradiation or chemical carcinogens. Since these lymphomas often show evidence of C-type viral expression, though not ecotropic virus production, it is very tempting to assume that the nonecotropic C-type virus in these mice is somehow etiologic. To challenge this assumption may seem to be a logician's nit-picking. However, since it is these virus-negative, low lymphoma mice which seem to be the closest model for the human disease, but not the florid infection of AKR mice, we must not take such a fundamental conclusion for granted.

In addition to the viral genomes that can act as leukemogenic genes, there are many other genetic traits that affect the development of murine leukemias. With the ability to detect, and if desired, genetically insert or eliminate the genes for production of ecotropic viruses, in either high- or low-inducible form, we may be able to define much more clearly the role of these other genes. For example, $Fv-1$, can act as a powerful antileukemic gene, but this is of little or no theoretical importance; it is acting only by suppressing the spread of ecotropic virus. I strongly suspect that it will have no influence on lymphomas in ecotropic virus-negative mice. It should now be possible to carry the genetic dissection of murine leukemogenesis a major step forward.

I would like to stress that my emphasis on chromosomal genomes is not meant to ignore the importance of horizontal spread of C-type viruses in their natural biology. In some species, particularly cats and fowl, horizontal spread is a major route of infection, in addition to the genetic route; but in laboratory mice this is probably a minor factor that needs further study. The distinction between horizontal and vertical transmission is crucial, however, in that eventual preventative vaccination against horizontally acquired C-type viruses is quite conceivable, but vaccination of man against his endogenous viruses, if such exist, would be criminal. The expression of viral antigens in tumors may represent a signal by which the immune system can recognize and destroy microfoci of transformed cells; if we should disturb this system, the consequences could be disastrous.

As a genetic system, the murine C-type viruses may offer completely unique tools for study of gene structure, regulation, and amplification. Given the long history of the bitter conflict between the proponents of the genetic and viral etiologies of murine leukemia, it has been a highly satisfying intellectual experience to have witnessed, and to have been a part of, the synthesis between the two.

REFERENCES

Aaronson, S. A. (1971). Proc. Natl. Acad. Sci. U.S.A. **68,** 3069–3072.

Aaronson, S. A., and Stephenson, J. R. (1973). *Proc. Natl. Acad. Sci. U.S.A.* **70,** 2055–2058.

Aaronson, S. A., Todaro, G. J., and Scolnick, E. M. (1971). *Science* **174,** 157–159.

Chattopadhyay, S. K., Lowy, D. R., Teich, N. M., Levine, A. S., and Rowe, W. P. (1974a). *Proc. Natl. Acad. Sci. U.S.A.* **71,** 167–171.

Chattopadhyay, S. K., Lowy, D. R., Teich, N. M., Levine, A. S., and Rowe, W. P. (1974b). *Cold Spring Harbor Symp. Quant. Biol.* **39,** 1085–1101.

Chattopadhyay, S. K., Rowe, W. P., Teich, N. M., and Lowy, D. R. (1975). *Proc. Natl. Acad. Sci. U.S.A.* **72,** 906–910.

Fekete, E., and Otis, H. K. (1954). *Cancer Res.* **14,** 445–447.

Gross, L. (1951). *Proc. Soc. Exp. Biol. Med.* **78,** 342–348.

Hartley, J. W., and Rowe, W. P. (1976). *J. Virol.* **19,** 19–25.

Huebner, R. J., Kelloff, G. J., Sarma, P. S., Lane, W. T., Turner, H. C., Gilden, R. V., Oroszlan, S., Meier, H., Myers, D. D., and Peters, R. L. (1970). *Proc. Natl. Acad. Sci. U.S.A.* **67,** 366–376.

Law, L. W. (1954). *Ann. N. Y. Acad. Sci.* **57,** 575–583.

Levy, J. A. (1973). *Science* **182,** 1151–1153.

Levy, J. A., and Pincus, T. (1970). *Science* **170,** 326–327.

Lilly, F. (1970). *J. Natl. Cancer Inst.* **45,** 163–169.

Lilly, F., Duran-Reynals, M. L., and Rowe, W. P. (1975). *J. Exp. Med.* **141,** 882–889.

Lowy, D. R., Rowe, W. P., Teich, N., and Hartley, J. W. (1971). *Science* **174,** 155–156.

MacDowell, E. C., and Richter, M. N. (1935). *Arch. Pathol* **20,** 709–724.

Pincus, T., Hartley, J. W., and Rowe, W. P. (1971). *J. Exp. Med.* **133,** 1219–1233.

Rasheed, S., Gardner, M. B., and Chan, E. (1976). *J. Virol.* **19,** 13–18.

Rowe, W. P. (1961). *Bacteriol. Rev.* **25,** 18–31.

Rowe, W. P. (1972). *J. Exp. Med.* **136,** 1272–1285.

Rowe, W. P. (1973). *Cancer Res.* **33,** 3061–3068.

Rowe, W. P., and Pincus, T. (1972). *J. Exp. Med.* **135,** 429–436.

Rowe, W. P., Huebner, R. J., and Hartley, J. W. (1961). *In* ''Perspectives in Virology - II'' (M. Pollard, ed.), pp. 177–190. Burgess, Minneapolis, Minnesota.

Rowe, W. P., Hartley, J. W., Lander, M. R., Pugh, W. E., and Teich, N. (1971). *Virology* **46,** 866–876.

Rowe, W. P., Hartley, J. W., and Bremner, T. (1972). *Science* **178,** 860–862.

Stephenson, J. R., and Aaronson, S. A. (1973). *Science* **180,** 865–866.

Stockert, E., Old, L. J., and Boyse, E. A. (1971). *J. Exp. Med.* **133,** 1334–1355.

Taylor, B. A., Meier, H., and Myers, D. D. (1971). *Proc. Natl. Acad. Sci. U.S.A.* **68,** 3190–3194.

Todaro, G. J., Arnstein, P., Parks, W. P., Lennette, E. H., and Huebner, R. J. (1973). *Proc. Natl. Acad. Sci. U.S.A.* **70,** 859–862.

GENE EXPRESSION IN NEOPLASIA AND DIFFERENTIATION*

BEATRICE MINTZ

*Institute for Cancer Research, Fox Chase Cancer Center,
Philadelphia, Pennsylvania*

I. INTRODUCTION

As differentiation normally unfolds in the organism, it encompasses a range of cell specializations, and levels of interaction and organization, unattainable in culture. Neoplasia, which may be essentially a derangement of differentiation, comprises some analogous features, not observable in "transformed" cultured cells. Thus, despite unique and invaluable experimental options *in vitro,* we are obliged to seek ways of analyzing some of the most complex, and least understood, aspects of these phenomena where they actually occur: *in vivo.* In the tradition pioneered by William Harvey, I have therefore sought experimental ways of probing, within the framework of the organism, the obscure formative events in mammalian development and neoplasia. As will become evident later in this lecture, I have also recently attempted to devise a versatile experimental situation, whereby the special virtues of *in vitro* and *in vivo* approaches could be combined.

The events of normal and abnormal differentiation are, in good part, initiated or controlled by genes acting within cells. I therefore decided, some time ago (Mintz, 1962), to "construct" artificial laboratory animals in which two cell populations of different genetic provenance coexisted from the outset and jointly participated in all of differentiation. The cellular genotypic differences were intended to serve several general purposes: They would generate alternative phenotypes that would function as contrasting cell "labels," permitting cell lineages, fusions, and deployments to be revealed, and allowing the underlying developmental organization of tissues—even those as intricate as the brain—to become analyzable. They could also be used to learn what cell

*Lecture delivered April 1, 1976.

193

interactions were critical for formation of tissue-specific products, such as immunoglobulins. And they would provide a means of identifying the primary tissue focus of gene action in clinically complex genetic diseases.

The contributing cells might thus both be from normal strains; or one might be from a normal and the other from a genetically defective strain or a strain susceptible to malignancy; or malignant cells might actually be one of the input strains. This work has been done largely in mice, whose inbred strains and known genes make it the species of choice. Each experimental individual has four natural parents and an "incubator mother" (Fig. 1). They are *allophenic* animals, in which two cellular phenotypes, ascribable to genotypic differences, coexist within tissues (Mintz, 1971a).

We will be chiefly concerned here with the developmental origins and the developmental potentialities of neoplastic cells. The relevance of experiments with allophenic mice rests on the peculiar characteristics of these animals; they will first be described. A series of questions regarding neoplasia will then be posed and discussed.

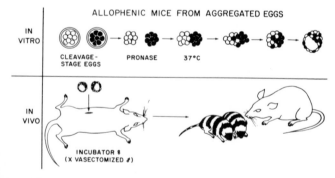

Fig. 1. Allophenic mice with two different cellular phenotypes, each attributable to a specific genotype, may be produced experimentally as shown in this diagram. Two cleavage-stage embryos of dissimilar genotypes (e.g., black and albino) are removed from the uteri of pregnant females and, after lysis of the acellular zona pellucida in Pronase, are placed in contact at 37°C. During a day in culture the cells form a spherical aggregate that develops into a normal, but double-size, blastocyst. Surgical transfer to the uterus of a pseudopregnant "incubator" mother (previously mated to a sterile male) results in restoration of normal embryo size and is generally followed by birth of normal, viable mosaic mice, in this case striped, as in Fig. 2. From Mintz (1967).

II. Characteristics of Allophenic Mice

The sustained developmental lability and totipotency of mammalian embryo cells, at least through the cleavage period, permits the blastomeres to be rearranged with impunity, as in the aggregations diagrammed in Fig. 1. When the aggregates include cells of different genotypes, integral animals with cells of both kinds are obtained (Fig. 2). Since the time when the first viable allophenic mice were produced by these methods (Mintz, 1965), thousands of such individually "assembled" laboratory artifacts have come into existence. They comprise many different paired combinations of cellular genotypes and have enabled experimental *in vivo* study of a wide range of questions (reviewed in Mintz, 1974) previously inaccessible to investigation.

A major feature of allophenic animals is that, while they are fully immunologically competent to reject foreign proteins, they are permanently immunologically tolerant of any immunogenetic differences in their component cell strains. This is documented by their capacity to retain skin grafts from parental strains having histocompatibility differences at the strong *H-2* locus (Fig. 3), and by the absence in them of graft-*vs*-host disease. As a consequence, virtually any cell strains may be developmentally conjoined irrespective of their genotypic disparities. The "intrinsic" (as opposed to "acquired") immunological tolerance of allophenic mice appears to be a valid model (Mintz and Silvers, 1967) of the ontogeny of normal self-tolerance (Burnet, 1959): In both cases, new proteins appearing prior to immune-system maturation are not later recognized as foreign by the lymphoid cells. According to another interpretation of the basis for self-tolerance in allophenic mice (Wegmann *et al.*, 1971), specific antiself lymphocytes directed against "foreign" cells are generated, but these are kept from attacking their targets by serum blocking factors. This hypothesis, which would require invoking many such blocking specificities during normal differentiation, appears not to have stood the test of further scrutiny (Brent *et al.*, 1972; Meo *et al.*, 1974; see review in Mintz, 1974).

Markers for *in situ* cell-strain visualization in the ontogeny of allophenic mice would be expected to reveal a highly ordered developmental history for each cell type. An example is seen in the retrospective visualization of the prenatal history of melanocytes, after the cells become melanized postnatally. In the case illustrated here (Fig. 2),

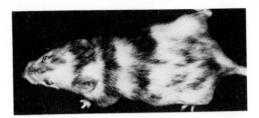

FIG. 2. A black-and-albino allophenic mouse produced as shown in Fig. 1. *Each transverse stripe of one or the other color, on the animal's left or right side, appears to be a clone formed during embryogenesis and descended from a single precursor melanoblast cell of that genotype; the cells are deployed mediolaterally as the clone expands.* From Mintz (1967).

genetically pigmented (*C/C*) and albino (*c/c*) cells have coexisted throughout the periods of pigment cell determination, proliferation, and migration. The mutually exclusive cell-color markers now bear witness to hitherto cryptic cell lineages and cell movements, and disclose the archetypal developmental events. An orderly arrangement of separate transverse pigmented or albino bands is readily apparent on the left and

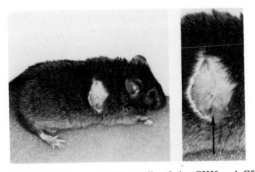

FIG. 3. An allophenic mouse comprising cells of the C3Hf and C57BL/6 inbred strains. Although the coat in this case is entirely of the C3Hf (agouti) color, analyses revealed C57BL/6 cells in some internal tissues. Immunological "self" tolerance of both strains, which differ in strong histocompatibility alleles, is shown by permanent retention of ear-skin grafts from the respective strains (on either side of the arrow, in the enlargement). From Mintz and Silvers (1967). Copyright 1967 by the American Association for the Advancement of Science.

right sides. In this individual, virtually all possible bands are evident; in some other animals, some bands appear wider, owing to the fortuitous occurrence of the same cell-strain in neighboring bands. Each unit-width transverse territory on each side is presumably a *clone* mitotically descended from a single primordial melanoblast cell (Mintz, 1967). Thirty-four of these clones, originating in the neural crest near the dorsal midline and migrating laterally, make up the entire definitive melanocyte population of the coat. Genes affecting melanoblast viability, mitosis, or movement, in one or both of the allophenic component lineages, are capable of modifying this underlying pattern in specific ways. Allophenic mice with such modifications have provided models of corresponding coat patterns in ordinary single-genotype mice. Thus, previously uninterpretable coat patterns due to particular genes are now understandable in terms of definable perturbations of a developmental archetype. Moreover, genes responsible for comparable patterns in nonexperimental mice appear to generate those patterns via production (by unknown means) of two phenotypically different melanocyte subpopulations (e.g., with respect to relative cell viabilities), despite the identical genotypes of the cells within each individual (Mintz, 1970b, 1971b).

Genotypic markers in other tissues of allophenic mice have brought to light a unique clonal history for each tissue. Tissues in which developmental lineages have been examined in allophenic models include muscle (Mintz and Baker, 1967; Gearhart and Mintz, 1972), retina (Mintz and Sanyal, 1970), brain (Dewey *et al.,* 1976), liver (Condamine *et al.,* 1971), vertebral column (Moore and Mintz, 1972), and hair follicles (Mintz, 1970b). Each specialized kind of cell seems to originate from a relatively small, tissue-specific number of clonal initiator cells (at least two in all cases). Various clues from the allophenic models suggest that for many cell types the time of initiation is very early, i.e., shortly after implantation, around day 6–7 of embryonic life (Mintz, 1970b, 1971b). Determination is normally stable and irreversible as the clones develop. Discovery of some of these clonal histories has supplied insights into the etiology of birth defects, as in the case of morphogenetic anomalies of the vertebral column (Moore and Mintz, 1972). Analyses of development from a clonal point of view have also suggested that clonal heterogeneity and selection *within* a tissue (already referred to above, in melanocyte differentiation) may be widespread in development and are not the exclusive province of the immune system. And a knowledge of clonal identities has provided a partial basis for identifying somatic cell mutations *in vivo,* by recognizing their occurrence in a known clonal territory (Mintz, 1969).

One of the most valuable characteristics of allophenic mice is that they vary greatly in the proportions and tissue distributions of their two genotypic cell strains (Mintz and Palm, 1969). This individual variability affords *in vivo* ways of detecting shared tissue derivations, primary tissue sites of gene expression, and interactions between cells or tissues. All three kinds of analyses will be illustrated from studies of hematopoiesis.

Several lines of earlier work had indicated the probability that multipotential hematopoietic stem cells give rise to myeloid blood cells, including erythrocytes, granulocytes, and megakaryocytes, and also to lymphoid cells. The question has more recently been examined in allophenic mice of appropriate normal strain combinations. The two genotypes of red blood cells, or of white blood cells, were distinguished from each other by their allelic electrophoretic differences for the ubiquitous enzyme glucosephosphate isomerase; erythrocyte strain identification was also made from allelic differences in electrophoretic patterns of hemoglobin; and the strain origin of immunoglobulin-producing lymphocytes was judged indirectly from Ouchterlony tests with antisera directed against their respective immunoglobulin variants. When these tissues, and many others, were analyzed for genotypic composition in individuals of several series, some of the other tissues often differed in their strain composition within individuals, as would be expected if they developed independently from separate precursor pools. But extremely high correlations were consistently found within individuals between the genotypic composition of their circulating erythrocytes and white blood cells (Fig. 4) (Mintz, 1971c), and between the genotypes of their crythrocytes and lymphocytes (or immunoglobulins) (Mintz and Palm, 1969; Wegmann and Gilman, 1970). Therefore, the data from allophenic mice strongly support the view that a pool of shared hematopoietic precursor cells gives rise eventually to erythrocytes, granulocytes, and lymphocytes.

Striking exceptions to these correlations in blood-cell genotypes occur in certain strain combinations involving genetic anemias; the exceptions serve to pinpoint the tissue focus of expression of the anemia-

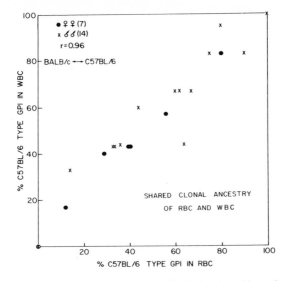

FIG. 4. In a group of 21 BALB/c ↔ C57BL/6 allophenic mice with varying cellular contributions from the two strains, the cellular genotypes of circulating red blood cells (RBC) and white blood cells (WBC) were compared within individuals, by means of their proportions of strain-specific allelic electrophoretic variants of glucosephosphate isomerase (GPI). The high correlation ($r = 0.96$) between RBC and WBC genotypes, despite lack of correlation between some other tissues in the same animals, is evidence for a shared developmental ancestry of the blood cells from a common hematopoietic stem-cell pool. Reprinted from Mintz (1971c), *Federation Proceedings* **30**, 935–943.

causing gene in blood development. In allophenic combinations of defective and normal cells, selection would be expected to replace the defective cells with normal ones after the locus in question was expressed, but not before; this should reveal the developmental stage and time in hematopoiesis when the mutant gene first becomes active. Genotypic analyses would also tell whether the defect is autonomous in the blood cells or is influenced by their tissue environment. In experiments involving cells of the lethal macrocytic hypoplastic W/W anemia, in combination with normal ($+/+$) cells, fully viable $W/W \leftrightarrow +/+$ adults were obtained. In them, not only red but also white blood cells were entirely of the normal strain (Mintz, 1971c), although W/W cells were well represented in other tissues. This suggests a possible early initial action of the gene, in the generalized hematopoietic stem cell stage, rather than exclusively in the erythroid line. In other experiments, normal cells were combined with cells of the microcytic *mk/mk* anemic genotype, which is characterized by an iron-absorption defect and is occasionally lethal but may be successfully compensated by increased formation of erythrocytes (Bannerman *et al.*, 1973). A number of viable *mk/mk* ↔ +/+ allophenics have been produced. All have entirely or largely +/+ red blood cells, along with both strains of white blood cells (data from Mintz and Custer, cited in Mintz, 1974). That the predominance of normal over *mk/mk* erythrocytes is achieved gradually (probably starting prenatally) is seen in repeated samplings over a period of time (Fig. 5). The results are consistent with expression of the locus only in the erythroid line, although the basis and mechanism of selection remain unknown.

Tissue genotypic variability in allophenic mice has also been useful in analyzing lymphoid cell interactions required for the immune response. T (thymus-derived) lymphocytes somehow help B (bone-marrow-derived) lymphocytes to become active in humoral antibody production. The ability of an animal to generate a strong immune response to a

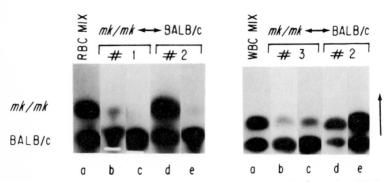

FIG. 5. The similarity in genotypic composition between red (RBC) and white (WBC) blood cells within all-normal-genotype individuals (see Fig. 4) is secondarily altered by selection if one of the strains is genetically anemic, as in the allophenic combination of *mk/mk* (*microcytic anemia*) and +/+ (*wild-type*) cells. Genotypic analyses of circulating blood with the strain-associated glucosephosphate isomerase marker show that the defective *mk/mk* red blood cells are gradually replaced by +/+ red cells as the animal ages (left), while no selection occurs in the white blood cell population (right) of the same individual.

specific antigen is controlled by the so-called immune response genes. A synthetic polypeptide affords a way of presenting the immune system with a highly specific challenge; different mouse strains differ quantitatively and genetically in their capacity to respond by making antibodies. A specific polypeptide was administered to allophenic mice derived from a combination of cells from a high-responder and a low-responder strain. It was reasoned that if the response-controlling gene were expressed solely in T cells, as suspected, some individuals with *low*-responder-strain B cells should show a specific antibody response higher than the low-strain controls. Results were consistent with this expectation and these animals were presumed (but not yet directly demonstrated) to have high-responder-strain helper T cells (Bechtol *et al.*, 1974). These experiments partly involve apparent cooperation between T and B cells with different histocompatibility (*H-2*) alleles. Some other experimental systems have yielded results indicating that such cooperation is not possible across an *H-2* barrier (Zinkernagel, 1976). The question continues to be investigated, especially in various kinds of mosaic animals containing allogeneic cells.

Some of the general characteristics of allophenic mice that have been described in this section have specific relevance for studies of neoplasia. These will be considered further at appropriate places in the following sections.

III. Is Tumor Susceptibility Localized or Systemic?

Strain-specific spontaneous or induced neoplasms in mice offer clear evidence of a genetic basis for some aspects of susceptibility to malignancy. As the term "susceptibility" indicates, the gene products need not themselves be causing the tumor. They may be implicated in regulating viral infectivity or expression of endogenous oncogenic viruses, in influencing the conversions of carcinogenic chemicals, in controlling chromosome stability, or in other phenomena. Allophenic mice composed of both susceptible and nonsusceptible cell strains provide an exceptional opportunity to identify the tissue(s) in which "susceptibility" genes are expressed. This is a first step toward defining more precisely the cell phenotypes leading to malignancy.

The variable tissue distribution of cellular genotypes, from one allophenic individual to another, creates a series of *in vivo* tests of the involvement of specific tissues. In each animal, the occurrence and genotype of a tumor, or its absence, may be evaluated in relation to the genotypes of its other tissues. If susceptible-strain cells in the target organ become malignant in individuals whose other test tissues are largely of nonsusceptible genotype, the relevant genes must be acting autonomously in that organ. If, however, transformation of susceptible-strain cells occurs only in allophenics having cells of that strain in another specific tissue, it is in the latter that these genes are expressed; tumor formation is then the result of indirect or systemic events. Still another possibility is that cells of *non*susceptible genotype might become tumorous in the allophenic situation, either because of transmission of viral or other tumor information from nearby transformed cells of the susceptible strain, or through an effect of gene action in susceptible cells of another tissue.

Among postulated indirect effects that might contribute to persistence *vs* disappearance of a tumor, one that has received particular attention is that immunological defense mechanisms might be crucial. According to this hypothesis of immunological surveillance (Burnet, 1970), tumors are generally immunogenic to their hosts, whose immune lymphocytes respond by obliterating the tumor cells or inhibiting their growth. Experiments (reviewed by Prehn, 1976) to test the hypothesis have relied heavily on transplantable tumors; they seemed able to immunize recipients against graft takes of subsequent tumor inocula. Artificially immunosuppressed animals have also been extensively used; the increase in their spontaneous tumors was attributed to lowered surveillance against tumor antigens. However, this increase may have resulted not from lack of response to antigens of the tumor cells but from lowered defense against tumor viruses. For other reasons as well, difficulties with the hypothesis have emerged in recent work. A cogent new observation is that primary spontaneous tumors (as opposed to tumors that have been retransplanted and may have undergone selection) in fact have little or no capacity to elicit a host reaction that can interfere with their growth. Another telling point is that congenitally athymic (*nude*) mice deficient in T-lymphocytes do not show an excess of any nonlymphoreticular neoplasms. Thus, a reevaluation is in progress of the question whether immunological surveillance effects any notable restraint on malignancy, as it ordinarily occurs.

If an insufficiency of such a surveillance mechanism were contributing appreciably to the growth of strain-specific neoplasms in mice, this should become evident from a correlation, in allophenic animals, between presence of lymphocytes of the susceptible strain and formation of a tumor in the target organ. Animals free of tumors should predominantly show the nonsusceptible or putatively protective cell-strain in the lymphoid population.

The various questions raised above have been examined in allophenic mice, in development of spontaneous mammary tumors (Mintz, 1970a), liver tumors (Mintz, 1970a; Condamine *et al.*, 1971), and lung tumors (Mintz *et al.*, 1971). Mammary tumors occur in virtually all females of the C3H control strain, in which the causal agent is the high-virulence, milk-transmitted mammary tumor virus. The tumors are less frequent (43%) in C3Hf controls, which carry a less virulent form of the agent, transmitted by the reproductive cells; and occur rarely in the C57BL/6 strain. They are moderately frequent (40%) if C57BL/6 controls are foster-nursed on C3H mothers (Table I). Thus, allophenic females of the C3H ↔ C57BL/6 and C3Hf ↔ C57BL/6 strain combinations pro-

TABLE I

INCIDENCE AND GENOTYPES OF MAMMARY TUMORS IN ALLOPHENIC
C3H(f) ↔ C57BL/6 AND CONTROL FEMALES[a]

Incidence	C3Hf controls	C57BL/6 controls	C3Hf ↔ C57BL/6	C3H controls[b]	C57BL/6 controls[b]	C3H ↔ C57BL/6[b]
Number with tumors/total	6/14	0/9	5/10	16/16	6/15	23/27
Percent with tumors	43	(Low)	50	100	40	85
Average age (months) at tumor	15	—	18	10	14	10
Number of tumors	7	—	6	30	8	42
Tumor genotypes	—	—	5 C3Hf, 1 C57	—	—	39 C3H, 3 C57

[a]From Mintz (1970a); and unpublished data.

[b]C3H controls (but not C3Hf or C57BL/6 controls) carry the high-virulence, milk-transmitted mammary tumor virus. In the C3H ↔ C57BL/6 experiment, allophenics and their C57BL/6 controls were foster-nursed by C3H mothers.

vide material for studies of autonomy *vs* nonautonomy of expression of
genetic susceptibility in mammary tumor formation. Allophenic males
of the same two paired strain combinations may be used to study
hepatoma formation, which is high (69%) in C3H male controls, somewhat less frequent (33%) in C3Hf controls, and virually absent in
C57BL/6 males. Lung tumor development has been investigated in both
males and females of another allophenic strain combination, BALB/c ↔
C57BL/6, because of the fairly high (56%) spontaneous incidence of
these tumors in BALB/c controls and their rarity or absence in the
C57BL/6 control strain. In each of these studies, the animals were kept
alive until tumors or other serious ailments developed. At autopsy,
tumor and other tissue samples were fixed for histopathologic inspection, and samples were prepared by suitable means for genotypic
analyses with strain-specific markers. Marker loci were used that coded
for electrophoretic allelic differences in enzymes, a few of which are
indicated in Table II; in histocompatibility (*H-2*) differences, detectable

TABLE II

MAMMARY TUMOR AND OTHER TISSUE GENOTYPES[a]
IN C3H(f) ↔ C57BL/6 ALLOPHENIC FEMALES[b]

Tissue:	Mammary tumor(s)	Normal mammary gland	7 S G2a immuno- globulins	Spleen cells	Red blood cells
Marker locus:	Mod-1	Mod-1	Ig-1	Gpd-1	H-2
Mouse no.					
1	100	100	50	90	50
2	100	—	50	—	50
3	100, 100	—	40	90	40
4	100, 100	—	40	85	40
5	100	66	—	50	—
6	100	—	15	40	0
7	100	15	0	0	—
8	0	—	33	66	33

[a] Data are given as approximate percentage of the tissue from the high-tumor C3H (or
C3Hf) strain. The tumor genotype may differ from genotypes of other tissues in the same
individuals.
[b] From Mintz (1970a).

by serology or graft tests; in immunoglobulin allotypes, and in many other phenotypes.

As shown (Table II) in some allophenic individuals of the mammary tumor experimental series, the sampled lymphoid tissue contained 10–100% of the *nonsusceptible* (C57BL/6) strain; 7 S G2a immunoglobulins also comprised a majority of the C57BL/6 genotypic class. Nevertheless, mammary tumors effectively grew in these same animals and were usually of the susceptible (C3H or C3Hf) genotype. Case No. 7 is particularly striking because of the extreme discordance of lymphoid and tumor genotypes. Thus, in development of strain-specific mammary tumors, lymphoid cells of the low-tumor genotype apparently afford no protection whatever against formation of a tumor. Similar results were obtained in the allophenic experiments on hepatomas (Mintz, 1970a) and on lung tumors (Mintz *et al.*, 1971). As already pointed out, the animals show normal competence to reject allogeneic skin grafts. Therefore, the observations support the conclusion that a deficiency in immunological surveillance against "tumor antigens" is not at issue in development of these types of spontaneous neoplasms. (The possibility is not excluded that immune response to oncogenic viruses may be important, though presence of the agents in the tolerizable early period of life could tend to lead to tolerance of them.)

Genotypic analyses of other tissues in the allophenics, in relation to the presence or the absence, and to the genotypes, of these tumors, also demonstrate that genetic expression resulting in susceptibility is largely localized to the cells of the potentially malignant tissue. This is seen in the fact that the genotypes of the tumors and of a variety of extrinsic tissues, e.g., blood (Table II), often differ from each other. In each animal, autonomous behavior of the two genotypes of target cells is occurring in the presence of shared systemic influences. Striking evidence not only of target-tissue autonomy, but also of cell-localized genetic specificity within that tissue, has been found in liver and mammary gland, in which the susceptible and nonsusceptible strains may be intimately admixed. This is especially striking in mammary tumor formation. When sections of hyperplastic premalignant mammary gland were histochemically stained to reveal genotypic cellular identities, through quantitative strain differences in β-glucuronidase activity, fine-grained interspersions of the two cell strains were often seen, even within single alveoli (Fig. 6). Yet it was the high-tumor-strain cells that

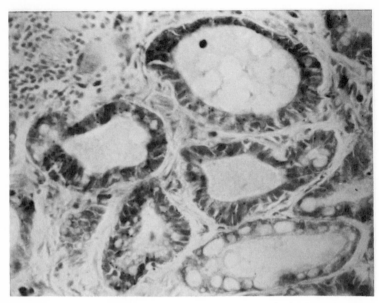

Fɪɢ. 6. A section of the hyperplastic, genetically mosaic mammary gland of a C3H ↔ C57BL/6 allophenic female. The pale C3H (high mammary-tumor-susceptible) alveolar cells are intimately intermingled with the darkly stained C57BL/6 (low-susceptibility) cells. Histochemical visualization of strain identity is due to an allelic strain difference governing activity of the enzyme β-glucuronidase.

usually proceeded to become malignant, as in the controls of that pure strain.

During this close association, when malignancy is beginning, the morphology of such mosaic hyperplastic alveolar nodules is indistinguishable from that of premalignant C3H pure-strain nodules (Fig. 7). This would appear to suggest, paradoxically, that the low-tumor-strain C57BL/6 cells have become transformed. But such has proved not to be the case: When halves of single nodules were grafted separately to pure-strain recipients, each recipient selectively recognized and rejected only those cells of the *H-2* antigenic type foreign to it. The surviving cells in each graft then grew out, forming, in the C57BL/6 case, a perfectly normal mammary tree and, in the C3H case, another premalignant nodule (Mintz and Slemmer, 1969). In some instances that were followed for a longer time, the C3H nodule became frankly malignant.

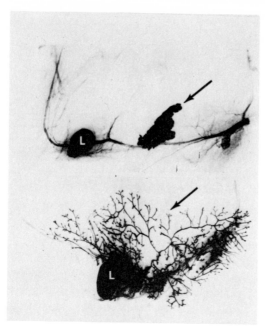

FIG. 7. Halves of a *single* mosaic hyperplastic alveolar nodule from a C3H ↔ C57BL/6 allophenic mouse after transplantation to cleared mammary fat pads in pure-strain recipients, whose strong histocompatibility alleles differ. In a C3H host (top), only the high mammary-tumor-susceptible (C3H) cell strain survives, and hyperplastic or premalignant alveolar growth (arrow) again occurs. In a C57BL/6 host (bottom), the C57BL/6 (low-susceptibility) cells, now liberated from their former entrapment with C3H, form an entirely normal-appearing mammary tree. From Mintz and Slemmer (1969).

Therefore, the preneoplastic appearance of the original mosaic nodule was attributable to its C3H cells, among which normal C57BL/6 cells were entrapped. Thus, nodules of similar appearance in single-genotype animals may be a phenotypic mosaic of hyperplastic and normal cells. From this model, and further experiments with genetically mosaic nodules, a hypothesis of early mammary tumor progression in ordinary single-genotype animals has been advanced. According to the hypothesis, the capacity of transformed cells in the early stages of malignancy to survive and go on to full tumor formation may actually depend upon a close association with normal cells. Possibly a similar indispensable supportive role of associated normal cells may also characterize the early stages of some other malignancies.

Tumors of the immune system itself, such as the spontaneous thymic lymphomas and leukemia of AKR mice or the neoplasms found in the autoimmune syndrome of NZB mice, are of course in a separate category from the other tumors discussed here. Cellular sites of active genetic mechanisms controlling transformation of lymphoreticular cells in inbred strains is one of the new and promising areas of investigation in allophenic mice.

IV. ARE TUMORS MONOCLONAL OR MULTICLONAL IN ORIGIN?

The significance of this question lies partly in its intimate relation to the question of mutational *vs* nonmutational mechanisms as the trigger in tumorigenesis (see Section V). If a tumor usually arises as the result of a mutation (spontaneous or induced) in a somatic cell, then the relative rarity of mutations would be expected to lead to single-clone tumors as a general rule (Burnet, 1974). However, any investigation of the problem is fraught with an insurmountable practical difficulty: By the time the tumor reaches macroscopic size, it has passed through many cell generations during which selection may have amplified some clones and diminished or eradicated others. Thus, a tumor that is monoclonal in *composition* may have been multiclonal in *origin*.

Most human tumors at the time of sampling are aneuploid and are highly individualized chromosomally. The karyotypically distinguishable tumor ''stemline'' is believed to have arisen clonally from a single genetically variant cell that made its appearance some time *after* tumor initiation and early growth (Makino, 1956; Hauschka and Levan, 1958). According to the stemline concept, the variant cell selectively survives because of superior proliferative or other adaptive properties, and it may give rise to subpopulations with further genetic changes. These variants supply the raw material for the stepwise appearance of new characteristics during tumor progression (Foulds, 1954; Nowell, 1974).

The well documented picture of tumor progression is consistent with many reports (reviewed by Friedman and Fialkow, 1976) that most human tumors are monoclonal in composition. These studies have been conducted on tumors from patients with cellular chromosomal mosaicism, or from women heterozygous for certain X-linked genes.

Activation of only one X-linked gene of a pair per somatic cell in heterozygous females creates a cellular mosaic of gene function, rather than gene structure, in all tissues. The presence of only one phenotype in the tumor has often been assumed, perhaps without complete justification, to indicate not merely monoclonal composition but also monoclonal *origin*. The human tumor studies have relied most heavily on electrophoretically variant forms of X-linked glucose-6-phosphate dehydrogenase (G-6-PD). Among the most extensively sampled monoclonal tumors are uterine leiomyomas, chronic lymphatic leukemia, and Burkitt's lymphoma. [Most of the other tumors considered to be monoclonal have thus far been examined in only small numbers of specimens (1–6) each; conclusions from them should perhaps be regarded as provisional.]

Apart from the difficulty of employing a postselection situation to discern obscured origins, there is the further complication that a marker sensitive enough to reveal a minor malignant clone in a tissue homogenate might also reveal, confusingly, the admixed nontumorous host cells, e.g., normal tissue parenchyma, stroma, blood vessels, and blood cells—all of them comprising two enzyme phenotypes. An example of the dilemma is seen in the fact that human hereditary trichoepitheliomas are mosaic for G-6-PD, but this is viewed as uninterpretable, on the ground that admixed nontumorous cells are conspicuous in histological sections (Friedman and Fialkow, 1976). At the same time, the two G-6-PD types in neurofibromas are taken as evidence of multiclonality, attributed to their hereditary basis, i.e., to an elevated tendency for all neural cells of that tumor-prone genotype to become tumorous in response to an inducing stimulus. It would be interesting to know whether these tumors of multiclonal composition have undergone less progression and selection since their origin than have single-clone tumors.

Allophenic mice have also furnished tumors in which cell lineages have been examined (Mintz, 1970a). In this case, the different genotypic populations may have any of a number of biochemical, chromosomal, or histocompatibility markers, on autosomes or sex chromosomes. With isozymic markers not detectable in blood and stroma (e.g., malate dehydrogenase electrophoretic variants), hepatomas, mammary tumors, and lymphoid tumors have all shown only one cell strain; but the methods are not sufficiently sensitive to reveal minor populations (less than approximately 5%) of malignant cells. With a ubiquitous and more sensitive marker (glucosephosphate isomerase electrophoretic variants), tumor homogenates generally show both variants, in those animals with blood mosaicism; but in poorly vascularized tumors—at least in the lung—it becomes apparent that the tumor itself is all or largely of one cell-strain (Mintz *et al.*, 1971).

Ambiguities due to normal-cell admixtures would be put to rest if histochemical visualization of each strain were possible; the normal or tumorous status of the same cells could then be visually assessed at the same time. At present, the sole histochemical marker available for tumor analyses is in allophenic mice. Activity of the enzyme β-glucuronidase varies in different inbred strains of mice, depending on alleles at a single locus. Hepatomas and mammary tumors may be analyzed histochemically for their strain composition because the malignant state does not markedly alter the relative enzyme activities in tumors of pure-strain controls. When 12 spontaneous hepatomas from a low- and high-activity allophenic strain combination were examined, the malignant cells of nine of the tumors were of only the low-activity strain and one had only high-activity-strain tumor cells. (Some contained normal reticuloendothelial cells of the opposite pure strain, or were surrounded by normal hepatocytes of both strains.) However, two of the 12 tumors were clearly mosaic, with malignant hepatic cells of both genotypes (Fig. 8) (Condamine *et al.*, 1971). Of special relevance to the present discussion is the fact that the mosaicism was not diagnosed when homogenates of samples from the same two tumors were typed electrophoretically for strain-specific isozymes. The fact of two multiclonal hepatomas among only 12 tumors examined histochemically is all the more noteworthy because in only one of the input strains (C3H) do the controls have a high hepatoma incidence; in the other (C57BL/6 or BALB/c), the control incidence is very low. The odds were thus decidedly against finding tumors of both genotypes. Therefore, multiclonality in hepatomas, and possibly in some other kinds of tumors, may be more common than results from allophenic mice have shown, but may usually go undetected because all clones are of the same (i.e., the more susceptible) genotype.

It is possible that a mosaic tumor may truly signify origin from two (or more) transformed cells; if such tumors are not a rarity, this would imply origin by nonmutational means. It is also admissable that a mosaic tumor may represent a fortuitous intercalation of two indepen-

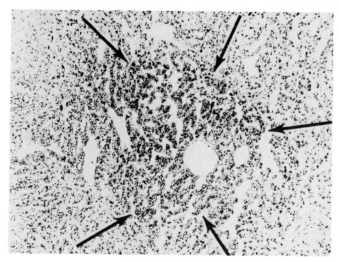

FIG. 8. A genetically mosaic hepatoma of multiclonal origin in a C3H ↔ C57BL/6 allophenic animal. The darkly stained core (arrows) of C57BL/6 cells is surrounded by C3H (unstained) tumor cells. Visualization of cell genotypes is due to their allelic strain differences in activity of β-glucuronidase. From Condamine *et al.* (1971).

dently originating tumors. Or, intercellular transmission of some form of tumor agent may have occurred, from a transformed single clone to a normal cell. In order to help distinguish among these alternatives by increasing the chances of mosaic tumors, we are extending the tumor studies in allophenic mice to strain combinations in which both members are of high-susceptibility genotypes and in which the histochemical marker is present. At the same time, strong histocompatibility strain differences are included, as in earlier mammary tumor experiments (Mintz and Slemmer, 1969), so that if both cell strains are malignant, each will survive and produce a tumor in the histocompatible strain after pieces are grafted to pure-strain recipients.

The caveat that emerges from the preceding summary is that extrapolations of tumor origins have been accompanied by unavoidable biological and technical ambiguities. If tumors are in fact largely monoclonal in composition at the time of their clinical detection, this is an important indication of how they have evolved and it may become an important clue as to how they should be treated. It need not necessarily mean that tumors generally originate from one cell, mutationally; nor that preventive measures should always be based on that assumption.

V. Do Tumors Arise through Genetic or Epigenetic Errors?

There has been increasingly expressed, in recent years, the view that neoplasia may be essentially a disease or derangement of cell differentiation and not merely of cell multiplication (e.g., Pierce, 1967; Markert, 1968). This suspicion has been fed by a variety of clues: Some tumors have been found to produce proteins ordinarily found only in fetal stages of the corresponding normal tissue; examples are fetal, rather than adult, liver isozymes (Schapira *et al.*, 1975), or α-fetoprotein (Abelev, 1974), in hepatomas. Moreover, tumors of certain tissues may display a "confusion" of tissue identity and form products usually associated with other tissues, as in the case of hormone secretion by tumors of nonendocrine origin (Lipsett, 1965). And, occasionally, there are tumors whose histological composition gradually shifts to a more differentiated or benign state, as in the change of a neuroblastoma into a ganglioneuroma (Cushing and Wolbach, 1927).

At the same time, the idea that cancer originates by somatic mutation (e.g., Burnet, 1974) has gained momentum. This has been strengthened by such lines of evidence as the mutagenic effects of carcinogens (McCann and Ames, 1976), by the mutational models consistent with incidence of certain childhood tumors (Knudson, 1973), by the chromosomal instability found in human tumor-prone Mendelian disorders (German, 1974), and by the apparently monoclonal composition of some tumors (already discussed in Section IV).

These two points of view seem to have become progressively polarized [e.g., see the exchange of letters between Rubin (1976) and Ames (1976)], thereby tending toward what I believe to be a false dichotomy, i.e., the mutually exclusive generalizations that all cancers are mutational ("genetic"), or that all are nonmutational ("epigenetic"), in origin. I propose instead that *all* involve derangements of differentiation; but that the critical *initiating* events in some cancers are nonmutational, whereas in some other cancers they are mutational genetic or chromosomal changes. Nonmutational cancers presumably result from physiological changes in the cell or tissue milieu. Conditions possibly conducive to cancers of this sort might include ectopic location of a tissue, local trauma, or hormonal imbalance. Agents capable of causing mutational cancers probably comprise radiation, chemical mutagens, and some viruses. However, some stimuli known to be carcinogenic, such as oncogenic viruses or chemical carcinogens, may act in diverse ways. For example, some oncogenic viruses may trigger nonmutational changes leading to neoplasia by disrupting the cellular environment; others may cause premalignant genetic changes by intercalating genetic material into the cell's own genome, or by otherwise altering the genetic organization of the cell. Similarly, some compounds might act as carcinogens in an essentially nonmutational fashion, by blocking a metabolic pathway or by binding to the cell's DNA, RNA, or other macromolecules; other carcinogens might be mutagens, causing substitutions or deletions in the DNA. In the sense that epigenesis seems normally to rest on nonmutational changes in gene expression, all cancers—even if triggered by mutation—may be considered epigenetic; that is, anomalies of gene expression may always be intimately involved (as will be discussed further in Section VI). Moreover, some genetic considerations may play important roles even in initially nonmutational cancers. For example, a "susceptible" genotype may be required for oncogenic viral infectivity (Rowe, 1973); or the genotype may determine the presence of enzymic mechanisms needed for conversion of certain carcinogens to their active forms (Miller, 1970). In addition, secondary chromosomal changes in the course of malignant progression may be virtually universal, supplying the material basis for selection of more rapidly dividing or metabolizing cells (Nowell, 1974).

The first unequivocal example of an animal malignancy of nonmutational origin has only recently been identified, by methods which now provide a paradigm for other nonmutational tumors. It is the mouse teratocarcinoma (Mintz and Illmensee, 1975), which will be discussed in greater detail in Section VII. This tumor has remained euploid, despite many years of *in vivo* transplantation, and we may presume that near-euploidy would be required for comparable tests of other tumors. The demonstration of its genomic normalcy was achieved by introducing the malignant stem cells—suspected of being developmentally totipotent—into the particular kind of environment appropriate for their normal totipotent counterparts, i.e., into a normal early embryo. There, restoration of an orderly sequence of gene expressions occurred in the tumor cells, resulting in their completely normal differentiation into all somatic tissues, and also functional gametes. This is compelling evidence for retention of an intact genome.

Such tumors seem to arise from parthenogenetically activated germ cells in the gonads, or from germ cells or early embryos located in ectopic sites. In either case, the developing embryo finds itself in an anomalous tissue environment incompatible with retention of normal organization. This fact, combined with successful induction of normal differentiation when the transformed cells are placed in the framework of a normal embryo, leads to the conclusion that the initial neoplastic conversion had probably been triggered by an abnormal environment. Inasmuch as the microenvironment of embryo cells seems to be critical in determining their genetic activities (Mintz, 1974), it is reasonable to expect that environmental disturbances (though still undefined) could promote aberrant gene expression leading, in some instances, to malignancy.

The ease with which teratocarcinomas may be experimentally produced in many inbred strains of mice (Stevens, 1970) is further evidence of their nonmutational initiation. Nevertheless, genetic "susceptibility" factors clearly play various roles, as they may in other cancers: These tumors are not inducible in all mouse strains. And in only the males of one strain (129) and the females of another (LT) do they tend to occur spontaneously, as gonadal tumors (Stevens, 1970; Stevens and Varnum, 1974). Teratomas in the human population may also show hereditary components, as in the six kindreds described by Ashcraft and Holder (1974). (There is no information on whether these or other human teratomas arise nonmutationally, as in the mouse.)

One may reasonably hypothesize that at least some other animal cancers originate without mutation, through environmentally caused, potentially reversible, aberrations of gene expression. This could be shown by their experimental normalization in the tissue environment appropriate for the normal stem cells from which the tumor originated. But a failure of normalization would fail to distinguish between possible genetic changes causal to the malignancy and those arising as a concomitant of its progression. While many or most tumors may be caused by somatic mutation, as is widely believed, the difficulty is that specific genetic changes can be demonstrated only through germ-line transmission and specific phenotype expression; evidence for mutation as the cause of a neoplasm is thus likely to be circumstantial.

Nevertheless, there is good reason to believe that primary gene or chromosome change is the most likely explanation for some cancers. Examples are the childhood malignancies of retinoblastoma, Wilms' tumor, and neuroblastoma. Statistical analyses of their occurrence have revealed the probability of two mutational events in each (Knudson, 1973). A hereditary (dominant) type is presumably due to a germ-line mutation, causing increased susceptibility in all potential target cells; but a somatic mutation must then ensue. In the nonhereditary type, the two events seem both to be somatic mutations. Bilateral tumors (arising independently from two or more cells) are in fact more common in the hereditary type, as this mutational model would predict.

Chromosome instability syndromes provide another class of possible mutational tumors. Several hereditary diseases of man involve chromosome breakage and rearrangement and are characterized by an increased predisposition to cancer. An example is Bloom's syndrome (German, 1974). Here the chromosome changes apparently antedate the cancers and hence may be causal to them. The picture is much less clear in the aneuploidy commonly seen in many nonhereditary tumors. There, the chromosomal changes may have been a consequence of malignant progression rather than a cause of the cancer. This possibility is realistic, especially as experimental tumors are often euploid in the early stages; and the emergence of variant subpopulations (Nowell, 1974) is a familiar feature of tumor "evolution." The common presence of a *specific* chromosomal change in a malignancy was first documented in human chronic myelogenous leukemia (Nowell and Hungerford, 1960). More recently, studies with new chromosome banding techniques suggest that some other malignancies may become characterizable by specific chromosomal deviations (Rowley, 1974). However, even in the case of specific changes, it is difficult to rule out the possibility that they are only consistent consequences of specific antecedent events which are themselves causal in that malignancy. An orderly series of consistent secondary changes, hence of epiphenomena, may in fact occur, judging from the regularities with which similar karyotype abnormalities have appeared among patients in terminal stages of chronic myelogenous leukemia (Prigogina and Fleischman, 1975). In general, inferences regarding tumor etiology remain ambiguous if they must be based solely on composition of the tumors, whether with respect to chromosomal, enzymic, antigenic, or other markers. The twin facts, that tumors undergo clonal selection, and that they are inevitably sampled only when they are macroscopic (i.e., when they have probably already undergone some selection), militate against a clear interpretation.

VI. How Is Neoplasia a Derangement of Differentiation?

The hypothesis that neoplasia (whether mutational or nonmutational in origin) is essentially a developmental disturbance, is in fact not one but many hypotheses. Under that broad umbrella are sheltered such partially diverse views of the ontogenic fault as: dedifferentiation, or loss of differentiated functions in specialized cells (Pitot, 1968); impairment of forward differentiation of stem cells (Pierce, 1974); misprogramming of gene function at any step in differentiation, from the least to the most differentiated cells, resulting in new patterns of gene expression (Markert, 1968); and selective reactivation of some genes involved in early development (Coggin and Anderson, 1973). It will not be possible in this brief account to expand and discuss most of these, or still other developmental hypotheses. The particular view that I hold, and will present here, owes much to previous students of the problem of neoplasia, and particularly to the studies of Pierce (1967, 1974).

The normal process of development proceeds from cells that divide and are relatively undifferentiated to cells that are terminally differentiated and can no longer divide. In only a few tissues has this progression been worked out in any detail. They are generally the ones in which the less differentiated source cells are readily recognizable because they continue to divide, sometimes throughout adult life. Included among them are the hematopoietic tissues, the germinal layers of the skin, the epithelium of the intestinal crypts, and the spermatogonial cells. These are "stem cell renewal" systems (Leblond and Walker, 1956), in which cell production continues to be balanced by cell loss. It seems likely that analogous *stem cell* systems, albeit without continuous renewal and thus with a much shorter proliferative history, characterize the differentiation of all tissues. Indeed, our understanding of normal differentiation would be greatly advanced if the stem cell populations could be recognized in all tissues, and if pure populations of these cells could be obtained for experimental purposes. In some tissues, there is only a limited capacity for growth in the adult, due to declining stem cell proliferation. In others, such as the brain, the stem cell pool may vanish in early postnatal life. The basic stem cell scheme of normal differentiation is diagrammed in the left-hand panel of Fig. 9. As shown, there is a hierarchy of stem cells of increasing degrees of differentiation, starting with the most primitive (i.e., totipotent) stem cells and proceeding through progressive levels of specialization to form the stem cells of a particular specialized tissue type. At any level, when a stem cell divides, its cellular progeny may themselves remain like the parent cell or may differentiate further.

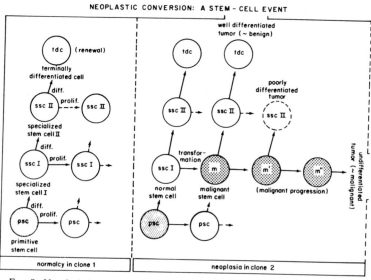

FIG. 9. Neoplasia is depicted as a change or diminution in progressive differentiation, as the result of transformation—through either mutational or nonmutational triggering events—of an initially normal stem cell. As a result, the normal balance between stem cell proliferation (prolif.) and hierarchical differentiation (diff.) (left panel) is altered, to varying degrees. Differentiation may then be slightly impaired, as in a well-differentiated benign tumor; or prevented, as in an undifferentiated malignant tumor. Selection for more rapidly proliferating variant cells may further reduce differentiation as malignancy progresses. tdc, terminally differentiated cell; ssc, specialized stem cell; psc, primitive stem cell.

A question of considerable importance concerns the channeling of stem-cell progeny into the old (proliferative stem cell) *vs* the new (differentiative) pathway. Is this an intrinsic event, resulting from a unique asymmetric division that yields unlike progeny cells (Rolshoven, 1951) or is it the result of local influences in different microenvironments, acting on initially similar progeny cells? This question, which remains an open one, is significant not only for stem-cell differentiation in normal ontogeny, but also for its aberration in neoplasia (as will be discussed presently). In studies of stem-cell renewal in the esophageal epithelium, Leblond (1964) found that if either or both of the mitotic products of a given stem cell happened to remain in the germinal layer, they became stem cells, whereas if either or both chanced to be pushed, by crowding, into the spinous layer, they would differentiate. Similarly, in analyses of myogenesis, Buckley and Konigsberg (1974) observed that uninucleated proliferative myoblasts do not fuse to form multinucleated myotubes as the result of some special terminal mitosis. Rather, they fuse as the consequence of a number of growth conditions (readily subject to experimental alteration *in vitro*); fusion then causes nuclear mitoses to cease within the syncytia, which continue their differentiation into muscle fibers.

The entire process of neoplasia is, in my view, likely to remain largely obscure unless the normal target cell can first be identified. It is here where matters first go awry and where the underlying molecular mechanisms may most profitably be sought. Further changes, however significant clinically, may be epiphenomena. Yet there has been relatively little attention given to this aspect of the problem. This may be partly because of experimental limitations posed by the fact that the progressive emergence of new cell types cannot be simulated *in vitro;* and *in vivo* experimentation on carcinogenesis relies on macroscopic tumors that, unlike transformed cells in culture, are often complex tissues. It may be claimed that virtually any cell may become malignant. Yet the evidence argues against that generalization: Neoplasms must all contain a population of proliferating cells, irrespective of their rates of proliferation; on this basis alone, it appears unlikely that terminally differentiated cells can undergo malignant conversion. While "dedifferentiation" of terminal cells might hypothetically account for resumption of mitosis, there is no persuasive documentation to support the view that malignant cells arise by such a process. Instead, the normal stem cells responsible for the growth and differentiation of tissues are the logical candidate target cells of neoplastic conversion. If this were in fact the case, it would account not only for the proliferative aspects of malignancy, but also for the common presence in tumors of a variety of cell types, the whole comprising a kind of aberrant or abortive differentiation of that tissue from its stem-cell population. Moreover, it would account for shifts toward a more benign or more malignant state. In this sense, neoplasia is indeed a derangement of differentiation.

The hypothesis is diagrammed in the right-hand panel of Fig. 9. Any normal stem cell (e.g., "specialized stem cell I") in the developmental hierarchy may undergo transformation, to become a malignant stem cell. As implied in the foregoing discussion on regulation of proliferation *vs* differentiation of stem cells, this means that the malignant stem cell progeny retain their proliferative option, but suffer *a diminution or loss of their differentiative option*. The diminution may come about in several ways: The stem cell itself may suffer the initial defect (e.g., due to mutation, viral infection, binding of macromolecules by exogenous compounds). Or the cells of the microenvironment may have secondarily become defective, for comparable reasons. Still another possibility is that the stem cells and their environmental tissues may both be essentially normal, but may fail to be brought into the proper association. The latter mechanism might be partly involved in teratocarcinoma formation (see Section VII) from embryos in ectopic sites: If the normal architecture is disrupted and the cells outwander, interactions critical for orderly differentiation of stem cells (in this instance, psc in Fig. 9) could fail.

Tumors are roughly characterizable histologically as undifferentiated (anaplastic), poorly differentiated, or well differentiated. As indicated in Fig. 9, these alternatives would arise as the result of varying degrees of differentiation of the malignant stem cells. If the latter (m) continue to undergo malignant progression, or natural selection for more rapidly dividing variants (m' and m''), the ultimate, highly modified neoplastic stem cell may have virtually no capacity for differentiation; the composition of the tumor may thus shift in time, perhaps along with karyotypic changes resulting in aneuploidy. At the other extreme, a relatively well differentiated tumor implies substantial retention of stem-cell differentiation, and is more likely to remain close to euploidy. If the stem cells are lost or retain a modest degree of proliferation, the tumor may become quite benign (although it may nevertheless cause severe mechanical interference with organ function).

Pierce (1967, 1974) has aptly termed tumorigenesis a "caricature of stem cell renewal" and has obtained *in vivo* experimental data in support of this interpretation. For example, when transplantable squamous cell carcinomas of rats were labeled with [³H]thymidine, labeled cells appeared first in the undifferentiated cells and only substantially later in the well-differentiated squamous cell "pearls" (Pierce and Wallace, 1971). Proliferative stem cells that migrated into the pearls had apparently become differentiated. They subsequently ceased mitosis and became benign, i.e., incapable of forming a tumor upon retransplantation.

There is increasing support for the idea that the varied populations of cells found in many tumors are most readily explained as the result of varying degrees of differentiation of the stem cells rather than varying degrees of dedifferentiation of specialized cells. Neural tumors are particularly instructive in this regard. These tumors tend to occur primarily in children and, when they appear in adults, to result from very slow growth (Willis, 1967), as would be expected if they form only from stem cells that are not normally retained in adult life. The histological changes observed in some of these tumors have been the subject of puzzlement (Rubinstein *et al.,* 1974), owing partly to our limited knowledge of the normal ontogeny of some of the neural and glial elements. Yet there is good evidence that some of the more primitive tumors, such as neuroblastomas of the sympathetic nervous system, may sometimes undergo a transition to a more highly differentiated tumor, such as a ganglioneuroma (Cushing and Wolbach, 1927). This phenomenon is understandable on the basis of gradual differentiation of stem-cell progeny.

In some tissues, it appears that differentiated cells are able to divide in the adult, as in the case of preexisting hepatocytes during liver regeneration. It cannot be excluded that the proliferation is restricted to a still unrecognized subpopulation of hepatocytes. In any case, there is good evidence (reviewed by Abelev, 1974) that hepatocarcinogenesis proceeds instead from proliferative "oval" precursor cells; these form small diploid hepatocytes which may develop into large, mainly polyploid, hepatocytes. Despite continuing uncertainty as to the target cell in transformation, the fact that experimental hepatomas are generally diploid lends support to the view that it is the precursor stem cells, not the mature differentiated hepatocytes, that are the target cells in malignant conversion. This interpretation is further strengthened by cell localization studies of α-fetoprotein, which is synthesized by fetal liver, regenerating adult liver, and hepatomas, but not by normal nonregenerating adult liver. The studies indicate that α-fetoprotein is a product of some but not all kinds of hepatocytes; and that its formation in liver tumors depends on the presence of tumor stem cells that retain the capacity for differentiating into hepatocytes, including those responsible for synthesis of this protein in normal ontogeny (Abelev, 1974).

The apparent origin of the relatively normal, more differentiated ("benign") cells of tumors from their malignant stem cells has prompted some generalizations that tumors are not due to mutation; and that it may become practicable to deal with them therapeutically by "directing" the differentiation of their stem cells (Pierce, 1967, 1974; Pierce and Johnson, 1971). With respect to the first point, I believe (as already stated in Section V) that it is unlikely that all tumors are nonmutational. I would also hesitate to base optimism for *universal* therapy on inducing differentiation of stem cells. While this approach may indeed be helpful in *some* cases, many tumors have already undergone progression toward aneuploidy by the time they are detected. It seems likely that other means will continue to be required in dealing clinically with cancers; and that the knowledge of target cell identity and stem cell behavior will be useful in recognizing causes of transformation and in defining preventive measures.

VII. WHAT ARE THE DEVELOPMENTAL POTENTIALITIES OF MALIGNANT TERATOCARCINOMA STEM CELLS?

The hypothesis that normal stem cells may sometimes become malignant as the result of nonmutational mechanisms would be validated if the malignant cells could be made to resume completely normal development. Failure of reversibility to normalcy would signify either that a genetic alteration had in fact caused the malignancy, or that cascades of errors had supervened and now obscured the primary cause.

The most rigorous possible demonstration of an intact genome in a cell is through the palpable expression of all of its genes, among its clonal normal descendants. Only limited numbers of genes would become functionally evident if the stem cells of a specific-tissue tumor were normalized; the full spectrum of gene expression could be tested solely if all specialized cell types were generated. This would require the differentiation of virtually an entire individual from totipotent stem cells. A malignancy of such primitive cells would therefore provide the most promising source of material for tests of nonmutational transformation.

Teratomas have for some time been suspected, but not known with certainty, of being tumors derived from such primitive stem cells. They are "neoplasms composed of multiple tissues of kinds foreign to the part in which they arise" (Willis, 1967). The most malignant and anaplastic of these tumors consist entirely or largely of relatively undifferentiated embryonal carcinoma (or teratocarcinoma) stem cells. The most benign have retained few if any stem cells and display a variety of differentiated tissues, chaotically arranged. Between these extremes are the most interesting teratomas—those in which there are substantial numbers of embryonal carcinoma stem cells, along with various differentiated tissues. These teratomas have been studied most extensively in the mouse (Stevens, 1967a; Pierce, 1967), where their maintenance by serial transplantation in the strain of origin is possible only by virtue of retention of a reservoir of proliferative stem cells. That the differentiated cell types in the tumors arise from the embryonal carcinoma cells was clearly shown in an experiment by Kleinsmith and Pierce (1964): When single stem cells were transplanted in mice, a multiplicity of tissues was generated within clonal tumors.

While the stem cells were thus shown to be developmentally multipotential, there was until recently no evidence that they might be totipotent. Indeed, totipotency seemed contraindicated by the incomplete differentiation of many tissues in teratomas, and by the consistent absence of certain tissues, including liver, kidney, lung, thymus, and immunocompetent cells (Stevens and Hummel, 1957; Stevens, 1970). Therefore, the possibility remained that some of the many genes required for differentiation of the deficient tissues may have been mutated or deleted when stem-cell transformation occurred.

A possible counterpoise to the mutational argument is that "teratoma-producing mutations" would have to be inducible with surprising ease, judging from the high frequency with which teratomas may be experimentally generated in mice. The tumors tend to occur spontaneously in only two inbred strains, either as testicular tumors in the 129 strain or as ovarian tumors in the LT strain. However, they are readily initiated in many strains simply by transplanting early-stage embryos, or germ-cell-containing fetal germinal ridges, to an ectopic site, such as the testis capsule or kidney capsule (Stevens, 1967a, 1970). There, the developing embryo soon becomes disorganized and a teratoma results. Those tumors that remain transplantable display the conventional attributes of malignancy: they may invade and metastasize, the stem cells divide rapidly, and the disease is fatal in about a month.

In choosing a source of teratocarcinoma stem cells for "normalization" attempts, it seemed reasonable to expect that cells grown only *in vivo* would be less likely to have undergone ancillary genetic or chromosomal changes than those adapted to long-term tissue culture. An appropriate tumor was the transplantable one experimentally produced by Stevens in 1967, by transferring a 6-day embryo beneath the testis capsule of an adult. The solid tumor formed there was transferred to the body cavity, where it grew as a modified ascites. At the start of our experiment, this tumor (OTT 6050) had been carried for over 200 transplant generations spanning 8 years (Fig. 10). Very little differentiation occurs in the ascites state; this may have had the salutary effect of diminishing competitive selection for rapidly growing, aneuploid, variants of the undifferentiated stem cells. More extensive differentiation occurs when the cells attach to a tissue substratum. The ascites contains multicellular "embryoid bodies," with some limited resemblance to early embryos. When still small, the embryoid bodies comprise only a "core" of embryonal carcinoma cells and a "rind" of yolk-sac-like epithelial cells. When we examined the chromosomal constitution of the *core* cells after enzymatically loosening the rind and stripping it away with needles, a high frequency of euploidy was found (Mintz *et al.*, 1975; Mintz and Illmensee, 1975).

Malignant teratocarcinoma stem cells would scarcely be expected to realize any prospects for fully normal differentiation in any environment other than that of a normal early embryo, as normal totipotent stem cells do not ultimately yield fully differentiated tissues in a nonembryo site or in culture. Thus, a version of the mosaic mouse experiment (Mintz, 1971a) seemed to be called for—this time by associating normal embryo cells with teratocarcinoma stem cells taken from embryoid body cores.

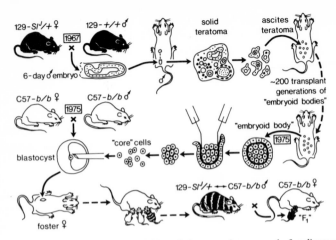

Fig. 10. The experiment diagrammed here led to complete reversal of malignancy in mouse teratocarcinoma cells, and their normal differentiation into somatic and germ-line tissues, after 8 years as a transplantable tumor. The teratoma was produced in 1967 by transplanting a 6-day chromosomally male (X/Y) 129-strain embryo under a testis capsule; it was converted to a modified ascites form consisting of "embryoid bodies." The malignant stem cells in the "cores" were separated from the yolk sac "rinds" and injected into blastocysts bearing coat-color and many other allelic differences from the tumor strain of origin. Such injected blastocysts, after transfer to the uterus of a surrogate mother, gave rise to live, healthy mosaic mice. Even when only a single teratocarcinoma cell had been injected, all somatic tissues analyzed were capable of comprising normal, functioning contributions derived from the tumor cell. Functional sperms were also produced in some mosaic males who thus fathered tumor-derived normal "F_1" progeny. Modified from Mintz and Illmensee (1975).

Cleavage-stage blastomeres and teratocarcinoma cells did not adhere well; therefore, the availability of a method (Lin, 1966) for microinjecting cells into the cavity of blastocysts made it possible to entrap the tumor cells where they might become integrated into the embryo-forming inner-cell-mass region (Mintz and Illmensee, 1975). Many genetic markers distinguishing the two input cell strains were used, as indicators of blastocyst- and tumor-derived cells in any tissues that might form; and as evidence that tumor-derived cells were able to synthesize tissue-specific normal products. Since the OTT 6050 teratoma arose in the inbred 129 strain, the alleles of that strain were tentatively assumed to be present.

The results of this experiment were dramatic and decisive. Normal, healthy, genetically mosaic mice were obtained (Mintz and Illmensee, 1975; Illmensee and Mintz, 1976). In the most successful cases, a single teratocarcinoma stem cell, after injection into a blastocyst, was able to give rise clonally to contributions in the full gamut of somatic tissues (Fig. 11). Inclusion of tumor-strain tissue-specific proteins was clear evidence of normal function. Tissue products coded for by 129-strain alleles in the tumor-derived cells included eumelanin and phaeomelanin pigments in the coat (Fig. 12), adult hemoglobin (Fig. 13), 7 S G1 and G2a classes of immunoglobulins (Fig. 14), and liver proteins (detected after excretion in the urine (Fig. 14). Inclusion of thymus, lung, kidney, and plasma cells was particularly noteworthy because of their complete absence from the tumors themselves. Differentiation of these tissues may possibly require inductive interactions between embryonic components which either fail to form in the tumors, or which fail to be brought into the proper associations.

Differentiation also uncovered, as an organismic phenotype, the presence of an unsuspected tumor-contributed coat color gene, *steel* (*Sl^J*) (Mintz and Illmensee, 1975), not previously known, from the published record (Stevens, 1970), to be present in the teratocarcinoma cells. From a retrospective search of the protocols (L. C. Stevens, personal communication), it was learned that the *steel* gene must have been transmitted from the mother of the 6-day embryo used to produce

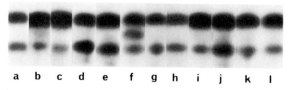

FIG 11. Glucosephosphate isomerase allelic strain variants in starch gel electrophoresis of tissue homogenates from a mosaic mouse produced by injecting a single teratocarcinoma stem cell into a blastocyst, as in Fig. 10. Slot (a) is a mixture of tumor-strain (slow-migrating) and blastocyst-strain types. Mosaic tissues with tumor-derived normal components include (b) blood; (c) brain; (d) spleen; (e) heart; (f) skeletal muscle, with a hybrid enzyme band due to heterokaryon formation; (g) kidneys; (h) reproductive tract; (i) liver; (j) gut and pancreas; (k) thymus; and (l) lungs. Mosaicism was verified by similar tests for allelic isozymes of isocitrate dehydrogenase, which is not expressed in blood cells. (Origin and anode are lowermost.) From Illmensee and Mintz (1976).

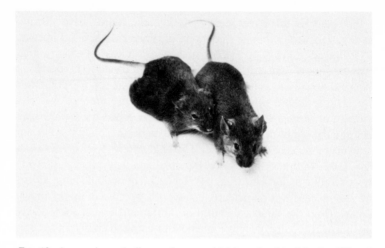

Fig. 12. A normal genetically mosaic mouse (right) produced by injecting 129-strain teratocarcinoma cells into a C57BL/6-*b/b* blastocyst. His tissues, including the largely agouti coat, are predominantly from the tumor-strain component. A control of that inbred strain (left) has been injected subcutaneously on the flank with teratocarcinoma cells; here, unlike the blastocyst injections, the cells form a huge tumor incompatible with survival.

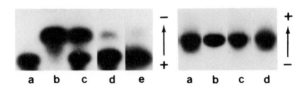

Fig 13. *Left:* Glucosephosphate isomerase starch gel electrophoretic analyses of blood cell lysates show the 129 teratoma-strain (a) and C57BL/6-*b/b* blastocyst-strain (b) controls, and a 1:1 control mixture (c). Red blood cells (d) and white blood cells (e) from the mosaic mouse in Fig. 12 are almost entirely of the tumor-strain type.

Right: Diffuse (129-type) (a) and allelic *single* (C57BL/6-*b/b*-type) (b) adult hemoglobins, and a 1:1 control mixture (c). The hemoglobin of the experimental mouse is largely producing the *diffuse* type (d), due to his tumor-strain red cells. From Mintz and Illmensee (1975).

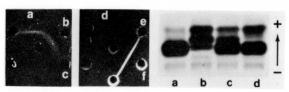

Fig. 14. *Left pair:* Ouchterlony double-diffusion analyses, showing only the tumor-strain specific allotypes of 7 S G1 and G2 immunoglobulin classes in the mosaic mouse in Fig. 12. Anti-129-type serum (left, center well) reacts with 129 control serum (a) and with a 1/20 dilution of serum from the mosaic mouse (b), but not with a C57 control (c). Anti-C57-type serum (right, center) reacts with a C57 control (f) but not with a 129 control (d) or undiluted serum from the experimental animal (e).

Right: Acrylamide gel electrophoresis of allelic strain variants of the major urinary protein complex in 129 (a) and C57 (b) controls and a 1:1 control mixture (c). The experimental mosaic mouse in Fig. 12 has a mixture of both strain types. He therefore has both cell strains of hepatocytes, in which the protein is produced. From Mintz and Illmensee (1975).

the tumor in 1967. (She had in fact been $Sl^J/+$, the Sl^J gene having been maintained in some animals of the strain by forced heterozygosity.) This gene, like many others, had remained silent and undetected for 8 years during the "malignant life" of the stem cells. Now, orderly expression in differentiation had revealed them.

The clonal origin, from a single teratocarcinoma stem cell, of the 129 cell-strain in all tested tissues is strong evidence for the developmental totipotency of the stem cells. In those GPI tests (Fig. 11) in which the animal's blood mosaicism might create an ambiguity in analyses of solid tissues, independent tests with a marker enzyme (isocitrate dehydrogenase) not expressed in blood confirmed the presence of both tumor- and blastocyst-derived cells in all tissues, irrespective of their vascular component (Illmensee and Mintz, 1976). Some animals had less extensive tissue derivatives from the tumor, as in the four cases shown in Table III. These results are not incompatible with stem-cell totipotency: here, the erratic distribution of the tumor cell-strain, often in developmentally unrelated tissues, implies delayed integration of the tumor lineage into the developing host embryo; the delay could result in a restricted distribution of the donor cells, and their differentiation according to their fortuitous locations.

TABLE III

NORMAL TISSUE CONTRIBUTIONS[a] CLONALLY DERIVED *in Vivo*
FROM SINGLE TERATOCARCINOMA CELLS INJECTED INTO BLASTOCYSTS[b]

Coat	Blood	Brain	Spleen	Heart	Muscle	Kidneys	Reproductive tract	Liver	Gut	Thymus	Lungs
—	0	0	0	0	0	50	0	60	33	0	25
0	0	0	0	5	0	0	0	0	5	10	0
0	0	0	0	0	60	0	0	0	0	0	40
—	0	—	—	40	0	0	—	0	0	—	50

[a] Data are given as approximate percentage of the tissue derived from the teratocarcinoma strain in each of 4 mosaic mice. Except for the coat color, tissues were biochemically analyzed for glucosephosphate isomerase electrophoretic allelic strain differences.

[b] Excerpted from Illmensee and Mintz (1976). These cases are selected to show contributions to developmentally unrelated tissues (see text).

In two other reports of teratocarcinoma cell injections into blastocysts, there is evidence in support of some donor cell participation in embryogenesis, albeit *not* of totipotency of the cells nor of their complete reversibility to normalcy. In one study (Brinster, 1974), only one genetic marker (pigmentation) was used, so that it was possible to test the differentiation only of a single cell type; one animal with a few pigmented stripes of the tumor-strain type was obtained. In the other study (Papaioannou *et al.,* 1975), the donor cells were all from cell culture lines, all of them aneuploid; only two genetic markers (pigmentation and GPI) were used. Because of the injection of large numbers (20–40) of embryonal carcinoma cells into each blastocyst, the developmental potentialities of stem cells could not be evaluated. The introduction of many malignant cells may also have prevented their integration, and may account for the fact that most of the animals developed one or more tumors. Some mosaic tissues were obtained, but no animal had tumor-strain contributions in all its tissues.

Even more striking than the full range of somatic differentiation, in the best of our own cases, was the formation in some individuals of fully functional sperms from the teratocarcinoma stem cells (Mintz and Illmensee, 1975). The OTT 6050 tumor was known, from karyotype analysis, to be of the X/Y, or male sex, chromosome type. [Earlier studies (reviewed in Mintz, 1974) have shown that functional gametes do generally develop in allophenic mice, even including X/X ↔ X/Y mosaics, but only from the germ cells whose sex chromosome type conforms to the morphological type of the individual.] The fertile males with germ cells derived from the X/Y teratocarcinoma were mated to normal females of the original blastocyst strain; their F_1 progeny exhibited many of the specific tumor-strain alleles, including the *steel* gene (Fig. 15), already detected phenotypically in the mosaic parent. Thus, final proof of genomic integrity was provided by silent transmission of the genes in the germ line, and their reexpression in the development of the next generation.

These experiments, demonstrating full realization of the totipotent developmental capacities of mouse embryonal carcinoma cells, furnish the first unequivocal case of complete reversal of an animal malignancy to normalcy. Whenever the injected cells were apparently successfully integrated into the developing embryo, they also were successfully normalized and remained normal, into old age, in the mosaic mice. In only a small minority, in which the carcinoma cells evidently *failed* to

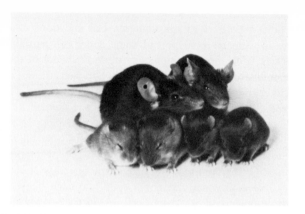

Fig. 15. A family portrait showing normal germ-cell differentiation, and transmission of genes, from formerly malignant teratocarcinoma cells. The normal mosaic male (rear, left) was derived from a WH-strain (black) blastocyst injected with teratocarcinoma stem cells. His coat is all-black, but he has both strains of sperms. A mating with a WH control female (rear, right) has produced two babies (front, left) from his tumor-derived (agouti) sperms and two (front, right) from his blastocyst-derived (black) sperms. The paler-coat agouti baby with the white head-spot and light feet (extreme left) has also received the *steel* (*Sl*) gene from the heterozygous (*Sl*/+) tumor cells, after meiosis in gametogenesis, while its darker agouti neighbor received the wild-type allele. From Mintz and Illmensee, unpublished data.

become integrated, did they continue their tumorous growth without contributing to normal embryogenesis, as in an ordinary tumor transplant situation (Mintz, Custer, and Illmensee, unpublished data).

The results, therefore, offer strong support for the interpretation that the initial conversion to malignancy in this tumor occurred in normal totipotent stem cells; and that it came about through induced changes in gene function, rather than gene structure. The changes were probably due to the anomalous environment in which the normal stem cells then found themselves. Normal gene function was restored when the malignant stem cells were returned to the proper environment.

A. Can Reversal of Malignancy Occur in Other Tumors?

If reversal of malignant stem cells to normal differentiation could be demonstrated in any other tumors, this would presumably identify them as additional examples of nonmutational stem-cell transformation. There have been numerous claims of clinical reversal to normalcy in other tumors. Upon closer scrutiny, it becomes difficult to sustain or even clarify most of these. Clinical remissions may result from loss or reduced division of malignant stem cells; these are of course not reversals in the sense of the mouse teratocarcinoma stem cells. Of particular interest is the fact, discussed in Section VI, that some clinical changes in tumors from the malignant to the benign state, as occasionally seen in human neuroblastomas (Cushing and Wolbach, 1927), seem to involve progression in stem-cell differentiation (Fig. 9).

One of the better known experimental cases of partial normalization occurs in Friend-virus-induced murine erythroleukemia cells. After their exposure to dimethyl sulfoxide *in vitro,* most of the erythroblasts undergo some maturation to normoblasts, and show increased hemoglobin synthesis (Friend *et al.,* 1971). Erythroleukemic stem cells also manifest an ability *in vivo* to respond favorably to a normal environment: When introduced into the spleens of irradiated nonleukemic hosts, they seem able to undergo apparently normal self-renewal and differentiation and, thereby, to rescue the host (Matioli, 1973). It remains to be determined whether reduction of malignancy under these circumstances is due primarily to a reversible change in properties of the causal viral agent, and whether heterogeneous cell populations may be involved.

In plant teratomas, complete phenotypic reversal to normalcy after transfer to a normal environment has clearly been obtained (Braun, 1959). This work has significantly underscored the possibility of an epigenetic, as opposed to a mutational, etiology, at least for some tumors. Nevertheless, different mechanisms appear to mediate reversal of plant as compared to animal teratomas. It is therefore questionable whether the plant reversal may be taken as a generalizable model of tumors or their potential reversal in animals, as has been suggested (Braun, 1969). Striking points of difference are seen in the normalization process: In the case of plant teratomas, a *series* of graftings to the growing tips of healthy host plants is required; recovery from the tumorous state is gradual; and it is compatible with marked departure from euploidy. In the mouse teratomas, a *single* transfer to the blastocyst cavity of a normal host embryo rapidly leads to normal participation of the donor cells in differentiation (Mintz and Illmensee, 1975), which is stable. (Only if the injected cells remain unassimilated into the embryo, as evidenced by their absence from specialized host tissues, do they continue their tumorous growth, as if in a culture chamber [Mintz,

Custer, and Illmensee, unpublished data].) Unlike the plant teratomas, successful participation of mouse teratoma cells in embryogenesis has thus far occurred solely with tumor cells close to euploidy. Apart from these differences, retrieval of normal totipotency is perhaps less surprising in plant than in animal teratomas, in light of the much greater general developmental lability of somatic cells in plants than in animals: The ordinary somatic cells of higher plants can give rise to an entire plant (Steward *et al.*, 1970), whereas normal developmental totipotency is restricted to early stem cells in higher animals.

The preceding statement is not contradicted by the results of nuclear transplantation studies in amphibians. There, a broadly expanded developmental repertoire is displayed by a specialized somatic cell nucleus only if it is transferred into the cytoplasm of an egg (Gurdon, 1962), not if it remains in its cell of origin, as in the present discussion of cellular reversibility. Even narrow-range developmental shifts in intact somatic cells are exceptional in higher vertebrates. Such rare changes, referred to as cellular metaplasia, are exemplified by the formation of a lens from pigmented cells at the margin of the iris when, after lentectomy in some species, the iris cells become depigmented and differentiate into lens cells.

Another tumor frequently cited—perhaps prematurely—as exhibiting reversibility and an epigenetic origin, is the Lucké renal adenocarcinoma, a malignancy of probable viral origin in the frog. When individual enucleated eggs from diploid donors were injected with several nuclei taken from tumors induced in triploid frogs, some triploid larvae that developed as far as the swimming stage were obtained (McKinnell *et al.*, 1969). Despite the intrinsic interest in these results, demonstrating as they do the multipotentiality of transplanted nuclei from the kidney, it is not yet possible to conclude that reversal of *malignant*-cell nuclei had taken place. Tumors are vascularized by nontumorous blood vessels, infiltrated by normal connective tissue, and often contain admixed normal parenchymal cells of the tumorous organ. In this experiment, all the possible normal cells of origin would have had triploid nuclei, along with the nuclei of the tumor cells; the question remains whether any such *normal* nuclei were among those introduced into any given egg.

The possibility of reversal in transformed cells has also been examined extensively in cultured cell lines. Those studies, which will not be reviewed here, show that cells may lose their transformed phenotypes if an oncogenic virus is lost, or if the cellular chromosome constitution changes in specific ways.

From the foregoing brief summary based on a survey of the extensive literature (see references listed by Willis, 1967; Braun, 1969; Friend *et al.*, 1971; Pierce, 1974), it appears that the mouse teratocarcinoma has, as already stated, furnished the first unequivocal case of complete and stable stem-cell reversal to normalcy in an animal malignancy (Mintz and Illmensee, 1975). No virus has been causally implicated in teratocarcinogenesis, so that viral loss or change is presumably not at issue. All the evidence, showing orderly somatic and germ-cell differentiation from the normalized tumor stem cells, points to an intact genome, hence to a nonmutational cause of the malignancy.

Despite the lack of other conclusive instances of reversal at the present time, there is no reason to think that the mouse teratocarcinoma is in fact unique. It provides a model that may well be applicable to some, though surely not all, malignancies of more specialized mammalian tissues. If a specialized tumor had arisen similarly, as the result of changes in the tissue milieu without production of mutations, its malignant stem cells might be induced to differentiate normally if placed in the normal stem-cell developmental environment of that particular tissue. In most cases, the appropriate environment would probably not be the blastocyst.

With this aim in view, I am screening primary and transplantable mouse tumors for "normalization" candidates. The more promising ones would be expected to be still fairly euploid, and well differentiated; the stem cells of undifferentiated tumors may have been so altered during tumor progression as to have virtually lost their differentiative capacity and their prospects for normalization. New microsurgical techniques will undoubtedly have to be devised for introduction of malignant cells in appropriate sites during relatively late stages of embryogenesis. These experiments, if successful, have no obvious clinical applicability, but will further document the role of differentiation in neoplasia.

B. When Does Conversion of Totipotent Stem Cells to Malignancy Occur?

Many kinds of stem cells, including totipotent ones as well as the stem cells of specific tissues, may have complex life histories. A well-

known example is found in spermatogonial stem-cell renewal. A
hypothesis meriting investigation therefore suggests itself—namely,
that conversion to malignancy may be possible in only a limited part of
that history.

The developmental sequence of totipotent mammalian cells does indeed appear to be complex. Totipotency characterizes not only germ
cells of several stages (which are able parthenogenetically to form embryos), but also zygotes, embryo cells in preimplantation stages (Mintz,
1974), and some embryo cells of the postimplantation egg cylinder
(Stevens, 1970; Levak-Svajger and Svajger, 1974). While the cells in
this long series share some ultrastructural, histochemical, and biochemical properties, they are clearly not identical. The ease with which
teratocarcinogenesis may be experimentally induced provides an opportunity to test the validity of the hypothesis under discussion, in the case
of totipotent stem cells. Is malignant conversion in fact possible in only
one "target" stage of the life history, as proposed here, or in many or
all stages?

A superficial examination of the evidence might be taken to signify that
teratocarcinogenesis may occur in virtually any stage: Primordial germ
cells, or embryos of any stage ranging up through the early egg cylinder,
may form teratocarcinomas if transplanted to an ectopic site (Stevens,
1967a,b, 1970); spontaneous testicular or ovarian tumors may form from
germ cells *in situ* (Linder, 1969; Stevens and Varnum, 1974); and spontaneous teratomas may also occasionally be found in other sites, after
having possibly arisen from "lost" germ cells or embryo cells (Willis,
1967). This ostensibly universal capacity for malignant transformation in
totipotent cells of all types may, however, be misleading; the actual
transformational event, as distinct from cell proliferation, may be occurring in only one developmental stage, shared ultimately by all.

In a controversy extending back at least a century, two schools of
thought have emerged. According to one, all teratomas come from germ
cells, whether gonadally or ectopically situated; according to the other,
the tumors come from somatic embryo cells (see the reviews by Stevens, 1967a, 1970; Pierce, 1967; Damjanov and Solter, 1974). As
Stevens (1970) has pointed out, the germinal and somatic viewpoints
converge, insofar as parthenogenetically developing germ cells (*in situ*
in the gonads or fetal germinal ridges, or in the transplanted germinal
ridges) form miniature embryos; and embryos that give rise to teratomas

may first have to form primordial germ cells. In an effort to break into this cycle, he ectopically transplanted fetal mouse genital ridges from matings in which the heterozygous ($Sl/+$) parents would be expected to yield 25% of embryos homozygous for a genetic condition (Sl/Sl) known to cause almost total absence of primordial germ cells (Stevens, 1967b). Failure of teratomas to form with approximately that frequency, in comparison with results of transplanting fertile-genotype control embryos, lent possible support to the view that germ cells are the initial target cell in teratocarcinogenesis. However, germ-cell absence in transferred germinal ridges of the homozygous Sl/Sl embryos leaves them with no alternative parthenogenetic source from which an embryo might develop, hence with no source of totipotent embryo cells, which might in fact be the real target cell. It thus appears that the question of a uniquely transformation-susceptible stage in teratocarcinogenesis is still unresolved.

We are attempting to clarify the issue by an experiment now in progress in my laboratory. Another place has been chosen to break into the cycle of events. Genetically sterile early embryos (rather than germinal ridges), and their presumptively fertile littermates, are being transplanted to an ectopic site *before* the time of normal primordial germ cell formation; the genetically sterile and fertile ones are specifically distinguishable by means of linked genetic markers. If those embryos individually identified as genetically incapable of germ cell formation do nevertheless form teratocarcinomas, this will constitute unequivocal proof that conversion to this malignancy is a somatic, not a germinal, event. Such a conclusion would not be surprising, in view of the fact that ectopically placed control embryos, up to 6 days of age, undergo teratocarcinogenesis (Stevens, 1970); these embryos are genetically capable of forming germ cells, but they have not yet done so at that age—at least not visibly (Mintz and Russell, 1957). The conclusion would also be compatible with all other observations and would mean that a stimulus capable of inciting germ cells to divide, either in early gonial phases (Stevens, 1967a) or postmeiotically in the gonad (Linder, 1969), merely potentiates embryogenesis, in which some still-totipotent somatic cells may then become transformed.

A possible further clue to the stage of inception of teratocarcinomas might be obtained by identifying the normal-cell stage to which the malignant stem cells most closely correspond. With this end in view, we have been comparing the soluble proteins of teratocarcinoma cells with those of normal early embryo cells of various stages. As the profiles from preliminary acrylamide gel electrophoretic separations show (Fig. 16), blastomeres in the morula stage have numerous differences from teratocarcinoma core cells (taken from embryoid bodies), although both are developmentally totipotent (Mintz *et al.*, 1975). We are presently refining the protein comparisons by the use of two-dimensional gels. Blastomeres and teratocarcinoma cells also differ in surface properties affecting adhesion (Mintz *et al.*, 1975) and in alkaline phosphatase levels (Damjanov and Solter, 1974).

The leading candidate for a stage-specific somatic target cell appears to be the so-called ectoderm of the egg cylinder (day 6) mouse embryo. Despite the restrictive connotation of classical germ layer nomenclature, these cells are most likely to be the ones terminally capable of conversion to malignancy. While there is as yet no direct evidence as to the duration of a totipotent cell population, transplanted embryos older than

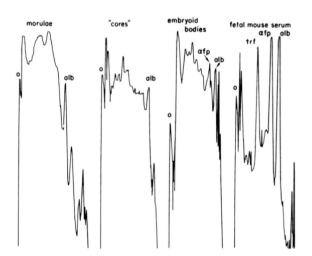

Fig. 16. Scans of acrylamide gel electrophoretic separations of soluble proteins from mouse morulae; teratocarcinoma stem cells from embryoid body "cores"; small-size whole embryoid bodies, with teratocarcinoma cells and yolk sac cells; and fetal mouse serum. Although morula and teratocarcinoma cells are developmentally totipotent, their protein profiles differ. αfp, α-fetoprotein; alb, albumin; trf, transferrin; o is the origin. From Mintz *et al.* (1975), reprinted with permission.

6.5 days can no longer form teratocarcinomas (Stevens, 1970); and lineages of specialized cells seem normally to be initiated at that time (Mintz, 1974). Thus, in teratomas induced by ectopic grafting of younger embryos (or germ cells that parthenogenetically form embryos), embryo development may continue, even if imperfectly, until stem cells of the stage appropriate for neoplastic conversion are present. Their terminally totipotent status in normal development suggests that *the critical time for susceptibility to transformation may occur relatively late in the life history of stem cells,* when the differentiative option is normally imposed, perhaps in a particular kind of local tissue environment.

The teratocarcinomas that form in different circumstances all have in common the fact that the embryo of origin is developing in an anomalous environment and becomes disorganized. How this disturbed milieu might trigger transformation is unknown, but the situation is not unique for these tumors. As pointed out earlier (Section VI), malignant conversion may occur if more specialized normal stem cells are placed in an unusual location. Bladder and intestinal carcinomas are examples (Zinzar *et al.,* 1976). If specific-stage restrictions on malignant transformation could be experimentally defined for the stem cells of such tissues, our understanding of cellular susceptibility to malignancy might be greatly enhanced.

VIII. PERSPECTIVES FOR RESEARCH

The ancestry of malignant stem cells from normal ones has been shown, in teratocarcinomas, by realization of their full developmental potentialities in a normal environment (Figs. 10–12). As a result, certain novel experimental potentialities, envisioned at the start of this work, have now become practicable.

In inquiring whether these malignant cells were totipotent, I had in mind two long-range experimental objectives. One, already elaborated here, concerned the problem of malignancy: Successful normalization in this malignancy would identify it as a nonmutational disturbance of differentiation, hence as a possible paradigm for some tumors of more specialized tissues. The other objective was directed at the problem of differentiation. Normalization would enable totipotency, in cells more readily available than are normal totipotent ones, to be exploited in a new genetic approach: Through mutagenesis and selection *in vitro,* followed by differentiation *in vivo,* experimentally useful genes could be introduced into mice. There, the full developmental consequences of specific gene mutations coding for biochemically identified changes could be brought to light.

In conventional mammalian genetics, e.g., in mice, germ cells (or embryos) are exposed to mutagenic agents and allowed to give rise to mutant animals—inevitably without prior selection, except for negatively self-selected lethals. The mutant individuals are usually recognized by gross deviations which are often parts of complex syndromes, rather than by biochemical features. Then, the primary molecular basis for the phenotypic change is sought; in most instances, it has remained unknown. It had seemed to me that such experiments were, in a manner of speaking, being conducted backwards, relative to those of bacterial genetics, in which biochemically definable heritable lesions were obtained virtually at will, by applying specific selective screens to mutagenized cultures.

Mammalian somatic cell geneticists have of course successfully availed themselves of some of the tools of microbial geneticists. Utilization of a variety of selective systems in mutagenized cell cultures (e.g., Puck, 1971) has yielded variant cell lines that have proved valuable in many ways. Nevertheless, the applicability of this approach to basic problems of differentiation in a multicellular species has been sharply circumscribed by the very limited developmental potentialities of even the most versatile cells hitherto used in such studies. A further restriction has been that the genetic status of variations presumed to be due to mutations in cultured cells is difficult to ascertain definitively in a purely mitotic somatic cell lineage, even with cell hybridization techniques. *In vivo,* transmission and orderly recombination during meiosis in the germ line enable mutant genes to be identified and mapped in detail.

Thus, there has largely been, by force of circumstance, a kind of separation of experimental assets: The *in vivo* mammalian work has had at its disposal the precision of genetic analysis and the organized full range of cellular differentiations and interactions; the *in vitro* work has had the important option of choosing biochemically specific variants, and the practicality of obtaining the cells in large numbers by clonal expansion. I therefore became interested in the possibility that teratocarcinoma cells, known to be multipotential, might actually be totipotential and convertible to normalcy. If so, they could—unlike zygotes—be grown in large numbers and cloned under selective conditions, and then be essentially "converted" into mice.

The new experimental system proposed here for the study of mammalian differentiation (Fig. 17), and briefly outlined previously (Mintz *et al.*, 1975; Mintz and Illmensee, 1975), does in fact combine the virtues of the *in vivo* and *in vitro* approaches. This is done, first, by mutageniz-

MUTANT MICE FROM MUTAGENIZED TERATOCARCINOMA CELLS

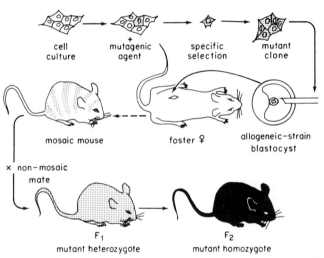

FIG. 17. A new scheme for generating definable genetic probes of mammalian differentiation, and for obtaining mouse models of human genetic diseases. Developmentally totipotent mouse teratocarcinoma stem cells are first mutagenized *in vitro,* where appropriate media or conditions may be used to select for survival of clones with specific biochemical (e.g., enzymatic) lesions, or for classes of alterations (e.g., changes in surface properties). A mutant cultured cell is then injected into a blastocyst of a genetically different strain, which continues its development in the uterus of a foster mother. In the resultant mosaic mouse, the effects of the specific mutation can be analyzed in the differentiation of somatic tissues derived from the mutant cell. Gametes may also be produced, enabling the mutation to be mapped through recombination during meiosis. Mice homozygous for a nonlethal autosomal mutation may be obtained in the F_2 generation.

ing cultures of totipotent malignant teratocarcinoma stem cells; by employing appropriately engineered media or conditions to screen for desired phenotypes; and by expanding the mutant cells into clones. Next, a mutant cell is introduced into a blastocyst of another strain and the blastocyst is surgically transferred to a foster mother. Some mosaic mice with both mutant (tumor-derived) and wild-type (blastocyst-derived) cells would be obtained. In such individuals, cells with mutations that might otherwise be lost through lethality to the organism might be ''rescued'' by coexistence with normal cells, as has already been shown in viable allophenic mice with both lethally anemic (W/W) and normal cells (Mintz, 1970b). The population of mosaic animals in the present experiment (Fig. 17), as in earlier allophenic ones, would undoubtedly vary considerably in the tissue distributions of their mutant cells. This would become an important adjunct enabling identification of the primary tissue in which mutant gene action is critical for the organismic phenotype. Animals with teratocarcinoma-derived germ cells would, in matings to mice of an appropriate (e.g., blastocyst) strain, yield F_1 progeny heterozygous for the mutation in all their diploid cells. Dominant or semidominant autosomal phenotypes could be studied in differentiation of the F_1; F_2 homozygous segregants could be produced for expression of recessive mutant genes. Mapping of the mutation in relation to known genes would be done through these transmission studies. Finally, some kinds of developing tissues or specialized cells (e.g., lymphocytes) from the mosaics or their F_1 or F_2 progeny might be explanted for short-term experiments or assays, thus completing the *in vitro–in vivo* cycle of available experimental options.

The proposed scheme (Fig. 17) would lend itself to analyses of numerous problems in mammalian differentiation, genetics, and metabolism. In the realm of differentiation, one could, through the use of mutations, learn the roles of specific enzymes or other proteins in cell differentiation and interactions. Cellular interactions could be illuminated by selecting for mutations affecting the cell surface. In the area of genetics, the increased availability of defined mutations, particularly in neighboring chromosomal regions, would greatly facilitate an analysis of gene control systems in mammals. Multigene effects might become apparent through fortuitous recombinations of genes. In problems of metabolism, the effects on development, of lesions in progressive parts of particular metabolic pathways (e.g., in purine metabolism) could be studied.

Perhaps one of the most promising experimental potentialities of this system is that it could be used to create animal models of human genetic diseases. Many serious human diseases for which no animal model is presently available are due to mutant genes which cause known enzymatic lesions. These diseases are often characterized by very complex syndromes, and the chain of events between the known molecular lesion and the final clinical picture has generally remained obscure. In at least some cases, this is undoubtedly because the primary difficulty arises during development, where it may lead to cascades of effects. Moreover, the clinically critical effect may in some diseases be tissue-localized, in others, systemic. Many of the relevant enzyme defects could probably be successfully selected for in mutagenized mouse teratocarcinoma cultures, from which mosaic mice could be produced. The fact that some mosaics would chance to have the mutant cells in only one, or another, of their tissues would—in relation to whether that animal showed the syndrome—indicate the primary focus of the disorder. In the F_1 or F_2 progeny, the entire animal would be a model of the human disease. Here, the primary and secondary developmental manifestations of the syndrome could be unraveled, and experimental cures could be attempted. An example of a human hereditary disorder that would lend itself to just such an analysis is the Lesch–Nyhan syndrome (Lesch and Nyhan, 1964), a metabolic derangement, with bizarre behavioral manifestations, due to deficiency of the X-linked enzyme hypoxanthine-guanine phosphoribosyltransferase.

It is also possible that some human normal or mutant genes could be successfully transferred, on small segments of their human chromosomes, into mouse teratocarcinoma cells, and could function during further differentiation into a mouse. This presumption is based on the notion that many mouse and human genes are likely to be evolutionarily homologous. Therefore, at least some human genes might express themselves, despite the different cellular environments and developmental timetables of the two species. Such studies could offer insights into various human disorders and would also be of intrinsic interest for genetics and evolution. Lederberg's remark, made in 1966, may have been prophetic: "Before long we are bound to hear of tests of the effect of dosage of the human twenty-first chromosome on the development of the brain of the mouse. . . ."

One piece of evidence indicating that the experimental system under discussion is indeed one capable of "reading" mutant genes during teratocarcinoma cell differentiation *in vivo* is the discovery, from the mosaic coat phenotype (Mintz and Illmensee, 1975), that the *steel* gene had been present in the tumor cells for 8 years, unexpressed and unsuspected. Although this was not, strictly speaking, a mutation, the process of *in vivo* detection was related to that for a new tumor-cell mutation.

Some hidden mutations, selectable in culture only with difficulty or not at all, may accompany the selected ones after *in vitro* mutagenesis of teratocarcinoma cells. Some of these could be routinely screened for in the mosaic mice or their progeny. Interesting examples of such "bonus" mutations would be changes in histocompatibility antigens or immunoglobulins.

Teratocarcinoma "*in vitro–in vivo*" experiments need not be confined to chromosomally male (X/Y) cells. Those were chosen for the initial blastocyst injections (Mintz *et al.*, 1975) partly because mosaic males with tumor-derived sperms from X/Y cells would supply many more progeny for genetic and other tests than would mosaic females with tumor-derived eggs from chromosmally female (X/X) teratocarcinoma cells. However, the latter offer another novel prospect: that of analyzing the time and mechanisms of single-allele activation of X-linked genes during differentiation. Optimal markers for this purpose are not yet available in the mouse and might be obtained in mutagenesis experiments. We have therefore undertaken, with promising preliminary results, blastocyst injections with the stem cells of a transplantable ovarian teratoma of the LT inbred strain.

This discussion of mutagenesis-plus-normalization has thus far been confined to teratocarcinoma cells. But the same principle could be applied to comparable new experiments with the malignant stem cells of some other tumors. The speculations have been advanced (in Section VII,A) that some tumors of specialized tissues might be further instances of nonmutational stem-cell malignant conversion; and that these stem cells might become normalized if introduced into a developmental environment (not necessarily the blastocyst) appropriate for the cells in question. If such cases are actually identified in this way, some of those stem cells might also be subjected to mutagenesis and specific selection *in vitro* before normalization. Mutant genes would then become available for studies focused on the differentiation of that particular tissue.

Thus, this view of cancer as a developmental aberration opens up complementary new possibilities of probing the nature of neoplasia, and of differentiation, within the framework of the organism: Normalization tests of tumor stem cells *in vivo* provide a means of exploring the role of genes and the control of their expression in malignancy. Development of mutagenized tumor stem cells *in vivo* offers expanded prospects for analyzing gene control of mammalian differentiation and disease. [See Note Added in Proof, p. 246.]

ACKNOWLEDGMENTS

It seems appropriate here to acknowledge, with affection, the lasting influence of my former teacher, the late Professor Emil Witschi. To his students he conveyed his boundless and contagious enthusiasm for science; a sense of wide horizons and the need to strike out in new directions, irrespective of the limitations of one's formal training; and the conviction that direct familiarity with biological material, more than with reports and interpretations thereof, should remain the principal source of inspiration.

I am grateful to the many colleagues with whom these studies were carried out. The names of some are cited here in joint publications with me; others are listed in the references of my 1974 review article referred to here.

The support and intellectual climate to The Institute for Cancer Research in Philadelphia have been indispensable in all of this work. The program has been generously funded by USPHS Grants HD-01646, CA-06927, and RR-05539, and by an appropriation from the Commonwealth of Pennsylvania.

REFERENCES

Abelev, G. I. (1974). *Transplant. Rev.* **20**, 3–37.

Ames, B. (1976). *Science* **191**, 241–244.

Ashcraft, K. W., and Holder, T. M. (1974). *J. Pediatr. Surg.* **9**, 691–697.

Bannerman, R. M., Edwards, J. A., and Pinkerton, P. H. (1973). *In* "Progress in Hematology," Vol. 8 (E. B. Brown, ed.), pp. 131–176. Grune & Stratton, New York.

Bechtol, K. B., Freed, J. H., Herzenberg, L. A., and McDevitt, H. O. (1974). *J. Exp. Med.* **140**, 1660–1675.

Braun, A. C. (1959). *Proc. Natl. Acad. Sci. U.S.A.* **45**, 932–938.

Braun, A. C. (1969). "The Cancer Problem: A Critical Analysis and Modern Synthesis." Columbia Univ. Press, New York.

Brent, L., Brooks, C., Lubling, N., and Thomas, A. V. (1972). *Transplantation* **14**, 382–387.

Brinster, R. L. (1974). *J. Exp. Med.* **140**, 1049–1056.

Buckley, P. A., and Konigsberg, I. R. (1974). *Dev. Biol.* **37**, 193–212.

Burnet, F. M. (1959). "The Clonal Selection Theory of Acquired Immunity." Vanderbilt Univ. Press, Nashville, Tennessee.

Burnet, F. M. (1970). "Immunological Surveillance." Pergamon, Oxford.

Burnet, M. (1974). *In* "Chromosomes and Cancer" (J. German, ed.), pp. 21–38. Wiley, New York.

Coggin, J. H., and Anderson, N. G. (1973). *Adv. Cancer Res.* **19**, 105–165.

Condamine, H., Custer, R. P., and Mintz, B. (1971). *Proc. Natl. Acad. Sci. U.S.A.* **68,** 2032–2036.

Cushing, H., and Wolbach, S. B. (1927). *Am. J. Pathol.* **3,** 203–220.

Damjanov, I., and Solter, D. (1974). *Curr. Top. Pathol.* **59,** 69–130.

Dewey, M. J., Gervais, A. G., and Mintz, B. (1976). *Dev. Biol.* **50,** 68–81.

Foulds, L. (1954). *Cancer Res.* **14,** 327–339.

Friedman, J. M., and Fialkow, P. J. (1976). *Transplant. Rev.* **28,** 2–33.

Friend, C., Scher, W., Holland, J. G., and Sato, T. (1971). *Proc. Natl. Acad. Sci. U.S.A.* **68,** 378–382.

Gearhart, J. D., and Mintz, B. (1972). *Dev. Biol.* **29,** 27–37.

German, J. (1974). *In* "Chromosomes and Cancer" (J. German, ed.), pp. 601–617. Wiley, New York.

Gurdon, J. B. (1962). *J. Embryol. Exp. Morphol.* **10,** 622–640.

Hauschka, T. S., and Levan, A. (1958). *J. Natl. Cancer Inst.* **21,** 77–111.

Illmensee, K., and Mintz, B. (1976). *Proc. Natl. Acad. Sci. U.S.A.* **73,** 549–553.

Kleinsmith, L. J., and Pierce, G. B., Jr. (1964). *Cancer Res.* **24,** 1544–1551.

Knudson, A. G., Jr. (1973). *Adv. Cancer Res.* **17,** 317–352.

Leblond, C. P. (1964). *J. Natl. Cancer Inst.* **14,** 119–150.

Leblond, C. P., and Walker, B. E. (1956). *Physiol. Rev.* **36,** 255–276.

Lederberg, J. (1966). *Bull. At. Sci.* **22,** 4–11.

Lesch, M., and Nyhan, W. L. (1964). *Am. J. Med.* **36,** 561–570.

Levak-Svajger, B., and Svajger, A. (1974). *J. Embryol. Exp. Morphol.* **32,** 445–459.

Lin, T. P. (1966). *Science* **151,** 333–337.

Linder, D. (1969). *Proc. Natl. Acad. Sci. U.S.A.* **63,** 699–704.

Lipsett, M. B. (1965). *Cancer Res.* **25,** 1068–1073.

McCann, J., and Ames, B. N. (1976). *Proc. Natl. Acad. Sci. U.S.A.* **73,** 950–954.

McKinnell, R. G., Deggins, B. A., and Labat, D. D. (1969). *Science* **165,** 394–396.

Makino, S. (1956). *Ann. N.Y. Acad. Sci.* **63,** 818–830.

Markert, C. L. (1968). *Cancer Res.* **28,** 1908–1914.

Matioli, G. (1973). *J. Reticuloendothel. Soc.* **14,** 380–386.

Meo, T., Matsunaga, T., and Rijnbeek, A. M. (1974). *Transplant. Proc.* **5,** 1607–1610.

Miller, J. A. (1970). *Cancer Res.* **30,** 559–576.

Mintz, B. (1962). *Am. Zool.* **2,** 432.

Mintz, B. (1965). *Science* **148,** 1232–1233.

Mintz, B. (1967). *Proc. Natl. Acad. Sci. U.S.A.* **58,** 344–351.

Mintz, B. (1969). *In* "Birth Defects: Orig. Art. Ser. 5" (D. Bergsma and V. McKusick, eds.), pp. 11–22. Nat. Found., New York.

Mintz, B. (1970a). *In* "Genetic Concepts and Neoplasia," *Symp. Fundam. Cancer Res.* **23,** 477–517.

Mintz, B. (1970b). *Symp. Int. Soc. Cell Biol.* **9,** 15–42.

Mintz, B. (1971a). *In* "Methods in Mammalian Embryology" (J. C. Daniel, Jr., ed.), pp. 186–214. Freeman, San Francisco.

Mintz, B. (1971b). *Symp. Soc. Exp. Biol.* **25,** 345–370.

Mintz, B. (1971c). *Fed. Proc., Fed. Am. Soc. Exp. Biol.* **30,** 935–943.

Mintz, B. (1974). *Annu. Rev. Genet.* **8,** 411–470.

Mintz, B., and Baker, W. W. (1967). *Proc. Natl. Acad. Sci. U.S.A.* **58**, 592–598.

Mintz, B., and Illmensee, K. (1975). *Proc. Natl. Acad. Sci. U.S.A.* **72**, 3585–3589.

Mintz, B., and Palm, J. (1969). *J. Exp. Med.* **129**, 1013–1027.

Mintz, B., and Russell, E. S. (1957). *J. Exp. Zool.* **134**, 207–238.

Mintz, B., and Sanyal, S. (1970). *Genetics* **64**, 43–44.

Mintz, B., and Silvers, W. K. (1967). *Science* **158**, 1484–1487.

Mintz, B., and Slemmer, G. (1969). *J. Natl. Cancer Inst.* **43**, 87–95.

Mintz, B., Custer, R. P., and Donnelly, A. J. (1971). *Int. Rev. Exp. Pathol.* **10**, 143.

Mintz, B., Illmensee, K., and Gearhart, J. D. (1975). *In* "Teratomas and Differentiation" (M. Sherman and D. Solter, eds.), pp. 59–82. Academic Press, New York.

Moore, W. J., and Mintz, B. (1972). *Dev. Biol.* **27**, 55–70.

Nowell, P. C. (1974). *In* "Chromosomes and Cancer" (J. German, ed.), pp. 267–285. Wiley, New York.

Nowell, P. C., and Hungerford, D. A. (1960). *Science* **132**, 1497.

Papaionnou, V. E., McBurney, M. W., Gardner, R. L., and Evans, M. J. (1975). *Nature (London)* **258**, 70–73.

Pierce, G. B. (1967). *Curr. Top. Dev. Biol.* **2**, 223–246.

Pierce, G. B. (1974). *In* "Developmental Aspects of Carcinogenesis and Immunity" (T. J. King, ed.), pp. 3–22. Academic Press, New York.

Pierce, G. B., and Johnson, L. D. (1971). *In Vitro* **7**, 140–145.

Pierce, G. B., and Wallace, C. (1971). *Cancer Res.* **31**, 127–134.

Pitot, H. C. (1968). *Cancer Res.* **28**, 1880–1887.

Prehn, R. T. (1976). *Transplant. Rev.* **28**, 34–42.

Prigogina, E. L., and Fleischman, E. W. (1975). *Humangen.* **30**, 113–119.

Puck, T. T. (1971). *In Vitro* **7**, 115–119.

Rolshoven, E. (1951). *Verh. Anat. Ges. Jena* **49**, 189–197.

Rowe, W. P. (1973). *Cancer Res.* **33**, 3061–3068.

Rowley, J. D. (1974). *J. Natl. Cancer Inst.* **52**, 315–320.

Rubin, H. (1976). *Science* **191**, 241.

Rubinstein, L. J., Herman, M. M., and Hanbery, J. W. (1974). *Cancer* **33**, 675–690.

Schapira, F., Hatzfeld, A., and Weber, A. (1975). *In* "Isozymes" (C. L. Markert, ed.), Vol. 3, pp. 987–1003. Academic Press, New York.

Stevens, L. C. (1967a). *Adv. Morphog.* **6**, 1–31.

Stevens, L. C. (1967b). *J. Natl. Cancer Inst.* **38**, 549–552.

Stevens, L. C. (1970). *Dev. Biol.* **21**, 364–382.

Stevens, L. C., and Hummel, K. P. (1957). *J. Natl. Cancer. Inst.* **18**, 719–747.

Stevens, L. C., and Varnum, D. (1974). *Dev. Biol.* **37**, 369–380.

Steward, F. C., Ammirato, P. V., and Mapes, M. O. (1970). *Ann. Bot.* **34**, 761–787.

Wegmann, T. G., and Gilman, J. G. (1970). *Dev. Biol.* **21**, 281–291.

Wegmann, T. G., Hellström, I., and Hellström, K. E. (1971). *Proc. Natl. Acad. Sci. U.S.A.* **68**, 1644–1647.

Willis, R. A. (1967). "Pathology of Tumours." Butterworth, London.

Zinkernagel, R. M. (1976). *J. Exp. Med.* **144**, 933–945.

Zinzar, S. N., Svet-Moldavsky, G. J., and Karmanova, N. V. (1976). *J. Natl. Cancer Inst.* **57**, 47–55.

Note Added in Proof

Since the time this lecture was presented, the first step has been successfully taken to implement the scheme shown in Fig. 17: Mosaic mice have been produced from blastocysts injected with mutagenized teratocarcinoma cells first selected *in vitro* for deficiency of hypoxanthine-guanine phosphoribosyltransferase (Lesch–Nyhan-type cells) [M. J. Dewey, D. W. Martin, Jr., G. R. Martin, and B. Mintz (1977) *Proc. Natl. Acad. Sci. USA* **74,** 5564–5568].

PROTECTION OF THE ISCHEMIC MYOCARDIUM*†

EUGENE BRAUNWALD

*Department of Medicine, Harvard Medical School,
and the Peter Bent Brigham Hospital,
Boston, Massachusetts*

I. INTRODUCTION

ISCHEMIC heart disease represents the most common serious health problem of contemporary Western society. It has been estimated that, in this country alone, more than 675,000 patients die each year from ischemic heart disease and its complications; approximately 1,300,000 patients develop myocardial infarction; and countless more suffer from congestive heart failure secondary to ischemic myocardial damage. Acute myocardial infarction thus remains the most common cause of in-hospital deaths in this country, indeed, in the Western World. In-hospital deaths in patients with acute myocardial infarction result mainly from primary arrhythmias and from pump failure (Harnarayan *et al.*, 1970). Whereas death due to arrhythmias has been reduced by modern monitoring techniques and more vigorous prophylaxis and treatment, the death rate following mechanical failure manifested by cardiogenic shock and/or pulmonary edema is still very high. These syndromes have been found to be associated with larger infarctions than those exhibited by other patients who succumbed to myocardial infarction, but did not die as a consequence of pump failure (Page *et al.*, 1971; Sobel *et al.*, 1972). In addition, the prognosis for patients with larger infarcts is distinctly worse than it is in those with smaller infarcts (Sobel *et al.*, 1972).

It had long been assumed that the myocardium in the vascular territory of a totally obstructed coronary artery rapidly becomes ischemic

*Lecture delivered May 20, 1976.

†This work was supported in part from Contract NO1 HV-53000 of the Division of Heart and Vascular Diseases, National Heart, Lung, and Blood Institute.

and that only a brief interval elapses before the damage becomes ir-reversible. Since it is now apparent that clinical prognosis following infarction depends directly on the quantity of residual viable, normally functioning myocardium, these widely held assumptions have taken on fresh significance. It would appear that if one could effectively limit tissue damage following coronary occlusion, pump failure and its con-sequences might be averted. Basic to any consideration of this problem is the progression of myocardial ischemic injury following coronary artery occlusion. In studies of experimentally induced infarcts in ani-mals, myocardial tissue supplied by an occluded vessel does not show an essentially homogeneous area of necrosis. Rather, after occlusion the affected myocardium is likely to manifest a region of central necrosis surrounded in patchy fashion by a substantial amount of abnormal but still viable tissue. Moreover, this ischemic zone may increase in size for some time, while the necrotic zone remains relatively small. Indeed, according to some studies, the ischemic zone may continue to enlarge for up to 18 hours after occlusion (Cox *et al.*, 1968); thereafter the region of central necrosis expands rapidly at the expense of ischemic tissue. The absence of a clear demarcation between normal and necrotic tissue on histologic examination of human hearts at autopsy has been noted repeatedly, and it appears likely that the progression from is-chemic damage to necrosis follows a time course in man similar to that in experimental animals.

Death from cardiogenic shock may now be viewed as the end result of a vicious cycle (Fig. 1) (Braunwald, 1976). Coronary obstruction leads to myocardial ischemia, which impairs myocardial contractility and ventricular performance; this, in turn, reduces arterial pressure and therefore coronary perfusion pressure, leading to further ischemia and extension of necrosis, until, in most cases, death occurs. There is some evidence that stasis in the smaller arteries and arterioles distal to a major proximal occlusion can result in secondary microvascular obstruction, further impairing myocardial perfusion.

Accordingly, a treatment that could decrease the extent of tissue death in the myocardium, and by this mechanism decrease the fre-quency of intractable cardiogenic shock and pulmonary edema, would be extremely useful, not only by reducing immediate mortality, but also by leaving the patient who had suffered a coronary occlusion with more viable myocardium. Such a patient would be expected to be less likely

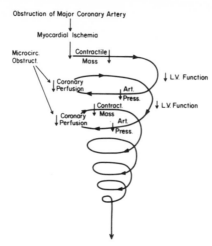

Fig. 1. Diagram depicting the sequence of events in the vicious cycle in which coronary artery obstruction leads to cardiogenic shock and progressive circulatory deterioration.

to develop chronic heart failure and would have a greater reserve of functioning myocardium should another coronary occlusion occur.

There is considerable evidence to suggest that factors that influence myocardial oxygen demands may aggravate or alleviate symptoms of myocardial ischemia. For example, in patients with angina and hyperthyroidism, treatment of the hypermetabolic state, and the associated reduction of myocardial oxygen needs, is often associated with relief of angina (Somerville and Kevin, 1950). Also, the reduction of myocardial oxygen needs by β-adrenergic blockade (Wolfson et al., 1966) or carotid sinus nerve stimulation (Braunwald et al., 1967) reduces symptoms of myocardial ischemia. Conversely, treatment of hypothyroidism or the development of tachycardia, influences that augment myocardial oxygen needs, increase the frequency and severity of myocardial ischemia in patients with coronary artery disease. The importance of the decreased availability of oxygen is apparent in cases where arterial hypotension and acute anemia may cause infarction in patients with coronary artery disease in the absence of coronary occlusion.

The above-mentioned clinical observations suggested to us in 1967 that the ultimate size of a myocardial infarct is not irrevocably determined by the site of coronary occlusion, but might be modified by other factors (Braunwald, 1967). We then proposed that when coronary occlusion occurs, the survival of the cardiac tissue normally perfused by the obstructed vessel depends on the balance between oxygen available to that segment of myocardium and its oxygen requirements and that the survival of the patient with coronary occlusion could, in large measure, be dependent on the balance between myocardial oxygen supply and demand (Braunwald *et al.*, 1969).

Our approach to this problem extended from a consideration of the determinants of myocardial oxygen consumption and how they are altered by some of the common interventions and drugs employed in the treatment of patients with acute myocardial infarction. These studies were based on the premise that an augmentation of myocardial oxygen requirements will, if other factors remain constant, tend to enlarge the area of ischemia and ultimately of necrosis, whereas a reduction of myocardial oxygen consumption will tend to have the opposite effect.

II. Determinants of the Heart's Oxygen Consumption

The determinants of myocardial oxygen consumption have been reviewed elsewhere (Braunwald, 1969, 1971), but will be briefly summarized here. It has been known for many years that the total metabolism of the arrested, quiescent heart is only a small fraction of that of the working organ. Thus, while the oxygen consumption of the beating mammalian heart ranges from 3 to 15 ml/min per 100 g of left ventricle, the oxygen consumption of the heart arrested with excess potassium is only about 1.3 ml/min per 100 g. Since the quantity of oxygen required for electrical activation of the heart is approximately 0.5% of the total O_2 consumed by the normally contracting organ (Klocke *et al.*, 1966), this difference between the arrested and beating heart results almost exclusively from the heart's contractile activity.

In studies in which the relative effects of aortic pressure, stroke volume and heart rate on the oxygen consumption of the isolated supported heart were determined, a close relation between myocardial oxygen consumption and the so-called tension-time index (TTI), that is, the area beneath the left ventricular pressure pulse per minute, was demonstrated (Sarnoff *et al.*, 1958). It was then emphasized that the tension of the myocardial wall is a more definitive determinant of myocardial energy utlization than is the developed pressure (Rodbard *et al.*, 1964) and that myocardial wall tension is a direct function of the radius and intraventricular pressure and is inversely related to ventricular wall thickness. Evidence was then provided that, in addition to developed tension, the peak velocity of contraction of the myocardium, reflecting the contractile or inotropic state of the heart, is also a major determinant of myocardial oxygen consumption (Ross *et al.*, 1965; Sonnenblick *et al.*, 1965). The basal metabolism of the organ, the activation of the heart, maintenance of the active state, and shortening against a load, all contribute to the heart's oxygen demands, but less so than the principal determinants, i.e., tension, contractility, and frequency of contraction (Braunwald, 1969, 1971).

It was proposed that since the blood supply to the ischemic zone surrounding the infarct is markedly reduced, the survival of this tissue may depend on its oxygen consumption. According to this concept, with occlusion of a coronary artery at any specific site, if the oxygen consumption of the myocardium were stimulated by factors such as increased rate, tension, and/or contractility, the viability of the ischemic border zone may be reduced and the size of the infarct enlarged. Furthermore, such an unfavorable alteration in the relationship between myocardial oxygen supply and demand could impair the contractile function of the ischemic myocardium at the margin of the infarct. This depression of left ventricular function could then result in enlargement of this chamber which, in accord with Laplace's law, will result in an augmentation of tension development at any level of ventricular pressure (Braunwald, 1974). An elevation of tension, in turn, leads to even higher levels of oxygen consumption, which could impair myocardial function further and thus lead to the vicious cycle of cardiogenic shock already referred to (Fig. 2).

III. ASSESSMENT OF ISCHEMIC INJURY

In order to study the effects of various physiologic and pharmacologic interventions on the myocardium following coronary occlusion, methods for recording myocardial ischemic injury and for predicting the subsequent development of myocardial necrosis had to be developed.

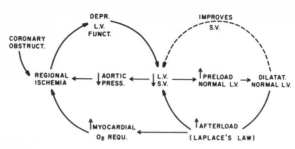

FIG. 2. Schema showing changes in circulatory regulation in ischemic heart disease. DEPR. L.V. FUNCT., depressed left ventricular function; S.V., stroke volume; DILATAT., dilatation; and O_2 REQU., oxygen requirements. Solid lines produce or intensify the effect, whereas a broken line diminished it. Reproduced, by permission, from Braunwald (1974).

Since it has long been appreciated that myocardial ischemia produces changes in the ST segment, it was natural to attempt to utilize this portion of the electrocardiogram as an index of ischemic injury (Braunwald and Maroko, 1976). The electrophysiologic bases of changes in the ST segment in myocardial ischemia have not been completely clarified, but it has been postulated that after repolarization of normal tissue the resting membrane potential of ischemic cells is lower than that of normal cells and that for this reason a "current of injury" flows across the boundary between the normally polarized region and the ischemic zone. According to this concept, this current disappears when the entire heart is depolarized during excitation, and the elevated ST segment really results from a depressed TQ segment (Nahum *et al.*, 1943). It has also been suggested that ST segment elevation may occur as a result of failure of the injured area to depolarize during excitation (Eyster *et al.*, 1938), which results in current flow during depolarization across the boundary between the partially polarized, injured region and the depolarized normal zone. A closely related possible mechanism of ST segment elevation is an altered wave form of the transmembrane action potential of ischemic tissue with loss of the normal plateau portion, so that current flows between such an area and normal tissue during inscription of the action potential (Samson and Scher, 1960; Cohen and Kaufman, 1975).

It is likely that alterations in the permeability of myocardial cell membranes—which modify ion transport and thereby alter the magnitudes of the resting potential, of the transmembrane potential inscribed during the plateau of the action potential, and of the voltage time course of repolarization—represent the ultimate cause of the ST segment shift during acute myocardial ischemia. However, it is critical to recognize that factors other than ischemia can also affect the ST segment. These changes in the electrical activity of nonischemic cells include, but are not limited to, alterations in pH and ion concentrations, temperature changes, drugs such as quinidine and digitalis, intraventricular conduction defects, sympathetic stimulation of the heart, and epicardial injury due to pericarditis (Braunwald and Maroko, 1976).

In 1949, Wegria first reported on the correlation in experimental animals between changes in the ST segment of the electrocardiogram and coronary blood flow (Wegria *et al.,* 1949). Reduction in flow by two-thirds or more always produced marked ST segment changes, while minor changes occurred when coronary blood flow was reduced by between one-third or two-thirds of control; no changes were noted with reductions in coronary flow by less than one-third. Becker *et al.* measured regional myocardial perfusion with radioactive microspheres and correlated the results with epicardial electrograms. ST segments were substantially elevated in most, though not all, sites overlying low flow zones (Becker *et al.,* 1973).

The correlations between ST segment changes and myocardial metabolism have been examined in several studies. When global ischemia of the left ventricle was produced, ST segment changes occurred almost simultaneously with the first biochemical indices of ischemia, i.e., reduction of myocardial lactate extraction, and efflux of K^+ from the heart (Scheuer and Brachfeld, 1966). In a correlation of epicardial ST segment changes with metabolic alterations in the underlying myocardium following occlusion of the anterior descending coronary artery in dogs, Karlsson found that biopsies of the myocardium subjacent to sites with epicardial ST segment elevations showed lactate accumulation, as well as depletion of ATP and creatine phosphate (Karlsson *et al.,* 1973), reflecting anaerobic myocardial metabolism. Sayen *et al.* using polarographic measurements of intramyocardial oxygen tension, found that ST segment elevations in the epicardial electrocardiogram promptly followed reduction of oxygen tension below

254   EUGENE BRAUNWALD

65% of control (Sayen *et al.*, 1973). More recently, Angell *et al.*
compared the magnitude of ST segment elevations in surface electrograms with the intramyocardial oxygen tension in the subjacent tissue
recorded by means of platinum–iridium electrodes. The ST map correlated closely with the oxygen tension as the latter was varied by altering
coronary perfusion pressure (Angell *et al.*, 1975). Also, Khuri and
associates varied coronary blood flow and recorded myocardial pO_2 and
pCO_2 using a mass spectrometer. When regional ischemia was produced, epicardial ST segment elevations correlated with changes in
myocardial gas tensions. However, intramyocardial ST segments
proved to be more sensitive than those recorded from the epicardium
(Khuri *et al.*, 1975).

We have noted consistently in the open-chest anesthetized dog that
epicardial ST segment elevation recorded shortly after occlusion of the
left anterior descending coronary artery, or one of its major branches, is
an excellent predictor of the loss of myocardial viability, as judged by
the depletion of cardiac creatine phosphokinase (CPK) activity in the
subjacent myocardium, as well as the histologic and electron microscopic appearance 24 hours (Khuri *et al.*, 1975; Maroko and Braunwald,
1973; Maroko *et al.*, 1971, 1972b) or 1 week (Ginks *et al.*, 1972) later
(Fig. 3). A linear inverse correlation was found between the log of
myocardial CPK activity and the degree of local ST segment elevation
(Fig. 4) (Maroko *et al.*, 1971; Maroko and Braunwald, 1973). In the

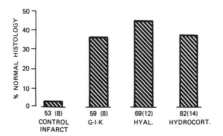

FIG. 3. Comparison of the effect of treatment on histology in areas with ST segment
elevations over 2 mV. First column: control group; second column: glucose–insulin–
potassium (G-I-K) group; third column: hyaluronidase group; fourth column: hydrocortisone group. Note that in all three treatment groups more than one-third of sites that were
expected to show early signs of myocardial infarction were spared. Reproduced by permission, from Maroko and Braunwald (1973).

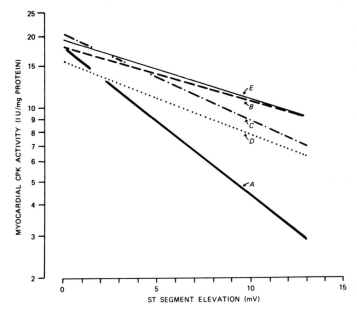

FIG. 4. Relationship between ST segment elevation 15 minutes after occlusion and log creatine phosphokinase (CPK) activity from the same specimens obtained 24 hours later. A: Control group (occlusion alone), 15 dogs, 101 biopsies; B: hyaluronidase, 13 dogs, 94 biopsies; C: propranolol; D: glucose 50%, 6 dogs, 46 biopsies; E: glucose–insulin-potassium infusion, 13 dogs, 96 biopsies. All interventions were started 30 minutes after coronary artery occlusion, i.e., 15 minutes after the epicardial mapping. There is a statistical difference ($P < 0.01$) between the slope of line A and the slopes of the other lines showing less CPK depression after treatment. Reproduced, by permission, from Maroko and Braunwald (1973).

absence of an intervention, myocardial CPK activity has always been found to be reduced 24 hours after sustained occlusion whenever epicardial ST segment elevation exceeds 2 mV 15 minutes after occlusion. However, a limitation of the epicardial ST segment measurement is its relative insensitivity to the more extensive subendocardial ischemic damage.

It was also observed, using multiple precordial electrodes in the dog, that changes in myocardial ischemic injury as measured by ST segment elevations parallel those observed on the epicardium (Muller *et al.*,

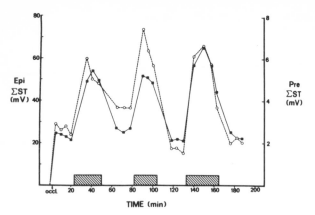

FIG. 5. An example of the correspondence between the Epi ΣST (○···○) and Pre ΣST (●———●) as ischemic injury following coronary artery occlusion was varied during intermittent intravenous infusions of isoproterenol (hatched rectangle). During the first and second infusions, isoproterenol was administered at the rate of 0.17 μg/kg per minute; during the third infusion isoproterenol was given at the rate of 4.0 μg/kg per minute following an intravenous bolus of 1 mg of propranolol per kilogram. Time, in minutes following coronary occlusion. Reproduced, by permission from Muller *et al.* (1975).

1975) (Fig. 5) and that both precordial and epicardial ST segment changes soon after coronary occlusion predict myocardial CPK activity measured 24 hours later. The exact relation between precordial and epicardial ST segment elevation varied for each dog, but in general the precordial electrocardiogram was less sensitive than the epicardial electrocardiogram in detecting ischemia (Muller *et al.*, 1975). This approach has been extended to precordial electrocardiograms in the closed-chest pig (Capone *et al.*, 1975).

It is clear from the experimental studies that in the absence of other changes capable of influencing the ST segment (e.g., electrolyte concentration, drugs, intraventricular conduction defects, sympathetic stimulation, and pericarditis), ST segment elevation recorded directly at a given epicardial site reflects ischemia of the subjacent myocardium, and that when such elevation is present 15–20 minutes after the onset of a permanent coronary occlusion, some degree of myocardial damage will be encountered 24 hours or more later unless a favorable intervention is interposed. In our studies, reviewed below, the efficacy of interventions designed to minimize myocardial ischemic damage following coronary occlusion has been based on observing significantly *less* morphologic damage and reduction of CPK activity 24 hours after coronary occlusion for any level of ST segment elevation occurring shortly after coronary occlusion, than in nontreated controls.

IV. Effects of Altering Myocardial Oxygen Balance

Using the technique of recording epicardial ST segments, it was found that a variety of interventions (Table I), notably those that increase myocardial oxygen consumption, such as isoproterenol (Fig. 6), digitalis, glucagon, bretylium, tosylate, and pacing-induced atrial tachycardia, all increase the severity and extent of myocardial injury (Maroko *et al.*, 1971). More recently, Redwood and associates, using subepicardial electrodes, studied the influence of atropine-induced tachycardia in conscious dogs and found a similar increase in myocardial injury, as reflected in ST segment elevations (Redwood *et al.*, 1972). Similarly, Shell and Sobel (1973), using serum creatine phosphokinase disappearance curves as an index of myocardial damage,

TABLE I

INTERVENTIONS THAT INCREASE MYOCARDIAL INJURY
FOLLOWING CORONARY ARTERY OCCLUSION

I. Increasing myocardial oxygen requirements
   A. Isoproterenol
   B. Digitalis (in the nonfailing heart)
   C. Glucagon
   D. Bretylium tosylate
   E. Tachycardia
   F. Hyperthermia
II. Decreasing myocardial oxygen supply
   A. Directly
      1. Hypoxemia
      2. Anemia
   B. Through collateral vessels—reducing coronary perfusion pressure
      1. Hemorrhage
      2. Sodium nitroprusside
      3. Minoxidil
III. Decreasing substrate availability—hypoglycemia

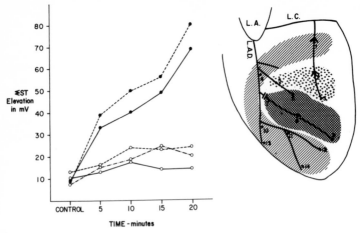

FIG. 6. Effects of occlusion alone (○) and occlusion after the infusion of isoproterenol (0.25 μg/kg per minute) (●). *Right:* Schematic representation of the anterior surface of the heart. The coronary arteries and branches, and sites of epicardial electrograms are marked. L.A.D., left anterior descending coronary artery; L.A., left atrial appendage; L.C., left circumflex coronary artery. Crosshatched area: area of injury after 15 minutes of occlusion. Stippled area: increase of area of injury when the occlusion was performed under the influence of isoproterenol. Diagonally lined area: area that showed no ST segment elevation under any circumstances. *Left:* ΣST in the same experiment after three simple occlusions and after two occlusions under the influence of isoproterenol. Time = minutes after occlusion. Runs: 1, ○———○; 2, ○– – –○; 3, ●———●; 4, ○–·–·–○; 5, ●– – –●. Reproduced, by permission, from Maroko *et al.* (1971).

have shown that pacing-induced atrial tachycardia results in an increase in serum CPK activity after each increase in heart rate.

If the increases in infarct size produced by these interventions were in fact related to the increased myocardial oxygen needs induced by their application, then the opposite effect should be achieved with interventions that reduce myocardial oxygen consumption (Table II). Therefore, the influence of the administration of two β-adrenergic blocking agents, propranolol (Maroko *et al.,* 1971) and practolol (Libby *et al.,* 1973b), which exert such an effect, were studied and were found to decrease myocardial injury after coronary artery occlusion (Figs. 7 and 8). Using histologic techniques, Sommers and Jennings (1972) also observed smaller infarctions following coronary occlusion after pretreatment with

TABLE II

INTERVENTIONS THAT REDUCE MYOCARDIAL INJURY
FOLLOWING CORONARY ARTERY OCCLUSION

I. Decreasing myocardial oxygen requirements
   A. Propranolol[a]
   B. Practolol[a]
   C. Digitalis (in the failing heart)
   D. Counterpulsation
      1. Intraaortic balloon[a]
      2. External[a]
   E. Nitroglycerin[a]
   F. Decreasing afterload in patients with hypertension[a]
   G. Reducing intracellular free fatty acid levels
      1. Antilipolytic agents—β-pyridylcarbinol
      2. Lipid-free albumin infusions
      3. Glucose–insulin–potassium[a] (presumed)
II. Increasing myocardial oxygen supply
   A. Directly
      1. Coronary artery reperfusion[a]
      2. Elevating arterial pO_2[a]
      3. Thrombolytic agents
      4. Heparin[a] (presumed)
   B. Through collateral vessels
      1. Elevation of coronary perfusion pressure by methoxamine, neosynephrine, or norepinephrine
      2. Intraaortic balloon counterpulsation[a]
      3. External counterpulsation[a]
      4. Hyaluronidase[a]
   C. Increasing plasma osmolality
      1. Mannitol
      2. Hypertonic glucose
III. Augmenting anaerobic metabolism (presumed)
   A. Glucose–insulin–potassium[a]
   B. Hypertonic glucose
   C. I-Carnitine
   D. Sodium dichloroacetate
IV. Protecting against autolytic and heterolytic processes (presumed)
   A. Corticosteroids[a]
   B. Cobra venom factor
   C. Aprotinin

[a] Intervention has been applied to patients.

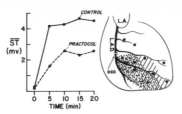

FIG. 7. *Left:* Average ST segment elevations in all sites ($\overline{ST}$) at various times after occlusion: ●———●, control occlusion; ●– – –●, occlusion after practolol. *Right:* Diagram of the heart showing the site of occlusion [occ], the area with ST segment elevation 15 minutes after control (diagonal lines) and after treatment (stippled area) of occlusions. L.A., left atrial appendage; L.A.D., left anterior descending coronary artery. Reproduced, with permission, from Libby *et al.* (1973).

propranolol, and, in recent experiments in our laboratory, Kloner has shown that β-adrenergic blockade reduces not only ischemic injury of myocardial cells, but microvascular injury as well (Kloner *et al.*, 1977b). Thus, in untreated dogs following coronary occlusion, electron microscopy showed swollen myocardial cells as well as endothelial gaps, blebs, and swelling. All these changes were reduced in propranolol-treated dogs.

Experiments by Mueller and associates in patients with acute myocardial infarction have shown that, while the infusion of iso-

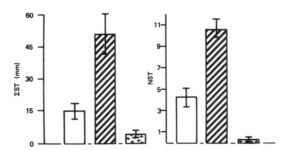

FIG. 8. Changes in average ΣST (left panel) and average NST (right panel) 15 minutes after occlusion alone (open bars), after occlusion during infusion of isoproterenol (hatched bars), and after occlusion after administration of propranolol (stippled bars) in closed-chest dogs. Brackets indicate $\pm$ 1 SEM. Reproduced, with permission, from Maroko *et al.* (1972d).

proterenol resulted in either increased lactate production or a shift from lactate extraction to production (Mueller *et al.,* 1970), the administration of propranolol shifted lactate production to extraction or increased lactate extraction (Mueller *et al.,* 1974). Thus, these clinical observations, which show the detrimental metabolic effect of isoproterenol and the beneficial effect of propranolol, also support the hypothesis that myocardial oxygen consumption is important in determining the outcome of myocardial tissue subjected to ischemia.

The effects of digitalis on the extent and magnitude of ischemic injury were then extended to studies in the failing heart (Watanabe *et al.,* 1972). Digitalis may reduce myocardial oxygen consumption in the failing heart by lowering wall tension consequent to the shortening of the ventricular radius, which overrides the increase in myocardial oxygen consumption resulting from increases in contractility. Thus, in the failing heart, digitalis reduced myocardial ischemic injury after coronary occlusion, even though the opposite effect had been observed in the nonfailing heart (Maroko *et al.,* 1971).

To study the importance of the oxygen supply to the ischemic myocardium, either hemorrhagic hypotension or arterial hypertension were induced after coronary occlusion (Maroko *et al.,* 1971). Arterial hypotension increased the area of myocardial ischemic injury, whereas raising arterial pressure by infusions of methoxamine or neosynephrine reduced myocardial ischemic injury. In these experiments the effect of arterial pressure on coronary blood flow and therefore on myocardial oxygen delivery appeared to be more important than the changes induced in myocardial oxygen demand as a consequence of altering wall tension. In addition, the inhalation of 40% oxygen significantly reduced electrocardiographic evidence of acute myocardial ischemic injury as well as the extent of subsequent myocardial necrosis (Maroko *et al.,* 1975a); the inhalation of 10% oxygen had the opposite effect (Fig. 9) (Radvany *et al.,* 1975b).

The effect of altering the balance between oxygen supply and demand by causing a redistribution of coronary blood flow was also studied with minoxidil and sodium nitroprusside, two potent vasodilators (Chiariello *et al.,* 1976; Radvany *et al.,* 1975a). Despite a marked increase in blood delivery to the nonischemic myocardium, the regional blood flow, both to the border zone and to the center of the ischemic zone, declined with both drugs. This effect caused an increase in ischemic injury, showing

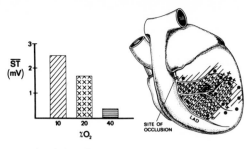

FIG. 9. An example of the effects of hyperoxia and hypoxia on acute myocardial ischemic injury. *Right:* Schematic representation of the heart and its arteries. The area with diagonal lines represents the area of ST segment elevation following coronary occlusion with FIO_2 of 0.10. The crosshatched area represents the area of injury with FIO_2 of 0.20. The area with horizontal lines represents the area of injury with FIO_2 of 0.40. *Left:* Average ST segment elevation ($\overline{ST}$) 15 minutes after occlusion with FIO_2 of 0.10 (diagonal lines), with FIO_2 of 0.20 (crosshatched bar), and with FIO_2 of 0.40 (horizontal lines).

the detrimental effect of this type of intervention. On the other hand, nitroglycerin was found to redistribute the flow to the ischemic area and thereby to reduce myocardial damage (Chiariello *et al.,* 1976).

Another more direct method of preserving myocardial cells would be to increase oxygen supply by restoring blood flow to the obstructed vessel (Maroko *et al.,* 1972e). This method not only is of theoretical importance, but is the basis of the surgical restoration of blood flow in patients with acute or impending myocardial infarction, Using the same method as that employed for the studies already discussed, and reperfusing the coronary artery 3 hours after occlusion, it was found that there was an acute and abrupt fall in ST segment elevation after the release of occlusion. Creatine phosphokinase activity and histological appearance both 24 hours (Maroko *et al.,* 1972e) and 7 days (Ginks *et al.,* 1972) later showed preservation of extensive portions of the myocardium otherwise expected to have lost their viability. In addition, ventricular function was investigated using radioopaque beads implanted in the inner third of the left ventricular wall (Ginks *et al.,* 1972), and the paradoxical movements of the ventricle, which were present after coronary occlusion, ceased or were reversed 0.5 hour after reperfusion. Thus, not only was there a reduction in myocardial damage anatomically, but the ultimate aim of restoring viable, normally functioning myocardium was achieved. It should be noted, however, that preliminary reports from several investigators, using different methods for assessing the viability of myocardial tissue after coronary artery reperfusion and after variable time intervals from the onset of coronary artery occlusion, have shown conflicting results. Indeed, in some studies reperfusion actually resulted in a hemorrhagic infarct, larger than would have been expected from simple coronary occlusion (Bresnahan *et al.*, 1974). Presumably, ischemic damage to the microvasculature can result in the extravasation of blood during reperfusion. Despite these deleterious results in some experiments, the clear-cut demonstration in others of myocardial salvage after several hours of ischemia indicate the clinical potential of myocardial salvage.

Another series of related experiments was performed using intraaortic balloon counterpulsation (Maroko *et al.*, 1972a). This intervention has the advantage of reducing the heart's need for oxygen while simultaneously increasing its supply (Braunwald *et al.*, 1969). As anticipated, with this intervention there was also a striking decrease in myocardial ischemic injury (Fig. 10).

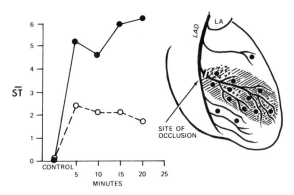

FIG. 10. *Left:* Average ST segment elevation ($\overline{\text{ST}}$) during occlusion alone (●———●) and during occlusion with counterpulsation (○– – –○). *Right:* Schematic representation of the heart, with circles (●) indicating sites where epicardial electrocardiograms were obtained. The area of ischemic injury after occlusion alone (S-T>2 mV) is depicted by the diagonally striped area, and during occlusion with counterpulsation by the stippled area. Note the reduction of the injured zone by counterpulsation. LA, = left atrial appendage; LAD, left anterior descending coronary artery. Reproduced, by permission, from Maroko *et al.* (1972a).

These experiments, taken as a group, showed that the balance between myocardial oxygen supply and demand is an important factor in
determining infarct size after coronary occlusion. They suggest that
tachycardia or arterial hypotension, or both, in a patient with an acute
coronary occlusion might extend the size of the ischemic zone and
thereby further impair left ventricular function, resulting in a vicious
cycle. They also point to the potential deleterious effects of the administration of positive inotropic agents such as isoproterenol, digitalis
glycosides, or glucagon to patients with acute myocardial infarction
without heart failure. All these positive inotropic agents augment
myocardial oxygen demands in the nonfailing heart, but do not necessarily exert such an effect in the presence of heart failure (Watanabe *et
al.*, 1972).

V. EFFECTS OF GLUCOSE–INSULIN–POTASSIUM

Analysis of the relationship between myocardial energy requirements
and supply was then extended to anaerobic myocardial metabolism.

FIG. 11. Representative photomicrographs from hematoxlin and eosin (H & E) sections (upper row, reduced from × 100) and oil red O fat-stained sections (lower row,
reduced from × 160). Insets in the panels on the upper row are epicardial ECG traces
obtained 15 minutes after occlusion from the same site from which the section shown in
the photomicrograph was obtained. Left-hand panels are H & E and oil red O-stained
sections obtained from a site without ST segment elevation. The myocardial fibers are
intact with oval nuclei and contain numerous cross striations. No fat granules are present
within the individual fibers. The middle panels are photomicrographs obtained from a site
with ST segment elevation from group 1 (occlusion alone). There is extensive fragmentation of the myocardial fibers and loss of the cross striations. The myocardial nuclei are
pyknotic and exhibit karyolysis, while an extensive polymorphonuclear cell infiltrate lies within the interstitial spaces. Oil red O fat stains demonstrate the presence of numerous massive
fat granules within the cytoplasm of most of the myocardial fibers undergoing ischemic
necrosis. Right-hand panels are photomicrographs obtained from a site with ST segment
elevation of the same magnitude as that in the middle column in a dog which had received
glucose–insulin–potassium infusion. The myocardial fibers are intact with normal cross
striations present. There is no evidence of fragmentation of the fibers or any cellular
infiltrate within the interstitial spaces. Glycogen stains of this section demonstrated the
presence of normal amounts of glycogen within the myocardial fibers. Oil red O stain
resembles the section observed in the control animal (lower left-hand panel) although an
occasional small fat granule is present within a myocardial fiber. Reproduced, by permission, from Maroko *et al.* (1972b).

Normally, the heart derives essentially all its energy from the oxidation of various substrates in the Krebs cycle; however, in the absence of oxygen, the myocardium possesses the capacity to derive significant quantities of energy from anaerobic glycolysis (Ballinger and Vollenweider, 1962). Experiments were therefore conducted to determine whether anaerobic glycolysis could provide sufficient energy to limit the extent of myocardial necrosis after coronary occlusion. It was reasoned that if the size of a myocardial infarct is dependent on the balance between the availability and the demand for the various compounds involved in energy production, then the anatomic and functional integrity of cardiac muscle might be preserved by increasing anaerobic glycolysis. Accordingly, the effects of the infusion of glucose–insulin–potassium and of hypertonic glucose alone were examined (Maroko *et*

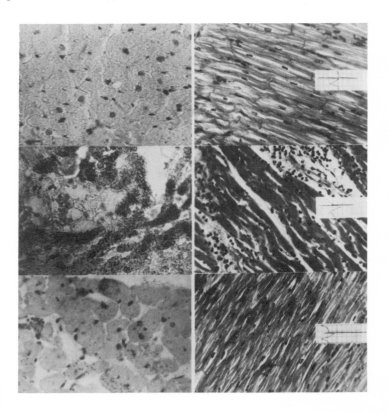

al., 1972b). It was found that, when administration was begun 30 minutes after coronary occlusion, glucose–insulin–potassium substantially decreased the quantity of necrosis, as reflected in CPK activity and histological as well as electron microscopic (Sybers *et al.,* 1973) appearance 24 hours later. A number of sites in the myocardium that were otherwise expected to develop necrosis, as predicted by ST segment elevation 15 minutes after occlusion, showed normal CPK activity 24 hours later, as a consequence of the administration of glucose–insulin–potassium. Furthermore, sites that were in the center of distribution of the occluded vessel and were expected to show very low CPK activity 24 hours later, exhibited only moderate reduction. This lesser depression of CPK activity was reflected in an altered regression line between the ST segment 15 minutes after occlusion and the CPK activity 24 hours later (Fig. 4). Histologically, 36% of biopsies expected to show signs of myocardial infarction 24 hours after occlusion were normal, substantiating the protective effect of the glucose–insulin–potassium mixture (Figs. 3 and 11). The beneficial effects of hypertonic glucose alone were similar to, but somewhat less marked than those of glucose–insulin–potassium.

VI. Effects of Hyaluronidase

Since hyaluronidase increases diffusion through the extracellular space and may thereby facilitate delivery of substrates to ischemic cells, its influence on the size of experimentally produced infarcts was also analyzed (Maroko *et al.,* 1972c). It was found in dogs with coronary occlusion that after the administration of this enzyme both the extent and magnitude of ST segment elevation were considerably reduced (Fig. 12). In related experiments, hyaluronidase, when administered 0.5 hour after coronary artery occlusion, decreased the depression of CPK activity predicted on the basis of ST segment elevation and also reduced the size of the infarct as evaluated histologically (Figs. 3 and 4). The sparing of CPK activity was similar in magnitude to that observed with glucose–insulin–potassium, as discussed above; in 45% of biopsies histologic examinations expected to show signs of myocardial infarction were normal as a consequence of the administration of hyaluronidase. In order to quantify directly the effects of hyaluronidase on infarct size after 2 and 21 days, without relying on electrophysiologic mea-

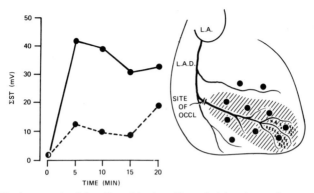

Fig. 12. An example of the effect of hyaluronidase administration on the sum of ST segment elevations (ΣST). *Right:* Schematic representation of the heart. Diagonally lined area = area of ST segment elevation 15 minutes after occlusion alone; crosshatched area = area of ST segment elevation 15 minutes after occlusion preceded by hyaluronidase administration; L.A., left atrium, L. A. D., left anterior descending coronary artery; SITE OF OCCL., site of occlusion; filled circles (●), sites where epicardial electrocardiograms were obtained. *Left:* Comparison between the sum of ST segment elevation (ΣST) in the same animal after the two occlusions. ●———●, ΣST just before and after the control occlusion; ●– – –●, ΣST just before and after occlusion with hyaluronidase pretreatment. Abscissa: Time in minutes after occlusion. Reproduced, by permission, from Maroko *et al.* (1972c).

surements, the left coronary artery was occluded in two groups of rats: they were either controls or received hyaluronidase shortly after coronary occlusion (Maclean *et al.,* 1976a). Infarct size was determined by planimetric measurements of histologic sections of serial slices of the left ventricle: after 2 days, infarct size averaged 52% of the left ventricle in control rats and significantly less, i.e., only 33%, in the hyaluronidase-treated rats, and after 21 days, infarct size was 38% in control rats and only 26% in the treated rats. In the second group of rats infarct size was calculated from total left ventricular CPK depression: after 2 days, infarct size in untreated rats averaged 50% of the left ventricle in the untreated animals and only 24% in the hyaluronidase-treated rats. Therefore, this enzyme clearly protects the ischemic myocardium from evolving to an irreversible phase of injury and subsequent necrosis. An important aspect of this investigation was the observation that myocardial tissue, otherwise destined to undergo necrosis, was permanently salvaged.

The precise mode of action of this enzyme in reducing infarct size is not known. However, it has been suggested that its action is based on its ability to depolymerize hyaluronic acid (Meyer, 1947; Hechter, 1950), to increase capillary permeability (Szabo and Magyar, 1958), and thereby to facilitate the transport of energy-producing substances from the blood stream through the interstitium to the myocardial cells. Using histochemical techniques and staining for hyaluronic acid (Alcian green and colloidal iron), it was observed that 24 hours after coronary occlusion the quantity of positively stained material in the interstitial space in the center of the infarct is clearly reduced by the administration of hyaluronidase. This observation is consistent with the hypothesis that hyaluronidase acts through its depolymerizing capabilities and demonstrates that hyaluronidase reaches the center of distribution of an occluded coronary artery. This action could be significant in the presence of coronary occlusion, when nutrients must be transported through longer extravascular pathways than when the coronary arteries are patent.

In other studies designed to study the mechanism by which hyaluronidase decreases myocardial injury after coronary artery occlusion, myocardial blood flow was determined using radiolabeled microspheres (Askenazi et al., 1977). Mean arterial pressure, heart rate, cardiac output, and flow in the nonischemic myocardium, both in the control (untreated) and the hyaluronidase-treated dogs, were similar 15 minutes and 6 hours after occlusion. Fifteen minutes after occlusion the flow to the ischemic myocardium in the two groups of dogs was similar. After 6 hours, flow in the ischemic zone fell in the untreated dogs. In contrast, hyaluronidase-treated dogs showed no fall in flow after 6 hours. Thus, salvage of ischemic myocardium by hyaluronidase may be explained by its beneficial effect on collateral blood flow to the injured area.

To obtain a further understanding of its mechanism of action, the nonperfused myocardium was examined by electron microscopy 3 hours after coronary occlusion (Kloner et al., 1977a). Morphometric analysis in untreated rats showed that 80% of myocardial cells and 49% of microvasculature had ischemic damage, while in hyaluronidase-treated rats only 50% of myocardial cells and 24% of the microvasculature exhibited ischemic changes. Thus, hyaluronidase protects the myocardium in the early phase of ischemia and also diminishes the damage to the microvasculature, which may result in improved collateral flow.

The administration of hyaluronidase offers several potential advantages compared with other interventions that reduce infarct size after experimental coronary occlusion: (1) Its application is simple and does not require any special equipment, as does intra-aortic balloon counterpulsation. (2) It does not depress cardiac contractility or cause hypotension, as does propranolol. (3) It does not have the intrinsic property of changing ST segments, as does glucose–insulin–potassium, and thus the electrocardiographic monitoring of ischemic injury may be used for monitoring the extent and severity of ischemic injury. (4) Most important, hyaluronidase has been widely used clinically, and its toxicity is extremely low. Allergic reactions are rare (0.08%), generally occurring only after frequent exposure, and may be avoided if a skin test is performed. Finally, in terms of effectiveness in reducing myocardial necrosis in the dog after coronary occlusion, hyaluronidase compared favorably with other interventions, such as propranolol and glucose–insulin–potassium.

VII. ANTI-INFLAMMATORY INTERVENTIONS

Following the initial damage caused directly by ischemia, many additional factors are responsible for myocardial cell injury. These include an increase in capillary permeability, interstitial edema, leukotaxis, phagocytosis, and nonspecific injury to cell membranes. Presumably, the boundary of the necrotic zone is defined not only by the ischemic stimulus per se, but also by many other influences that may result either in definite irreversible damage or the sparing of these cells in the border zone.

Accordingly, the influence of interventions that can limit these reactions have been examined. The activation of the complement system, which may occur during ischemic damage, releases leukotactic factors and may be responsible for increases in capillary permeability and interstitial edema, and complement may contribute substantially to the injury to cell membranes. Accordingly, the action of cobra venom factor, a protein that enzymically cleaves C3 and thus inhibits the action of the complement system, (Maroko and Carpenter, 1974; Maroko and

Braunwald, 1976). Also, the effects on infarct size of aprotinin, an inhibitor of the kallikrein system, have been studied, since activation of the kallikrein system also may enhance leukotactic activity, capillary permeability, interstitial edema, and proteolytic activity (Diaz and Maroko, 1975). Moreover, the effects of pharmacologic doses of glucocorticoids, which may stabilize lysosomal and other cellular membranes were also examined (Libby *et al.*, 1973a). All three of these interventions, i.e., cobra venom factor, aprotinin, and glucocorticoids, were shown to be beneficial, limiting substantially the extent of myocardial ischemic injury following experimental coronary artery occlusion in the dog. Preliminary studies in the rat model have shown their effectiveness as well (Maclean *et al.*, 1976b). It may be postulated that, by limiting the inflammatory responses of the organism to ischemic injury, additional damage of myocardial cells is avoided and thus the cells that are only reversibly damaged may recover, since the development of the collateral circulation occurs relatively soon following the ischemic stimulus provided by coronary occlusion.

VIII. Effects of Delayed Interventions

The direct clinical application of the above-cited interventions on infarct size might be limited to patients who had experienced an infarct under observation in hospitals or those who might be treated for impending myocardial infarction unless these interventions showed effects for several hours after coronary occlusion. It was found in a group of scattered observations that isoproterenol, propranolol, methoxamine, phenylephrine, norepinephrine (Maroko *et al.*, 1971), the combination of glucose–insulin–potassium and propranolol (Maroko *et al.*, 1972b), hydrocortisone (Libby *et al.*, 1973a), and intra-aortic balloon counterpulsation (Maroko *et al.*, 1972a) can change the extent and magnitude of myocardial ischemic injury when administered 3–6 hours after coronary occlusion. However, more systematic studies were recently carried out with hyaluronidase (Hillis *et al.*, 1977). When hyaluronidase was given 20 minutes, 3 hours, or 6 hours after coronary occlusion, myocardial salvage was reflected by less CPK depletion for any degree of ST segment elevation than was observed in control (untreated) dogs. However, this effect decreased progressively after coronary occlusion; when administered 9 hours after coronary occlusion, hyaluronidase had no detectable effect, suggesting irreversible injury at this time.

IX. CLINICAL OBSERVATIONS

One of the most formidable barriers to the clinical application of the information obtained in the laboratory is the lack of a suitable technique to assess the efficacy, or lack thereof, of these interventions. The ideal technique for assessing the effectiveness of interventions designed to protect injured but potentially salvageable myocardium in patients would be: (1) safe and noninvasive; (2) capable of predicting the extent of necrosis to be expected if no interventions were employed; (3) capable of assessing the extent of necrosis that actually develops; (4) capable of providing the data in items 2 and 3 accurately and in quantitative terms, i.e., in grams; (5) effective if applied immediately upon the patient's admission, so that the intervention under study can be promptly applied, since delay in treatment may be expected to reduce the population of injured cells that are salvageable; (6) relatively simple, easy to apply, and inexpensive, so that its use will not be limited to specialized centers; and (7) applicable to all patients with acute myocardial infarction. Items 2 and 3 are of particular importance, since they would allow each patient to be used as his own control.

One such technique is based on examining the rate of resolution of ST segment elevation in precordial leads. The interpretation of altered rates of resolution of ST segment elevations in patients by various modes of treatment will ultimately require correlation with other measurements of the size of the damaged region. One such measure that is readily available clinically is the QRS complex. A reduction in the electromotive force of the epicardial R wave within 4 hours of experimental coronary occlusion was first demonstrated by Wilson and his associates (Wilson *et al.,* 1933). Later it was demonstrated that a reduction in epicardial R wave voltage was found at sites where ischemia produced a mixture of viable and necrotic myocardium, as determined by histologic study (Shaw *et al.,* 1954).

To apply this method clinically, we would propose to use the precordial ST segment early after the onset of the clinical event as a predictor of the ultimate fate of the tissue, in a manner analogous to the epicardial ST segment in the experimental animal. This precordial ST segment, recorded soon after the clinical event, may then be compared to the changes in the QRS complex that occur subsequently, such as the development or deepening of Q waves and the reduction of R waves; these changes in the QRS complex could then be employed in a manner analogous to the alterations in CPK activity or histological appearance of the myocardium subjacent to the epicardial electrode in the experimental animal.

Recent experiments in our laboratory have confirmed the existence of a very close correlation between changes in the QRS complex of epicardial leads and of myocardial CPK activity (Hillis *et al.*, 1976). In these experiments, unipolar electrograms, recorded from 10–16 epicardial sites in open-chest dogs before occlusion and 15 minutes and 24 hours later, were analyzed for ST segment elevation and changes in Q and R waves. Transmural myocardial specimens were obtained 24 hours after occlusion from the same sites at which the ECGs had been recorded. Both in control (untreated) dogs and in the hyaluronidase-treated dogs, the development of Q waves, the fall in R waves, and their combination ($\Delta R + \Delta Q$) at 24 hours correlated well with the final depression of myocardial creative phosphokinase activity depression. In addition ($\Delta R + \Delta Q$) correlated well with the extent of necrosis present on histologic examination (Fig. 13). From these investigations it is concluded that (1) Q-wave development and R-wave fall 24 hours after occlusion accurately reflect myocardial necrosis, as measured by CPK activity and by histologic appearance; (2) ST segment elevation 15 minutes after occlusion predicts subsequent changes in Q and R waves; (3) hyaluronidase and propranolol, agents shown by a variety of other techniques to reduce myocardial necrosis following coronary artery occlusion, can be detected by a diminution in the changes in QRS morphology (i.e., less Q-wave development and smaller fall in R-wave voltage).

This method of electrocardiographic mapping can be adapted for clinical use by utilizing ST segment elevation in the precordial leads, when the patient is first admitted to the Coronary Care Unit, as a predictor of the ultimate fate of the myocardium, in a manner analogous to that of the epicardial ST segment in the experimental animal. The evolution of the QRS complex in those leads which demonstrate initial ST segment elevation can then be compared in a control and a treated group of patients. These precordial QRS changes can be used in place of the analysis of changes in CPK activity and histologic appearance of myocardial specimens (Askenasi *et al.*, 1975).

The analysis of changes in the QRS complex, if applied to multiple precordial leads, potentially fulfills five of the seven aforementioned criteria for assessing the efficacy of interventions designed to protect the ischemic myocardium. Although it is *not* capable of expressing the mass

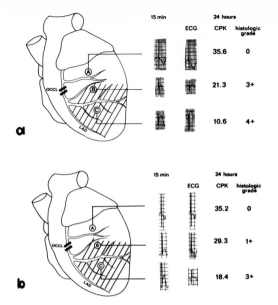

FIG 13. (a) *Left:* A schematic representation of the heart and its arteries. The left anterior descending (LAD) was occluded at its midpoint (OCCL). Diagonal lines indicate the zone of ST segment elevation 15 minutes after occlusion. *Right:* Examples of epicardial electrograms, myocardial creatine phosphokinase (CPK) values (in IU/mg protein), and histologic grades from a control dog. Site A (from nonischemic myocardium) exhibited no ST segment elevation at 15 minutes. At 24 hours it had no changes in QRS configuration and normal CPK activity, and it appeared normal histologically. Site B (border zone) showed moderate ST_{15m} while at 24 hours there was a significant Q wave and partial loss of R wave voltage. The CPK activity was moderately depressed, and the histologic section was graded 3+ (51–75%) necrosis. Site C (center of the ischemic zone) had marked ST_{15m}, and at 24 hours it demonstrated a total loss of R wave with a QS complex. The myocardial CPK activity was greatly depressed, and the histologic section was graded 4+ (>75%) necrosis.

(b) Examples of epicardial electrograms, myocardial CPK activity, and histologic grades in a dog which received hyaluronidase 20 minutes after occlusion. Site A (from nonischemic myocardium) exhibited no ST segment elevation at 15 minutes, and at 24 hours there were no changes in QRS configuration. The myocardial CPK was normal, and the specimen appeared normal histologically. Site B (border zone) showed moderate ST_{15m}; at 24 hours, the specimen did not exhibit the expected loss of CPK activity, was graded 1+ (1–25% necrosis) histologically, and did not show extensive changes in QRS configuration, indicating that hyaluronidase acted to reduce necrosis in the border zone. Site C (center of the ischemic zone) had marked ST_{15m}, while at 24 hours the QRS configuration and CPK activity were moderately altered; the histologic section was graded 3+ (51–75% ncrosis). Note, in comparing sites B and C in this figure with those in Fig. 13A, that for similar degrees of ST segment elevation, hyaluronidase reduces necrosis, as measured electrically (QRS complex), biochemically (CPK activity), and histologically. Reproduced, by permission, from Hillis *et al.* (1976).

of infarcted myocardium in quantitative terms, and its use is restricted to patients with anterior or lateral transmural myocardial infarctions, this method (1) is safe and atraumatic; (2) can predict the extent of necrosis to be expected at a time when much of the myocardial injury is still in a reversible phase (ST segment elevations); (3) is capable of assessing the extent of necrosis that actually develops (QRS changes); (4) can be applied immediately and need not delay therapy; and (5) is simple to apply, easy to interpret, and inexpensive. These advantages support the use of precordial QRS mapping for clinical studies of interventions designed to limit infarct size in man.

In view of the apparent lack of toxicity of hyaluronidase and the impressive experimental results with this agent, a pilot study was undertaken to examine its effectiveness in patients with acute myocardial infarction (Maroko et al., 1975b). Twenty-four patients who had suffered a typical transmural myocardial infarction, as determined by history, enzyme changes and electrocardiographic criteria, were studied. The 11 patients who did not receive hyaluronidase served as control subjects, and the 13 patients who received the drug constituted the experimental group. Although these patients were not assigned to one of the two groups in a randomized manner and the design of the study was not blind, there was no attempt to preselect the patients on the basis of the severity of their disease. All patients had acute myocardial infarction involving the anterior or lateral walls of the left ventricle, and the onset of chest pain occurred less than 8 hours before the beginning of the study. Patients more than 75 years of age and others with disease of kidney or liver, pregnancy, neoplasms, or infections were excluded. Patients received hyaluronidase, 500 National Formulary units per kilogram intravenously in a bolus injection, followed by additional identical doses at 2 and 6 hours, and then every 6 hours until 42 hours after the initial dose.

The precordial electrocardiograms were recorded with 35 unipolar leads (Maroko et al., 1972d). The precordial leads were in a fixed position in a blanket covering the precordium distributed in five rows of seven electrodes each. Average levels of ΣST and of the number of electrodes showing ST elevations greater than 1 mm (NST) before administration of hyaluronidase in this group were not statistically different from values in the control group. However, at all times after treatment with hyaluronidase, average ST and NST were significantly lower ($P < 0.05$) than in the control group (Figs. 14 and 15).

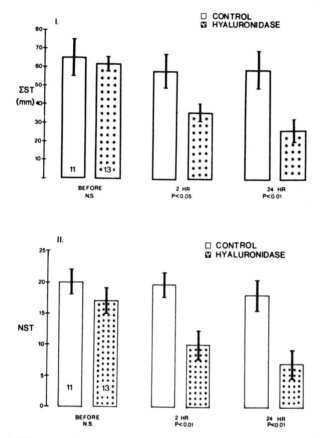

Fig. 14. The sum of ST segment elevations (ΣST) in control patients and in hyaluronidase-treated patients at zero time (before treatment), and at 2 and 24 hours after treatment. Note that before treatment both groups had similar values of ΣST. However, in the treated, ΣST dropped significantly more rapidly than in the control group. Panel II: Number of electrodes showing ST segment elevations exceeding 1 mm (NST) in control patients and in hyaluronidase-treated patients at zero time (before treatment), and at 2 and 24 hours after treatment. Note that before treatment both groups had similar values of NST. However, in the treated group NST dropped significantly more rapidly than in the control group. Reproduced, with permission, from Maroko *et al.* (1975b).

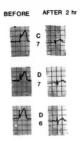

FIG 15. Three leads from a 35-lead precordial map in a patient with acute myocardial infarction showing ST segment elevations in these leads before hyaluronidase administration (left) and the striking reduction in ST segment elevation 2 hours after its administration (right). Reproduced, by permission, from Maroko *et al.* (1975b).

The results of this investigation showed that the reduction in the magnitude and extent of ST segment elevations was greater in the group treated with hyaluronidase than in the control group at various times during the 24 hours after treatment. This more rapid decline in the electrocardiographic indexes of injury was already evident 2 hours after drug administration. Also, although several patients in the untreated control group demonstrated an increase in ST segment elevation in sequential electrocardiograms, suggesting an extension of the infarction, this situation did not occur in any of the hyaluronidase-treated patients. Therefore, on the basis of studies in experimentally produced coronary occlusion, we suggest that this reduction in acute myocardial ischemic injury produced by hyaluronidase may reflect a reduction in the quantity of myocardium that eventually becomes necrotic.

In a subsequent study, which is still ongoing and is being caried out in a separate group of patients, the effects of a similar regimen of administration of hyaluronidase on the development of Q waves in 35 precordial electrocardiographic leads was examined (Maroko *et al.*, 1977). Preliminary results indicate that in 39 control (untreated) patients with acute anterior myocardial infarction significant changes in the QRS complex indicative of myocardial necrosis developed within 5 days in 72.4% of leads with ST segment elevation of 0.15 mV of more. Also, the sum of R-wave heights (ΣR) fell by 70.3% in these leads within the same time interval. In 39 hyaluronidase-treated patients these two indexes were both reduced significantly, to 59.3% and 55.8%, respectively ($P < 0.025$).

When they are all considered together, the observations on the effects of hyaluronidase on the extent of myocardial necrosis in dogs (Maroko *et al.*, 1972c) and rats (Maclean *et al.*, 1976a) with experimentally produced coronary occlusion, the two pilot clinical trials demonstrating the effects of this agent on the rate of resolution of abnormally elevated precordial ST segments (Maroko *et al.*, 1975b), and the development of electrocardiographic changes indicative of necrosis in the QRS complex (Maroko *et al.*, 1977), all suggest that this agent may be effective in reducing the quantity of myocardium that eventually becomes necrotic after coronary occlusion. Its low level of toxicity and its ease of administration suggest that expanded and rigorous clinical trials with hyaluronidase should now be undertaken.

A number of other pilot studies in patients with acute myocardial infarction have supported the hope that significant myocardium can be salvaged by the application of an intervention several hours after the clinical event (Table II). A number of agents, including propranolol (Gold *et al.*, 1976), oxygen (Madias *et al.*, 1976), nitroglycerin (Borer *et al.*, 1975; Come *et al.*, 1975; Flaherty *et al.*, 1975), and glucose–insulin–potassium (Russell *et al.*, 1976), appear to be efficacious in limiting ischemic injury in patients whose therapy is begun several hours after the onset of symptoms. Although the results of these pilot studies are encouraging and exciting, the overall clinical utility of interventions designed to limit myocardial necrosis can be assessed only through carefully and rigorously conducted clinical trials.

Recognition of the importance of the mass of myocardium undergoing necrosis as a determinant of prognosis and the efforts to preserve ischemic tissue may drastically alter the therapeutic approach to acute myocardial infarction. Rather than simply maintaining the patient's vital signs, the physician may now direct his attention toward preseving the myocardium as well as maintaining perfusion of peripheral organs. However, these two objectives may sometimes conflict. In the first hours following the onset of the clinical event, while the ultimate size of the infarct is not yet established, myocardial preservation might be given the highest priority. Later, once the size of the infarct is fixed and if heart failure supervenes, it may be more appropriate to stimulate the heart with positive inotropic agents and to reduce afterload, i.e., to employ interventions that may increase infarct size if given at an earlier time.

Recent observations by Reid *et al.* (1974) suggest that significant extensions of myocardial necrosis occur during apparently uneventful convalescence in a large fraction of patients with acute myocardial infarction. Also, in many patients previously classified as having acute myocardial infarction, tissue damage occurs in a slow, "stuttering" manner, rather than abruptly, a condition that might more properly be termed subacute infarction. These considerations greatly expand the horizon for what can be accomplished by techniques to prevent myocardial necrosis, since the interventions designed to limit infarct size could then be applied prophylactically, when they are most likely to be effective. The interesting observation by Cox *et al.* (1976) that the incidence of ventricular arrhythmia is a function of the size of the infarct, adds yet another dimension to the benefit that can potentially be derived from protection of jeopardized myocardium.

It is not possible, at present, to identify the specific intervention likely to be most effective in reducing infarct size. Indeed, there may not be a single treatment; rather, it seems more likely that, in the future, patients will be carefully but rapidly subdivided and categorized according to their clinical, electrocardiographic, hemodynamic, and perhaps coronary arteriographic findings, and the intervention will be tailored appropriately. For example, in hypertensive patients, afterload reduction may be effective; in patients without any evidence of myocardial depression, cardiospecific β-adrenergic blockade may be the treatment of choice; in normotensive or hypotensive patients with pump failure, circulatory support may be in order. All patients with acute infarction, regardless of their hemodynamic state, may benefit from the administration of an anti-inflammatory agent, such as aprotinin, or from a drug such as hyaluronidase.

Acute myocardial infarction continues to be the most common cause of death in the United States today, and, of those patients who survive the infarct, the quantity of viable, contractile myocardium with which they are left is critical to their well being. Considering the frequency of ischemic heart disease, the potential benefits from interventions designed to salvage ischemic tissue, and the encouraging preliminary results obtained thus far, continued intensive research in this field appears to be especially desirable.

ACKNOWLEDGMENT

The important contributions of Dr. Peter R. Maroko to this work are gratefully acknowledged.

REFERENCES

Angell, C. S., Lakatta, E. G., Weisfeldt, M. L., and Shock, N. W. (1975). *Cardiovasc. Res.* **9**, 12–18.

Askenazi, J., Dye, R., Hubbard, F., Lesch, M., Braunwald, E., and Maroko, P. R. (1975). *Circulation* **52**, Suppl. 2, 423 (Abstr.).

Askenazi, J., Hillis, L. D., Diaz, P. E., Davis, M. A., Braunwald, E., and Maroko, P. R. (1977). *Circ. Res.* **40**, 566–571.

Ballinger, W. F., II, and Vollenweider, H. (1962). *Circ. Res.* **11**, 681–685.

Becker, L. C., Ferreira, R., and Thomas, M. (1973). *Cardiovasc. Res.* **7**, 391–400.

Borer, J. S., Redwood, D. R., Levitt, B., Cagin, N., Bianchi, C., Vallin, H., and Epstein, S. E. (1975). *N. Engl. J. Med.* **293**, 1008–1012.

Braunwald, E. (1967). *Johns Hopkins Med. J.* **121**, 421–429.

Braunwald, E. (1969). *Physiologist* **12**, 65–93.

Braunwald, E. (1971). *Am. J. Cardiol.* **27**, 416–432.

Braunwald, E. (1974). *N. Engl. J. Med.* **290**, 1124–1129, 1420–1425.

Braunwald, E., ed. (1976). "Symposium on Protection of the Ischemic Myocardium." *Circulation* **53**, Suppl. 3, 1–217.

Braunwald, E., and Maroko, P. R. (1976). Editorial. *Circulation* **54**, 529–532.

Braunwald, E., Epstein, S. E., Glick, G., Wechsler, A., and Braunwald, N. S. (1967). *N. Engl. J. Med.* **277**, 1278–1283.

Braunwald, E., Covell, J. W., Maroko, P. R., and Ross, J., Jr. (1969). *Circulation* **40**, Suppl. 4, 220–228.

Bresnahan, G. F., Roberts, R., Shell, W. E., Ross, J., Jr., and Sobel, B. E. (1974). *Am. J. Cardiol.* **33**, 82–86.

Capone, R. J., Most, A. S., and Sydlik, P. A. (1975). *Chest* **67**, 577–582.

Chiariello, M., Gold, H. K., Leinbach, R. C., Davis, M. A., and Maroko, P. R. (1976). *Circulation* **54**, 766–773.

Cohen, D., and Kaufman, L. A. (1975). *Circu. Res.* **36**, 414–424.

Come, P., Flaherty, J. T., Weisfeldt, M. L., Greene, L., Becker, L., and Pitt, B. (1975). *N. Engl. J. Med.* **293**, 1003–1007.

Cox, J. L., McLaughlin, V. W., Flowers, N. C., and Horan, L. G. (1968). *Am. Heart J.* **76**, 650.

Cox, J. R., Jr., Roberts, R., Ambox, H. D., Oliver, C., and Sobel, B. E. (1976). *Circulation* **53**, Suppl. 1, 150–155.

Diaz, P. E., and Maroko, P. R. (1975). *Clin. Res.* **23**, 108A (Abstr.).

Eyster, J. A. E., Meek, W. J., Goldberg, H., and Gilson, W. E. (1938). *Am. J. Physiol.* **125**, 717–728.

Flaherty, J. T., Reid, P. R., Kelly, D. T., Taylor, D. R., Weisfeldt, M. L., and Pitt, B. (1975). *Circulation* **51**, 132–139.

Ginks, W. R., Sybers, H. D., Maroko, P. R., Covell, J. W., Sobel, B. E., and Ross, J., Jr. (1972). *J. Clin. Invest.* **51**, 2717–2723.

Gold, H. K., Leinbach, R. C., and Maroko, P. R. (1976). *Am. J. Cardiol.* **38,** 689–695.

Harnarayan, C., Bennett, M. S., Pentecost, B. L., and Brewer, D. B. (1970). *Br. Heart J.* **32,** 728.

Hechter, O. (1950). *Ann. N. Y. Acad. Sci.* **52,** 1028–1040.

Hillis, L. D., Askenazi, J., Braunwald, E., Radvany, P., Muller, J. E., Fishbein, M. C., and Maroko, P. R. (1976). *Circulation* **54,** 591–598.

Hillis, L. D., Fishbein, M. C., Braunwald, E., and Maroko, P. R. (1977). *Circ. Res.* **41,** 26–31.

Karlsson, J., Templeton, G. H., and Willerson, J. T. (1973). *Circ. Res.* **32,** 725–730.

Khuri, S. F., Flaherty, J. T., O'Riordan, J. B., Pitt, B., Brawley, R. L., Donahoo, J. W., and Gott, V. L. (1975). *Circ. Res.* **37,** 455–464.

Klocke, F. J., Braunwald, E., and Ross, J., Jr. (1966). *Circ. Res.* **18,** 357–365.

Koner, R. A., Fishbein, M. C., Maclean, D., Braunwald, E., and Maroko, P. R. (1977a). *Am. J. Cardiol.* **40,** 43–49.

Kloner, R. A., Fishbein, M. C., Cotran, R. S., Braunwald, E., and Maroko, P. R. (1977b). *Circulation* **55,** 872–880.

Libby, P., Maroko, P. R., Bloor, C. M., Sobel, B. E., and Braunwald, E. (1973a). *J. Clin. Invest.* **52,** 599–607.

Libby, P., Maroko, P. R., Covell, J. W., Malloch, C. I., Ross, J., Jr., and Braunwald, E. (1973b). *Cardiovasc. Res.* **7,** 167–173.

Maclean, D., Fishbein, M. C., Maroko, P. R., and Braunwald, E. (1976a). *Science* **194,** 199–200.

Maclean, D., Maroko, P. R., Fishbein, M. C., Carpenter, C. B., and Braunwald, E. (1976b). *Circulation* **54,** Suppl. 2, 628.

Madias, J. E., Madias, N. E., and Hood, W. B., Jr. (1976). *Circulation* **53,** 411–417.

Maroko, P. R., and Braunwald, E. (1973). *Ann. Intern. Med.* **79,** 720–733.

Maroko, P. R., and Braunwald, E. (1976). *In* "Experimental and Clinical Aspects on Preservation of the Ischemic Myocardium," (A. Hjalmarson and L. Werko, eds.), pp. 125–136. Molndal, Sweden.

Maroko, P. R., and Carpenter, C. B. (1974). *Clin. Res.* **22,** 289A (Abstr.).

Maroko, P. R., Kjekshus, J. K., Sobel, B. E., Watanabe, T., Covell, J. W., Ross, J., Jr., and Braunwald, E. (1971). *Circulation* **43,** 67–82.

Maroko, P. R., Bernstein, E. F., Libby, P., DeLaria, G. A., Covell, J. W., Ross, J., Jr., and Braunwald, E. (1972a). *Circulation* **45,** 1150–1159.

Maroko, P. R., Libby, P., Sobel, B. E., Bloor, C. M., Sybers, H. D., Shell, W. E., Covell, J. W., and Braunwald, E. (1972b). *Circulation* **45,** 1160–1175.

Maroko, P. R., Libby, P., Bloor, C. M., Sobel, B. E., and Braunwald, E. (1972c). *Circulation* **46,** 430–437.

Maroko, P. R., Libby, P., Covell, J. W., Sobel, B. E., Ross, J., Jr., and Braunwald, E. (1972d). *Am. J. Cardiol.* **29,** 223–230.

Maroko, P. R., Libby, P., Ginks, W. R., Bloor, C. M., Shell, W. E., Sobel, B. E., and Ross, J., Jr. (1972e). *J. Clin. Invest.* **51,** 2710–2716.

Maroko, P. R., Davidson, D. M., Libby, P., Hagan, A. D., and Braunwald, E. (1975). *Ann. Intern. Med.* **82,** 516–520.

Maroko, P. R., Radvany, P., Braunwald, E., and Hale, S. L. (1975). *Circulation* **52,** 360–368.

Maroko, P. R., Hillis, L. D., Miller, J. E., Tavazzi, L., Heyndrickx, G. R., Ray, M., Chiariello, M., Distante, A., Askenazi, J., Salerno, J., Carpentier, J., Reshetnaya, N. I., Radvany, P., Libby, P., Raabe, D. S., Chazov, E. I., Bobba, P., and Braunwald, E. (1977). *N. Engl. J. Med.* **296,** 898–903.

Meyer, K. (1947). *Physiol. Rev.* **27,** 335–359.

Mueller, H. S., Ayers, S. M., Gregory, J. J., Giannelli, S., Jr., and Grace, W. J. (1970). *J. Clin. Invest.* **49,** 1885–1902.

Mueller, H. S., Ayres, S. M., Religa, A., and Evans, R. G. (1974). *Circulation* **49,** 1078–1087.

Muller, J. E., Maroko, P. R., and Braunwald, E. (1975). *Circulation* **52,** 16–27.

Nahum, L. H., Hamilton, W. F., and Heff, H. E. (1943). *Am. J. Physiol.* **139,** 202–207.

Page, D. L., Caulfield, J. B., Kastor, J. A., DeSanctis, R. W., and Sanders, C. A. (1971). *N. Engl. J. Med.* **285,** 133.

Radvany, P., Davis, M. A., Muller, J. E., and Maroko, P. R. (1975a). *Clin. Res.* **23,** 203A (Abstr.).

Radvany, P., Maroko, P. R., and Braunwald, E. (1975b). *Am. J. Cardiol.* **35,** 795–800.

Redwood, D. R., Smith, E. R., and Epstein, S. E. (1972). *Circulation* **46,** 323.

Reid, P. R., Taylor, D. R., Kelly, D. T., Weisfeldt, M. L., Humphries, J. O., Ross, R. S., and Pitt, B. (1974). *N. Engl. J. Med.* **290,** 123–128.

Rodbard, S., Williams, C. B., Rodbard, D., and Berglund, E. (1964). *Circ. Res.* **14,** 139.

Ross, J., Jr., Sonnenblick, E. H., Kaiser, G. A., Frommer, P. L., and Braunwald, E. (1965). *Circ. Res.* **16,** 332.

Russell, R. O., Jr., Rogers, W. J., Mantle, J. A., McDaniel, H. G., and Rackley, C. E. (1976). *Circulation* **53,** Suppl. 1, 207–209.

Samson, W. E., and Scher, A. M. (1960). *Circ. Res.* **8,** 780–787.

Sarnoff, S. J., Braunwald, E., Welch, G. H., Jr., Case, R. B., Stainsby, W. N., and Macruz, R. (1958). *Am. J. Physiol.* **192,** 148–156.

Sayen, J. J., Peirce, G., Katcher, A. H., and Sheldon, W. F. (1973). *Circ. Res.* **32,** 725–730.

Scheuer, J., and Brachfeld, M. (1966). *Circ. Res.* **18,** 178–189.

Shaw, C. McK., Jr., Goldman, A., Kennamer, R., Kimura, N., Lindgren, I., Maxwell, M. H., and Prinzmetal, M. (1954). *Am. J. Med.* **16,** 490.

Shell, W. E., and Sobel, B. E. (1973). *Am. J. Cardiol.* **31,** 474–479.

Sobel, B. E., Bresnahan, G. F., Shell, W. E., and Yoder, R. D. (1972). *Circulation* **46,** 640–648.

Somerville, W., and Kevin, S. A. (1950). *Br. Heart J.* **12,** 245.

Sommers, H. M., and Jennings, R. B. (1972). *Arch. Intern. Med.* **129,** 780–789.

Sonnenblick, E. H., Ross, J., Jr., Covell, J. W., Kaiser, G. A., and Braunwald, E. (1965). *Am. J. Physiol.* **209,** 919.

Sybers, H. D., Maroko, P. R., Ashraf, M., Libby, P., and Braunwald, E. (1973). *Am. J. Pathol.* **70,** 401–420.

Szabo, G., and Magyar, S. (1958). *Nature (London)* **182,** 377–379.

Watanabe, T., Covell, J. W., Maroko, P. R., Braunwald, E., and Ross, J., Jr. (1972). *Am. J. Cardiol.* **30,** 371–377.

Wegria, R., Segers, M., Keating, R. P., and Ward, H. P. (1949). *Am. Heart J.* **38,** 90–96.

Wilson, F. N., MacLeod, A. G., Barker, P. S., Johnston, F. D., and Klostermeyer, L. L. (1933). *Heart* **16,** 155.

Wolfson, S., Heinle, R. A., Herman, M. V., *et al.* (1966). *Am. J. Cardiol.* **18,** 345.

FORMER OFFICERS OF THE HARVEY SOCIETY

1905–1906

President: GRAHAM LUSK
Vice-President: SIMON FLEXNER
Treasurer: FREDERIC S. LEE
Secretary: GEORGE B. WALLACE

Council:
   C. A. HERTER
   S. J. MELTZER
   EDWARD K. DUNHAM

1906–1907

President: GRAHAM LUSK
Vice-President: SIMON FLEXNER
Treasurer: FREDERIC S. LEE
Secretary: GEORGE B. WALLACE

Council:
   C. A. HERTER
   S. J. MELTZER
   JAMES EWING

1907–1908

President: GRAHAM LUSK
Vice-President: JAMES EWING
Treasurer: EDWARD K. DUNHAM
Secretary: GEORGE B. WALLACE

Council:
   SIMON FLEXNER
   THEO. C. JANEWAY
   PHILIP H. HISS, JR.

1908–1909

President: JAMES EWING
Vice-President: SIMON FLEXNER
Treasurer: EDWARD K. DUNHAM
Secretary: FRANCIS C. WOOD

Council:
   GRAHAM LUSK
   S. J. MELTZER
   ADOLPH MEYER

1909–1910*

President: JAMES EWING
Vice-President: THEO. C. JANEWAY
Treasurer: EDWARD K. DUNHAM
Secretary: FRANCIS C. WOOD

Council:
   GRAHAM LUSK
   S. J. MELTZER
   W. J. GIES

1910–1911

President: SIMON FLEXNER
Vice-President: JOHN HOWLAND
Treasurer: EDWARD K. DUNHAM
Secretary: HAVEN EMERSON

Council:
   GRAHAM LUSK
   S. J. MELTZER
   JAMES EWING

---

*At the Annual Meeting of May 18, 1909, these officers were elected. In publishing the 1909–1910 volume their names were omitted, possibly because in that volume the custom of publishing the names of the incumbents of the current year was changed to publishing the names of the officers selected for the ensuing year.

1911–1912

President: S. J. MELTZER
Vice-President: FREDERIC S. LEE
Treasurer: EDWARD K. DUNHAM
Secretary: HAVEN EMERSON

Council:
GRAHAM LUSK
JAMES EWING
SIMON FLEXNER

1912–1913

President: FREDERIC S. LEE
Vice-President: WM. H. PARK
Treasurer: EDWARD K. DUNHAM
Secretary: HAVEN EMERSON

Council:
GRAHAM LUSK
S. J. MELTZER
WM. G. MACCALLUM

1913–1914

President: FREDERIC S. LEE
Vice-President: WM. G. MACCALLUM
Treasurer: EDWARD K. DUNHAM
Secretary: AUGUSTUS B. WADSWORTH

Council:
GRAHAM LUSK
WM. H. PARK
GEORGE B. WALLACE

1914–1915

President: WM. G. MACCALLUM
Vice-President: RUFUS I. COLE
Treasurer: EDWARD K. DUNHAM
Secretary: JOHN A. MANDEL

Council:
GRAHAM LUSK
FREDERIC S. LEE
W. T. LONGCOPE

1915–1916

President: GEORGE B. WALLACE*
Treasurer: EDWARD K. DUNHAM
Secretary: ROBERT A. LAMBERT

Council:
GRAHAM LUSK
RUFUS I. COLE
NELLIS B. FOSTER

1916–1917

President: GEORGE B. WALLACE
Vice-President: RUFUS I. COLE
Treasurer: EDWARD K. DUNHAM
Secretary: ROBERT A. LAMBERT

Council:
GRAHAM LUSK†
W. T. LONGCOPE
S. R. BENEDICT
HANS ZINSSER

1917–1918

President: EDWARD K. DUNHAM
Vice-President: RUFUS I. COLE
Treasurer: F. H. PIKE
Secretary: A. M. PAPPENHEIMER

Council:
GRAHAM LUSK
GEORGE B. WALLACE
FREDERIC S. LEE
PEYTON ROUS

---

*Dr. William G. MacCallum resigned after election. On Doctor Lusk's motion Doctor George B. Wallace was made President—no Vice-President was appointed.

†Doctor Lusk was made Honorary permanent Counsellor.

1918–1919

President: GRAHAM LUSK
Vice-President: RUFUS I. COLE
Treasurer: F. H. PIKE
Secretary: K. M. VOGEL

Council:
GRAHAM LUSK
JAMES W. JOBLING
FREDERIC S. LEE
JOHN AUER

1919–1920

President: WARFIELD T. LONGCOPE
Vice-President: S. R. BENEDICT
Treasurer: F. H. PIKE
Secretary: K. M. VOGEL

Council:
GRAHAM LUSK
HANS ZINSSER
FREDERIC S. LEE
GEORGE B. WALLACE

1920–1921*

President: WARFIELD T. LONGCOPE
Vice-President: S. R. BENEDICT
Treasurer: A. M. PAPPENHEIMER
Secretary: HOMER F. SWIFT

Council:
GRAHAM LUSK
FREDERIC S. LEE
HANS ZINSSER
GEORGE B. WALLACE

1921–1922

President: RUFUS I. COLE
Vice-President: S. R. BENEDICT
Treasurer: A. M. PAPPENHEIMER
Secretary: HOMER F. SWIFT

Council:
GRAHAM LUSK
HANS ZINSSER
H. C. JACKSON
W. T. LONGCOPE

1922–1923

President: RUFUS I. COLE
Vice-President: HANS ZINSSER
Treasurer: CHARLES C. LIEB
Secretary: HOMER F. SWIFT

Council:
GRAHAM LUSK
W. T. LONGCOPE
H. C. JACKSON
S. R. BENEDICT

1923–1924

President: EUGENE F. DUBOIS
Vice-President: HOMER F. SWIFT
Treasurer: CHARLES C. LIEB
Secretary: GEORGE M. MACKENZIE

Council:
GRAHAM LUSK
ALPHONSE R. DOCHEZ
DAVID MARINE
PEYTON ROUS

---

*These officers were elected at the Annual Meeting of May 21, 1920 but were omitted in the publication of the 1919–1920 volume.

1924–1925

President: EUGENE F. DUBOIS
Vice-President: PEYTON ROUS
Treasurer: CHARLES C. LIEB
Secretary: GEORGE M. MACKENZIE

Council:
  GRAHAM LUSK
  RUFUS COLE
  HAVEN EMERSON
  WM. H. PARK

1925–1926

President: HOMER F. SWIFT
Vice-President: H. B. WILLIAMS
Treasurer: HAVEN EMERSON
Secretary: GEORGE M. MACKENZIE

Council:
  GRAHAM LUSK
  EUGENE F. DUBOIS
  WALTER W. PALMER
  H. D. SENIOR

1926–1927

President: WALTER W. PALMER
Vice-President: WM. H. PARK
Treasurer: HAVEN EMERSON
Secretary: GEORGE M. MACKENZIE

Council:
  GRAHAM LUSK
  HOMER F. SWIFT
  A. R. DOCHEZ
  ROBERT CHAMBERS

1927–1928

President: DONALD D. VAN SLYKE
Vice-President: JAMES W. JOBLING
Treasurer: HAVEN EMERSON
Secretary: CARL A. L. BINGER

Council:
  GRAHAM LUSK
  RUSSEL L. CECIL
  WARD J. MACNEAL
  DAVID MARINE

1928–1929

President: PEYTON ROUS
Vice-President: HORATIO B. WILLIAMS
Treasurer: HAVEN EMERSON
Secretary: PHILIP D. MCMASTER

Council:
  GRAHAM LUSK
  ROBERT CHAMBERS
  ALFRED F. HESS
  H. D. SENIOR

1929–1930

President: G. CANBY ROBINSON
Vice-President: ALFRED F. HESS
Treasurer: HAVEN EMERSON
Secretary: DAYTON J. EDWARDS

Council:
  GRAHAM LUSK
  ALFRED E. COHN
  A. M. PAPPENHEIMER
  H. D. SENIOR

1930–1931

President: ALFRED E. COHN
Vice-President: J. G. HOPKINS
Treasurer: HAVEN EMERSON
Secretary: DAYTON J. EDWARDS

Council:
  GRAHAM LUSK
  O. T. AVERY
  A. M. PAPPENHEIMER
  S. R. DETWILER

1931–1932

President: J. W. JOBLING
Vice-President: HOMER W. SMITH
Treasurer: HAVEN EMERSON
Secretary: DAYTON J. EDWARDS

Council:
GRAHAM LUSK
S. R. DETWILER
THOMAS M. RIVERS
RANDOLPH WEST

1932–1933

President: ALFRED F. HESS
Vice-President: HAVEN EMERSON
Treasurer: THOMAS M. RIVERS
Secretary: EDGAR STILLMAN

Council:
GRAHAM LUSK
HANS T. CLARKE
WALTER W. PALMER
HOMER W. SMITH

1933–1934

President: ALFRED HESS*
Vice-President: ROBERT K. CANNAN
Treasurer: THOMAS M. RIVERS
Secretary: EDGAR STILLMAN

Council:
STANLEY R. BENEDICT
ROBERT F. LOEB
WADE H. BROWN

1934–1935

President: ROBERT K. CANNAN
Vice-President: EUGENE L. OPIE
Treasurer: THOMAS M. RIVERS
Secretary: RANDOLPH H. WEST

Council:
HERBERT S. GASSER
B. S. OPPENHEIMER
PHILIP E. SMITH

1935–1936

President: ROBERT K. CANNAN
Vice-President: EUGENE L. OPIE
Treasurer: THOMAS M. RIVERS
Secretary: RANDOLPH H. WEST

Council:
ROBERT F. LOEB
HOMER W. SMITH
DAVID MARINE

1936–1937

President: EUGENE L. OPIE
Vice-President: PHILIP E. SMITH
Treasurer: THOMAS M. RIVERS
Secretary: MCKEEN CATTELL

Council:
GEORGE B. WALLACE
MARTIN H. DAWSON
JAMES B. MURPHY

1937–1938

President: EUGENE L. OPIE
Vice-President: PHILIP E. SMITH
Treasurer: THOMAS M. RIVERS
Secretary: MCKEEN CATTELL

Council:
GEORGE B. WALLACE
MARTIN H. DAWSON
HERBERT S. GASSER

---

*Dr. Hess died December 5, 1933.

1938–1939

President: PHILIP E. SMITH
Vice-President: HERBERT S. GASSER
Treasurer: KENNETH GOODNER
Secretary: MCKEEN CATTELL

Council:
   HANS T. CLARKE
   JAMES D. HARDY
   WILLIAM S. TILLETT

1939–1940

President: PHILIP E. SMITH
Vice-President: HERBERT S. GASSER
Treasurer: KENNETH GOODNER
Secretary: THOMAS FRANCIS, JR.

Council:
   HANS T. CLARKE
   N. CHANDLER FOOT
   WILLIAM S. TILLETT

1940–1941

President: HERBERT S. GASSER
Vice-President: HOMER W. SMITH
Treasurer: KENNETH GOODNER
Secretary: THOMAS FRANCIS, JR.

Council:
   N. CHANDLER FOOT
   VINCENT DU VIGNEAUD
   MICHAEL HEIDELBERGER

1941–1942

President: HERBERT S. GASSER
Vice-President: HOMER W. SMITH
Treasurer: KENNETH GOODNER
Secretary: JOSEPH C. HINSEY

Council:
   HARRY S. MUSTARD
   HAROLD G. WOLFF
   MICHAEL HEIDELBERGER

1942–1943

President: HANS T. CLARKE
Vice-President: THOMAS M. RIVERS
Treasurer: KENNETH GOODNER
Secretary: JOSEPH C. HINSEY

Council:
   ROBERT F. LOEB
   HAROLD G. WOLFF
   WILLIAM C. VON GLAHN

1943–1944

President: HANS T. CLARKE
Vice-President: THOMAS M. RIVERS
Treasurer: COLIN M. MACLEOD
Secretary: JOSEPH C. HINSEY

Council:
   ROBERT F. LOEB
   WILLIAM C. VON GLAHN
   WADE W. OLIVER

1944–1945

President: ROBERT CHAMBERS
Vice-President: VINCENT DU VIGNEAUD
Treasurer: COLIN M. MACLEOD
Secretary: JOSEPH C. HINSEY

Council:
   WADE W. OLIVER
   MICHAEL HEIDELBERGER
   PHILIP D. MCMASTER

1945–1946

President: ROBERT CHAMBERS
Vice-President: VINCENT DU VIGNEAUD
Treasurer: COLIN M. MACLEOD
Secretary: EDGAR G. MILLER, JR.

Council:
   PHILIP D. MCMASTER
   EARL T. ENGLE
   FRED W. STEWART

1946-1947

President: VINCENT DU VIGNEAUD
Vice-President: WADE W. OLIVER
Treasurer: COLIN M. MACLEOD
Secretary: EDGAR G. MILLER, JR.

Council:
   EARL T. ENGLE
   HAROLD G. WOLFF
   L. EMMETT HOLT, JR.

1947-1948

President: VINCENT DU VIGNEAUD
Vice-President: WADE W. OLIVER
Treasurer: HARRY B. VAN DYKE
Secretary: MACLYN MCCARTY

Council:
   PAUL KLEMPERER
   L. EMMETT HOLT, JR.
   HAROLD G. WOLFF

1948-1949

President: WADE W. OLIVER
Vice-President: ROBERT F. LOEB
Treasurer: HARRY B. VAN DYKE
Secretary: MACLYN MCCARTY

Council:
   PAUL KLEMPERER
   SEVERO OCHOA
   HAROLD L. TEMPLE

1949-1950

President: WADE W. OLIVER
Vice-President: ROBERT F. LOEB
Treasurer: JAMES B. HAMILTON
Secretary: MACLYN MCCARTY

Council:
   WILLIAM S. TILLETT
   SEVERO OCHOA
   HAROLD L. TEMPLE

1950-1951

President: ROBERT F. LOEB
Vice-President: MICHAEL HEIDELBERGER
Treasurer: JAMES B. HAMILTON
Secretary: LUDWIG W. EICHNA

Council:
   WILLIAM S. TILLETT
   A. M. PAPPENHEIMER, JR.
   DAVID P. BARR

1951-1952

President: RENÉ J. DUBOS
Vice-President: MICHAEL HEIDELBERGER
Treasurer: JAMES B. HAMILTON
Secretary: LUDWIG W. EICHNA

Council:
   DAVID P. BARR
   ROBERT F. PITTS
   A. M. PAPPENHEIMER, JR.

1952-1953

President: MICHAEL HEIDELBERGER
Vice-President: SEVERO OCHOA
Treasurer: CHANDLER MCC. BROOKS
Secretary: HENRY D. LAUSON

Council:
   ROBERT F. PITTS
   JEAN OLIVER
   ALEXANDER B. GUTMAN

1953-1954

President: SEVERO OCHOA
Vice-President: DAVID P. BARR
Treasurer: CHANDLER MCC. BROOKS
Secretary: HENRY D. LAUSON

Council:
   JEAN OLIVER
   ALEXANDER B. GUTMAN
   ROLLIN D. HOTCHKISS

1954–1955

President: DAVID P. BARR   *Council:*
Vice-President: COLIN M. MACLEOD   ALEXANDER B. GUTMAN
Treasurer: CHANDLER MCC. BROOKS   ROLLIN D. HOTCHKISS
Secretary: HENRY D. LAUSON   DAVID SHEMIN

1955–1956

President: COLIN M. MACLEOD   *Council:*
Vice-President: FRANK L. HORSFALL, JR.   ROLLIN D. HOTCHKISS
Treasurer: CHANDLER MCC. BROOKS   DAVID SHEMIN
Secretary: RULON W. RAWSON   ROBERT F. WATSON

1956–1957

President: FRANK L. HORSFALL, JR.   *Council:*
Vice-President: WILLIAM S. TILLETT   DAVID SHEMIN
Treasurer: CHANDLER MCC. BROOKS   ROBERT F. WATSON
Secretary: RULON W. RAWSON   ABRAHAM WHITE

1957–1958

President: WILLIAM S. TILLETT   *Council:*
Vice-President: ROLLIN D. HOTCHKISS   ROBERT F. WATSON
Treasurer: CHANDLER MCC. BROOKS   ABRAHAM WHITE
Secretary: H. SHERWOOD LAWRENCE   JOHN V. TAGGART

1958–1959

President: ROLLIN D. HOTCHKISS   *Council:*
Vice-President: ANDRE COURNAND   ABRAHAM WHITE
Treasurer: CHANDLER MCC. BROOKS   JOHN V. TAGGART
Secretary: H. SHERWOOD LAWRENCE   WALSH MCDERMOTT

1959–1960

President: ANDRE COURNAND   *Council:*
Vice-President: ROBERT F. PITTS   JOHN V. TAGGART
Treasurer: EDWARD J. HEHRE   WALSH MCDERMOTT
Secretary: H. SHERWOOD LAWRENCE   ROBERT F. FURCHGOTT

1960–1961

President: ROBERT F. PITTS   *Council:*
Vice-President: DICKINSON W. RICHARDS   WALSH MCDERMOTT
Treasurer: EDWARD J. HEHRE   ROBERT F. FURCHGOTT
Secretary: ALEXANDER G. BEARN   LUDWIG W. EICHNA

1961–1962

President: DICKINSON W. RICHARDS   *Council:*
Vice-President: PAUL WEISS   ROBERT F. FURCHGOTT
Treasurer: I. HERBERT SCHEINBERG   LUDWIG W. EXICHNA
Secretary: ALEXANDER G. BEARN   EFRAIM RACKER

1962–1963

President: PAUL WEISS
Vice-President: ALEXANDER B. GUTMAN
Treasurer: I. HERBERT SCHEINBERG
Secretary: ALEXANDER G. BEARN

Council:
LUDWIG W. EICHNA
EFRAIM RACKER
ROGER L. GREIF

1963–1964

President: ALEXANDER B. GUTMAN
Vice-President: EDWARD L. TATUM
Treasurer: SAUL J. FARBER
Secretary: ALEXANDER G. BEARN

Council:
EFRAIM RACKER
ROGER L. GREIF
IRVING M. LONDON

1964–1965

President: EDWARD TATUM
Vice-President: CHANDLER McC. BROOKS
Treasurer: SAUL J. FARBER
Secretary: RALPH L. ENGLE, JR.

Council:
ROGER L. GREIF
LEWIS THOMAS
IRVING M. LONDON

1965–1966

President: CHANDLER McC. BROOKS
Vice-President: ABRAHAM WHITE
Treasurer: SAUL J. FARBER
Secretary: RALPH L. ENGLE, JR.

Council:
IRVING M. LONDON
LEWIS THOMAS
GEORGE K. HIRST

1966–1967

President: ABRAHAM WHITE
Vice-President: RACHMIEL LEVINE
Treasurer: SAUL J. FARBER
Secretary: RALPH L. ENGLE, JR.

Council:
LEWIS THOMAS
GEORGE K. HIRST
DAVID NACHMANSOHN

1967–1968

President: RACHMIEL LEVINE
Vice-President: SAUL J. FARBER
Treasurer: PAUL A. MARKS
Secretary: RALPH L. ENGLE, JR.

Council:
GEORGE K. HIRST
DAVID NACHMANSOHN
MARTIN SONENBERG

1968–1969

President: SAUL J. FARBER
Vice-President: JOHN V. TAGGART
Treasurer: PAUL A. MARKS
Secretary: ELLIOTT F. OSSERMAN

Council:
DAVID NACHMANSOHN
MARTIN SONENBERG
HOWARD EDER

1969–1970

President: JOHN V. TAGGART
Vice-President: BERNARD L. HORECKER
Treasurer: PAUL A. MARKS
Secretary: ELLIOTT F. OSSERMAN

Council:
MARTIN SONENBERG
HOWARD A. EDER
SAUL J. FARBER

1970–1971

President: BERNARD L. HORECKER
Vice-President: MACLYN McCARTY
Treasurer: EDWARD C. FRANKLIN
Secretary: ELLIOTT F. OSSERMAN

Council:
   HOWARD A. EDER
   SAUL J. FARBER
   SOLOMON A. BERSON

1971–1972

President: MACLYN McCARTY
Vice-President: ALEXANDER BEARN
Treasurer: EDWARD C. FRANKLIN
Secretary: ELLIOTT F. OSSERMAN

Council:
   SAUL J. FARBER
   SOLOMON A. BERSON
   HARRY EAGLE

1972–1973

President: ALEXANDER BEARN
Vice-President: PAUL MARKS
Treasurer: EDWARD C. FRANKLIN
Secretary: JOHN ZABRISKIE

Council:
   HARRY EAGLE
   JERARD HURWITZ

1973–1974

President: PAUL A. MARKS
Vice-President: IGOR TAMM
Treasurer: EDWARD C. FRANKLIN
Secretary: JOHN B. ZABRISKIE

Council:
   HARRY EAGLE
   CHARLOTTE FRIEND
   JERARD HURWITZ

1974–1975

President: IGOR TAMM
Vice-President: GERALD M. EDELMAN
Treasurer: STEPHEN I. MORSE
Secretary: JOHN B. ZABRISKIE

Council:
   JERARD HURWITZ
   H. SHERWOOD LAWRENCE
   CHARLOTTE FRIEND

CUMULATIVE AUTHOR INDEX*

Dr. John J. Abel, 1923–24 (d)
Prof. J. D. Adami, 1906–07 (d)
Dr. Roger Adams, 1941–42 (d)
Dr. Thomas Addis, 1927–28 (d)
Dr. E. D. Adrian, 1931–32 (h)
Dr. Fuller Albright, 1942–43 (h)
Dr. Franz Alexander, 1930–31 (h)
Dr. Frederick Allen, 1916–17 (a)
Dr. John F. Anderson, 1908–09 (d)
Dr. R. J. Anderson, 1939–40 (d)
Dr. Christopher H. Andrews, 1961–62 (h)
Dr. Christian B. Anfinsen, 1965–66 (h)
Prof. G. V. Anrep, 1934–35 (h)
Dr. Charles Armstrong, 1940–41 (d)
Dr. Ludwig Aschoff, 1923–24 (d)
Dr. Leon Asher, 1922–23 (h)
Dr. W. T. Astbury, 1950–51 (h)
Dr. Edwin Astwood, 1944–45 (h)
Dr. Joseph C. Aub, 1928–29 (h)
Dr. Julius Axelrod, 1971–72 (h)
Dr. E. R. Baldwin, 1914–15 (d)
Dr. David Baltimore, 1974–75 (h)
Prof. Joseph Barcroft, 1921–22 (d)
Dr. Philip Bard, 1921–22 (h)
Dr. H. A. Barker, 1949–50 (h)
Prof. Lewellys Barker, 1905–06 (d)
Dr. Julius Bauer, 1932–33 (d)
Prof. William M. Bayliss, 1921–22 (d)
Dr. Frank Beach, 1947–48 (h)
Dr. George W. Beadle, 1944–45 (h)
Dr. Alexander G. Bearn, 1974–75 (a)
Dr. Albert Behnke, 1941–42 (h)
Dr. Baruj Benacerraf, 1971–72 (a)
Prof. F. G. Benedict, 1906–07 (d)
Dr. Stanley Benedict, 1915–16 (d)
Prof. R. R. Bensley, 1914–15 (d)
Dr. Seymour Benzer, 1960–61 (h)
Dr. Paul Berg, 1971–72 (h)
Dr. Max Bergmann, 1935–36 (d)

Dr. Sune Bergström, 1974–75 (h)
Dr. Robert W. Berliner, 1958–59 (h)
Dr. Solomon A. Berson, 1966–67 (a)
Dr. Marcel C. Bessis, 1962–63 (h)
Dr. C. H. Best, 1940–41 (h)
Dr. A. Biedl, 1923–24 (h)
Dr. Rupert E. Billingham, 1966–67 (h)
Dr. Richard J. Bing, 1954–55 (a)
Dr. John J. Bittner, 1946–47 (d)
Prof. Francis G. Blake, 1934–35 (d)
Dr. Alfred Blalock, 1945–46 (d)
Dr. Konrad Bloch, 1952–53 (a)
Dr. Walter R. Bloor, 1923–24 (d)
Dr. David Bodian, 1956–57 (h)
Dr. James Bonner, 1952–53 (h)
Dr. Jules Bordet, 1920–21 (h)
Dr. William T. Bovie, 1922–23 (d)
Dr. Edward A. Boyse, 1971–72, 1975–76 (h)
Dr. Stanley E. Bradley, 1959–60 (a)
Dr. Armin C. Braun, 1960–61 (h)
Dr. Eugene Braunwald, 1975–76 (h)
Prof. F. Bremer, (h)†
Prof. T. G. Brodie, 1909–10 (d)
Dr. Detlev W. Bronk, 1933–34 (d)
Dr. B. Brouwer, 1925–26 (d)
Dr. Wade H. Brown, 1928–29 (d)
Dr. John M. Buchanan, 1959–60 (h)
Dr. John Cairns, 1970–1971 (h)
Prof. A. Calmette, 1908–09 (d)
Dr. Melvin Calvin, 1950–51 (h)
Prof. Walter B. Cannon, 1911–12 (d)
Prof. A. J. Carlson, 1915–16 (d)
Dr. William H. Castle, 1934–35 (h)
Prof. W. E. Castle, 1910–11 (d)
Dr. I. L. Chaikoff, 1951–52 (h)
Dr. Robert Chambers, 1926–27 (d)
Dr. B. Chance, 1953–54 (h)
Dr. Charles V. Chapin, 1913–14 (d)
Dr. Erwin Chargaff, 1956–57 (h)

*(h), honorary; (a), active; (d) deceased.
†Did not present lecture because of World War II.

ACTIVE MEMBERS

Dr. Bent Aasted
Dr. Harold Abramson*
Dr. Ruth Gail Abramson
Dr. Frederic J. Agate
Dr. Edward H. Ahrens
Dr. Philip Aisen
Dr. Salah Al-Askari
Dr. Anthony A. Albanese
Dr. Michael Harris Alderman
Dr. Benjamin Alexander
Dr. Robert Alexander
Dr. Emma Gates Allen
Dr. Fred H. Allen, Jr.
Dr. Jona Allerhand
Dr. Fred Allison, Jr.
Dr. Norman R. Alpert
Dr. Aaron A. Alter
Dr. Norman Altszuler
Dr. Burton M. Altura
Dr. J. Burns Amberson*
Dr. Richard P. Ames
Dr. A. F. Anderson*
Dr. Charles Anderson
Dr. Helen M. Anderson
Dr. Rubert S. Anderson*
Dr. Giuseppe A. Andres
Dr. Muriel M. Andrews
Dr. Alfred Angrist*
Dr. Henry Aranow, Jr.
Dr. Reginald M. Archibald
Dr. Diana C. Argyros
Dr. Irwin M. Arias
Dr. Donald Armstrong
Dr. Philip B. Armstrong*
Dr. Aaron Arnold
Dr. Robert B. Aronson
Dr. Paul W. Aschner*
Dr. Amir Askari
Dr. Muvaffak A. Atamer
Dr. Dana W. Atchley*
Dr. Kimball Chase Atwood

Dr. Joseph T. August
Dr. Peter A. M. Auld
Dr. Felice B. Aull
Dr. Robert Austrian
Dr. Avram Avramides
Dr. D. Robert Axelrod
Dr. Stephen M. Ayres
Dr. L. Fred Ayvazian
Dr. Henry A. Azar
Dr. Radoslav Bachvaroff
Dr. Mortimer E. Bader
Dr. Richard A. Bader
Dr. George Baehr*
Dr. Silvio Baez
Dr. John C. Baiardi
Dr. Robert D. Baird*
Mrs. Katherine J. Baker
Dr. Sulamita Balagura
Dr. David S. Baldwin
Dr. Horace S. Baldwin*
Dr. M. Earl Balis
Dr. S. Banerjee
Dr. Arthur Bank
Dr. Norman Bank
Dr. Alvan L. Barach*
Dr. Michael Barany
Dr. W. H. Barber*
Dr. Marion Barclay
Dr. S. B. Barker*
Dr. Lane Barksdale
Dr. Peter Barland
Dr. W. A. Barnes
Dr. Harry Baron
Dr. Howard Baron
Dr. Jeremiah A. Barondess
Dr. David P. Barr*
Dr. Bruce A. Barron
Dr. Guy T. Barry
Dr. Claudio Basilico
Dr. C. Andrew L. Bassett
Dr. Bruce Batchelor

*Life member.

301

Dr. Jeanne Bateman*
Dr. Jack R. Battisto
Dr. Stephen G. Baum
Dr. Leona Baumgartner*
Dr. Eliot F. Beach*
Dr. Joseph W. Beard*
Dr. Alexander G. Bearn
Dr. Carl Becker
Dr. David Becker
Dr. E. Lovell Becker
Dr. Joseph W. Becker
Dr. William H. Becker
Dr. Paul B. Beeson*
Dr. Jeannette Allen Behre
Dr. Richard E. Behrman
Dr. Julius Belford
Dr. A. L. Loomis Bell
Dr. Bertrand Bell
Dr. Fritz Karl Beller
Dr. Baruj Benacerraf
Dr. Morris Bender*
Dr. Aaron Bendich
Dr. Bernard Benjamin*
Dr. Bry Benjamin
Dr. Ivan L. Bennett
Dr. Thomas P. Bennett
Dr. Harvey L. Benovitz
Dr. Gordon Benson
Dr. Benjamin N. Berg*
Dr. Kare Berg
Dr. Stanley S. Bergen
Dr. Adolph Berger
Dr. Eugene Y. Berger
Dr. Lawrence Berger
Dr. Ingemar Berggard
Dr. Edward H. Bergofsky
Dr. James Berkman
Dr. Alice R. Bernheim*
Dr. Alan W. Bernheimer
Dr. Harriet Bernheimer
Dr. Leslie Bernstein
Dr. Stanley Bernstein
Dr. Carl A. Berntsen

Dr. George Packer Berry*
Dr. John F. Bertles
Dr. Otto A. Bessey*
Dr. Joseph J. Betheil
Dr. Margaret Bevans
Dr. Sherman Beychok
Dr. Rajesh M. Bhatnagar
Dr. Celso Bianco
Dr. Edward Bien
Dr. John T. Bigger, Jr.
Dr. R. J. Bing*
Dr. Carl A. L. Binger*
Dr. Francis Binkley
Dr. Robert M. Bird
Dr. LeClair Bissell
Dr. Mark W. Bitensky
Dr. Maurice M. Black
Dr. William A. Blanc
Dr. Kenneth C. Blanchard*
Dr. David H. Blankenhorn
Dr. Sheldon P. Blau
Dr. Sheldon J. Bleicher
Dr. Richard W. Blide
Dr. Konrad E. Bloch
Dr. Arthur D. Bloom
Dr. Barry Bloom
Dr. Oscar Bodansky*
Dr. Diethelm Boehme
Dr. Bruce I. Bogart
Dr. Alfred J. Bollet
Dr. Richard J. Bonforte
Dr. Roy W. Bonsnes
Dr. Robert M. Bookchin
Dr. A. Bookman*
Dr. Frank Boschenstein
Dr. Max Bovarnick
Dr. John Z. Bowers
Dr. Barbara H. Bowman
Dr. Linn J. Boyd*
Dr. Richard C. Bozian
Dr. Stanley Bradley
Dr. Thomas B. Bradley
Dr. Leon Bradlow

*Life member.

Dr. J. Leonard Brandt
Dr. Jo Anne Brasel
Dr. Goodwin Breinin
Dr. Esther Breslow
Dr. Robin Briehl
Dr. Stanley A. Briller
Dr. Anne E. Briscoe
Dr. Susan Broder
Dr. Felix Bronner
Dr. Chandler McC. Brooks
Dr. Dana C. Brooks
Dr. D. E. S. Brown*
Dr. John Lyman Brown
Dr. Howard C. Bruenn*
Dr. Joseph Brumlik
Dr. J. Marion Bryant
Dr. J. Robert Buchanan
Dr. Nancy M. Buckley
Dr. Joseph A. Buda
Dr. Elmer D. Bueker
Dr. George E. Burch*
Dr. Joseph H. Burchenal
Dr. Richard Burger
Dr. Dean Burk*
Dr. Edward R. Burka
Dr. E. A. Burkhardt*
Dr. John J. Burns
Dr. Earl O. Butcher*
Dr. Vincent P. Butler, Jr.
Dr. Joel N. Buxbaum
Dr. Abbie Knowlton Calder
Dr. Peter T. B. Caldwell
Dr. Lawrence A. Caliguiri
Dr. Berry Campbell
Dr. Robert E. Canfield
Dr. Paul Jude Cannon
Dr. Guilio L. Cantoni
Dr. Charles R. Cantor
Dr. Eric T. Carlson
Dr. Peter Wagner Carmel
Dr. Fred Carpenter
Dr. Malcolm B. Carpenter
Dr. Hugh J. Carroll

Dr. Steven Carson
Dr. Anne C. Carter
Dr. Sidney Carter
Dr. J. Casals-Ariet*
Dr. Albert E. Casey*
Dr. Joan I. Casey
Dr. William D. Cash
Dr. McKeen Cattell*
Dr. William Caveness*
Dr. Peter P. Cervoni
Dr. R. W. Chambers
Dr. Philip C. Chan
Dr. W. Y. Chan
Dr. J. P. Chandler*
Dr. Merrill W. Chase*
Dr. Norman E. Chase
Dr. Herbert Chasis*
Dr. Kirk C. S. Chen
Dr. Theodore Chenkin
Dr. Norman L. Chernik
Dr. Marie T. Chiao
Dr. Shu Chien
Dr. C. Gardner Child
Dr. Francis P. Chinard
Dr. Yong Sung Choi
Dr. Purnell W. Choppin
Dr. Charles L. Christian
Dr. Ronald V. Christie*
Dr. Judith K. Christman
Dr. Nicholas P. Christy
Dr. Jacob Churg
Dr. Louis J. Cizek
Dr. Duncan W. Clark
Dr. Delphine H. Clarke
Dr. Frank H. Clarke
Dr. Albert Claude*
Dr. Hartwig Cleve
Dr. Leighton E. Cluff
Dr. Jaime B. Coelho
Dr. Bernard Cohen
Dr. Michael I. Cohen
Dr. Sidney Q. Cohlan
Dr. Cal K. Cohn

*Life member.

Dr. Mildred Cohn
Dr. Zanvil A. Cohn
Dr. Henry Colcher
Dr. Morton Coleman
Dr. Neville Colman
Dr. Spencer L. Commerford
Dr. Richard M. Compans
Dr. Neal J. Conan, Jr.
Dr. Lawrence A. Cone
Dr. Stephen C. Connolly
Dr. James H. Conover
Dr. Jean L. Cook
Dr. John S. Cook
Dr. Stuart D. Cook
Dr. George Cooper
Dr. Norman S. Cooper
Dr. Jack M. Cooperman
Dr. W. M. Copenhaver*
Dr. George N. Cornell
Dr. James S. Cornell
Dr. George Corner*
Dr. Armand F. Cortese
Dr. Thomas Costantino
Dr. Richard Costello
Dr. Lucien J. Cote
Dr. George Cotzias
Dr. Andre Cournand*
Dr. David Cowen
Dr. Herold R. Cox*
Dr. Rody P. Cox
Dr. George Craft
Dr. Francis N. Craig
Dr. John P. Craig
Dr. B. B. Crohn*
Dr. Richard J. Cross
Dr. Bruce Cunningham
Dr. Dorothy J. Cunningham
Dr. Edward C. Curnen*
Dr. Mary G. McCrea Curnen
Dr. T. J. Curphey*
Dr. Samuel W. Cushman
Dr. Samuel Dales
Dr. Marie Maynard Daly

Dr. Joseph Dancis
Dr. Betty S. Danes
Dr. Farrington Daniels, Jr.
Dr. R. C. Darling
Dr. James E. Darnell, Jr.
Dr. Fred M. Davenport
Dr. Charles M. David
Dr. John David
Dr. Leo M. Davidoff*
Dr. Murray Davidson
Dr. Jean Davignon
Dr. Bernard D. Davis
Dr. Robert P. Davis
Dr. Emerson Day
Dr. Noorbibi K. Day
Dr. Stacey B. Day
Dr. Peter G. Dayton
Dr. Norman Deane
Dr. Robert H. De Bellis
Dr. Vittorio Defendi
Dr. Paul F. de Gara*
Dr. Thomas J. Degnan
Dr. A. C. DeGraff*
Dr. John E. Deitrick*
Dr. C. E. de la Chapelle*
Dr. Nicholas Delhias
Dr. R. J. Dellenback
Dr. Felix E. Demartini
Dr. Quentin B. Deming
Dr. Felix de Narvaez
Dr. Miriam de Salegue
Dr. Ralph A. Deterling, Jr.
Dr. Wolf-Dietrich Dettbarn
Dr. Ingrith J. Deyrup
Dr. Elaine Diacumakos
Dr. Herbert S. Diamond
Dr. Leroy S. Dietrich
Dr. George W. Dietz, Jr.
Dr. Mario Di Girolamo
Dr. Alexander B. Dimich
Dr. Peter Dineen
Dr. J. R. Di Palma
Dr. Nicholas Di Salvo

*Life member.

Dr. P. A. Di Sant'Agnese
Dr. Zacharias Dische
Dr. Charles A. Doan*
Dr. William Dock*
Dr. Alvin M. Donnenfeld
Dr. Philip J. Dorman
Dr. Louis B. Dotti*
Dr. Joseph C. Dougherty
Dr. Gordon W. Douglas
Dr. Steven D. Douglas
Dr. Charles V. Dowling
Dr. Alan W. Downie*
Dr. Cora Downs*
Dr. Arnold Drapkin
Dr. Paul Driezen
Dr. David T. Dresdale
Dr. Lewis M. Drusin
Dr. René J. Dubos*
Dr. Allan Dumont
Dr. John H. Dunnington*
Dr. Vincent Du Vigneaud*
Dr. Murray Dworetzky
Dr. D. Dziewiatkowski
Dr. Harry Eagle
Dr. Lila W. Easley
Dr. Paul Ebert
Dr. Gerald M. Edelman
Dr. Chester M. Edelmann, Jr.
Dr. Howard A. Eder
Dr. Adrian L. E. Edwards
Dr. Richard M. Effros
Dr. Hans J. Eggers
Dr. Kathryn H. Ehlers
Dr. Klaus Eichmann
Dr. Ludwig W. Eichna*
Dr. Max Eisenberg
Dr. Moises Eisenberg
Dr. William J. Eisenmenger
Dr. Robert P. Eisinger
Dr. Borje Ejrup
Dr. Daniel Elbaum
Dr. Stuart D. Elliott
Dr. Robert J. Ellis

Dr. John T. Ellis
Dr. Rose-Ruth Tarr Ellison
Dr. Peter Elsbach
Dr. Samuel K. Elster
Dr. Charles A. Ely
Dr. Kendall Emerson, Jr.*
Dr. Morris Engelman
Dr. Mary Allen Engle
Dr. Ralph L. Engle, Jr.
Dr. Yale Enson
Dr. Leonard Epifano
Dr. Joseph A. Epstein
Dr. Bernard F. Erlanger
Dr. Solomon Estren
Dr. Hugh E. Evans
Dr. John Evans
Dr. Henry E. Evert
Dr. Stanley Fahn
Dr. Gordon F. Fairclough, Jr.
Dr. Saul J. Farber
Dr. Mehdi Farhangi
Dr. Peter B. Farnsworth
Dr. John W. Farquhar
Dr. Lee E. Farr*
Dr. Don W. Fawcett
Dr. Aaron Feder
Dr. Martha E. Fedorko
Dr. Muriel F. Feigelson
Dr. Philip Feigelson
Dr. Maurice Feinstein
Dr. Daniel Feldman
Dr. Colin Fell
Dr. Bernard N. Fields
Dr. Ronald R. Fieve
Dr. Laurence Finberg
Dr. Bruno Fingerhut
Dr. Louis M. Fink
Dr. Stanley R. Finke
Dr. John T. Finkenstaedt
Dr. Edward E. Fischel
Dr. Vincent A. Fischetti
Dr. Arthur Fishberg*
Dr. Saul Fisher

*Life member.

Dr. Alfred P. Fishman
Dr. Patrick J. Fitzgerald
Dr. Martin FitzPatrick
Dr. Charles Flood*
Dr. Alfred Florman
Dr. Jordi Folch-Pi*
Dr. Conrad T. O. Fong
Dr. Vincent Fontana
Dr. Joseph Fortner
Dr. Arthur C. Fox
Dr. Charles L. Fox, Jr.
Dr. Lewis M. Fraad*
Dr. Charles W. Frank
Dr. Harry Meyer Frankel
Dr. Edward C. Franklin
Dr. Richard C. Franson
Dr. Andrew G. Frantz
Dr. Carl E. Frasch
Dr. Blair A. Fraser
Dr. Aaron D. Freedman
Dr. Michael L. Freedman
Dr. Alvin Freiman
Dr. Matthew Jay Freund
Dr. Richard H. Freyberg*
Dr. Henry Clay Frick, II
Dr. Arnold J. Friedhof
Dr. Ralph Friedlander
Dr. Eli A. Friedman
Dr. Charlotte Friend
Dr. George W. Frimpter
Dr. William Frisell
Dr. Harry Fritts
Dr. Joseph S. Fruton*
Dr. Fritz F. Fuchs
Dr. Mildred Fulop
Dr. Robert F. Furchgott*
Dr. J. Furth*
Dr. Palmer H. Futcher*
Dr. Jacques L. Gabrilove
Dr. Morton Galdston
Dr. W. Einar Gall
Dr. Henry Gans
Dr. G. Gail Gardner

Dr. William A. Gardner*
Dr. Martin Gardy
Dr. Lawrence Gartner
Dr. Nancy E. Gary
Dr. Jerald D. Gass
Dr. Mario Gaudino
Dr. Malcolm Gefter
Dr. Walton B. Geiger
Dr. Jack Geller
Dr. Lester M. Geller
Dr. Jeremiah M. Gelles
Dr. Dorothy S. Genghof
Dr. Donald Gerber
Dr. James L. German, III
Dr. Edward L. Gershey
Dr. E. C. Gerst
Dr. Menard Gertler
Dr. Melvin Gertner
Dr. Norman R. Gevirtz
Dr. Nimai Ghosh
Dr. Stanley Giannelli, Jr.
Dr. Lewis I. Gidez
Dr. Gerhard H. Giebisch
Dr. Harriet S. Gilbert
Dr. Helena Gilder
Dr. Alfred Gilman
Dr. Sid Gilman
Dr. Charles Gilvarg
Dr. H. Earl Ginn
Dr. Harold S. Ginsberg
Dr. Isaac F. Gittleman
Dr. Sheldon Glabman
Dr. Philip R. Glade
Dr. Herman Gladstone
Dr. Warren Glaser
Dr. George B. Jerzy Glass
Dr. Ephraim Glassmann
Dr. Vincent V. Glaviano
Dr. Frank Glenn*
Dr. Seymour M. Glick
Dr. Marvin L. Gliedman
Dr. David L. Globus
Dr. Martin J. Glynn, Jr.

*Life member.

Dr. David J. Gocke
Dr. Gabriel C. Godman
Dr. Walther F. Goebel*
Dr. Robert B. Golbey
Dr. Allen M. Gold
Dr. Allan R. Goldberg
Dr. Burton Goldberg
Dr. Henry P. Goldberg
Dr. Anna Goldfeder
Dr. Martin G. Goldner
Dr. Roberta M. Goldring
Dr. William Goldring*
Dr. Edward I. Goldsmith
Dr. Eli D. Goldsmith*
Dr. Jack Goldstein
Dr. Marvin H. Goldstein
Dr. Robert Goldstein
Dr. Julius Golubow
Dr. Peter John Gomatos
Dr. Robert A. Good
Dr. Robert Goodhart*
Dr. DeWitt S. Goodman
Dr. Laurance D. Goodwin
Dr. Norman L. Gootman
Dr. Albert S. Gordon*
Dr. Alvin J. Gordon
Dr. Harry H. Gordon*
Dr. Irving Gordon
Dr. Emil Claus Gotschlich
Dr. Eugene Gottfried
Dr. Dicran Goulian, Jr.
Dr. Arthur W. Grace*
Dr. Irving Graef*
Dr. William R. Grafe
Dr. Samuel Graff*
Dr. Frank A. Graig
Dr. Jose Luis Granda
Dr. Lester Grant
Dr. Arthur I. Grayzel
Dr. Jack Peter Green
Dr. Robert H. Green
Dr. Saul Green
Dr. Lowell M. Greenbaum

Dr. Elias L. Greene
Dr. Lewis J. Greene
Dr. Olga Greengard
Dr. Ezra M. Greenspan
Dr. Isidor Greenwald*
Dr. Robert A. Greenwald
Dr. Mary R. Greenwood
Dr. John R. Gregg
Dr. Gregory Gregariadis
Dr. John D. Gregory
Dr. Roger I. Greif
Dr. Ira Greifer
Dr. Joel Grinker
Dr. Arthur Grishman
Dr. William R. Griswold
Dr. David Grob
Dr. Howard S. Grob
Dr. Arthur P. Grollman
Dr. Milton M. Gross
Dr. Paul Gross*
Dr. Lionel Grossbard
Dr. Carlo E. S. Grossi
Dr. Melvin Grumbach
Dr. Dezider Grunberger
Dr. Harry Grundfest*
Dr. Alan B. Gruskin
Dr. Richard S. Gubner
Dr. Peter Guida
Dr. Guido Guidotti
Dr. Connie M. Guion*
Dr. Stephen J. Gulotta
Dr. Sidney Gutstein
Dr. David V. Habif
Dr. John W. Hadden
Dr. Susan Jane Hadley
Dr. Hanspaul Hagenmaier
Dr. Jack W. C. Hagstrom
Dr. Richard G. Hahn*
Dr. Seymour P. Halbert
Dr. Bernard H. Hall
Dr. David Hamerman
Dr. James B. Hamilton*
Dr. Leonard Hamilton

*Life member.

Dr. Paul B. Hamilton*
Dr. Warner S. Hammond*
Dr. Chester W. Hampel*
Dr. Roger P. Hand
Dr. Eugene S. Handler
Dr. Evelyn E. Handler
Dr. Leonard C. Harber
Dr. James D. Hardy*
Dr. Kendrick Hare*
Dr. Ken Harewood
Dr. Joseph Harkavy*
Dr. Peter Cahners Harpel
Dr. Albert H. Harris*
Dr. Ruth C. Harris
Dr. Benjamin Harrow*
Dr. Una Hart
Dr. Donald H. Harter
Dr. ReJane Harvey
Dr. Rudy Haschemeyer
Dr. George A. Hashim
Dr. Sam A. Hashim
Dr. George M. Hass*
Dr. William K. Hass
Dr. A. Baird Hastings*
Dr. Victor Hatcher
Dr. A. Daniel Hauser
Dr. Teru Hayashi
Dr. Arthur H. Hayes
Dr. Richard M. Hays
Dr. Robert M. Heggie*
Dr. Michael Heidelberger*
Dr. Henry Heinemann
Dr. William Carroll Heird
Dr. Leon Hellman
Dr. Milton Helpern*
Dr. Lawrence Helson
Dr. Walter L. Henley
Dr. Philip H. Henneman
Dr. Victor Herbert
Dr. Robert M. Hearbst*
Dr. Morris Herman*
Dr. Frederic P. Herter
Dr. Robert B. Hiatt

Dr. Margaret Hilgartner
Dr. Charles H. Hill
Dr. Lawrence E. Hinkle, Jr.
Dr. Joseph C. Hinsey*
Dr. Christophe H. W. Hirs
Dr. Jacob Hirsch
Dr. James G. Hirsch
Dr. Jules Hirsch
Dr. Robert L. Hirsch
Dr. Kurt Hirschhorn
Dr. George K. Hirst*
Dr. Paul Hochstein
Dr. Paul F. A. Hoefer*
Dr. Thomas I. Hoen*
Dr. Joseph Hoffman
Dr. Lee Hoffman
Dr. Alan F. Hofmann
Dr. Frederick G. Hofmann
Dr. Duncan A. Holaday
Dr. Raymond F. Holden*
Dr. Charles S. Hollander
Dr. Vincent Hollander
Dr. J. H. Holmes*
Dr. Donald A. Holub
Dr. Robert S. Holzman
Dr. Edward W. Hook
Dr. Bernard L. Horecker
Dr. William H. Horner
Dr. Marshall S. Horwitz
Dr. Verne D. Hospelhorn
Dr. Rollin D. Hotchkiss*
Dr. S. S. Hotta
Dr. Michael Luray Howe
Dr. Howard H. T. Hsu
Dr. Konrad Chang Hsu
Dr. Mon-Tuan Huang
Dr. William N. Hubbard, Jr.
Dr. L. E. Hummel*
Dr. George H. Humphreys*
Dr. Jerard Hurwitz
Dr. Dorris Hutchinson
Dr. Thomas H. Hutteroth
Dr. Michale Iacobellis

*Life member.

Dr. Genevieve S. Incefy
Dr. Harry L. Ioachim
Dr. Henry D. Isenberg
Dr. Raymond S. Jackson
Dr. Richard W. Jackson*
Dr. Jerry C. Jacobs
Dr. Ernst R. Jaffe
Dr. Herbert Jaffe
Dr. S. Jakowska
Dr. George James
Dr. James D. Jamieson
Dr. Aaron Janoff
Dr. Alfonso H. Janoski
Dr. Henry D. Janowitz
Dr. Saul Jarcho*
Dr. Jamshid Javid
Dr. Norman B. Javitt
Dr. Graham H. Jeffries
Dr. Alan J. Johnson
Dr. Dorothy D. Johnson
Dr. Walter D. Johnson, Jr.
Dr. Barbara Johnston
Dr. Kenneth H. Johnston
Dr. Thomas Jones
Dr. Alan S. Josephson
Dr. Austin L. Joyner*
Dr. Elvin A. Kabat*
Dr. Lawrence J. Kagen
Dr. Melvin Kahn
Dr. Thomas Kahn
Dr. Alfred J. Kaltman
Dr. William Kammerer
Dr. Yoshinobu Kanno
Dr. Thomas G. Kantor
Dr. F. F. Kao
Dr. Barry H. Kaplan
Dr. David Kaplan
Dr. Attallah Kappas
Dr. Arthur Karanas
Dr. Arthur Karlin
Dr. Simon Karpatkin
Dr. Maxwell Karshan*
Dr. Arnold M. Katz

Dr. Michael Katz
Dr. Robert Katzman
Dr. George L. Kauer, Jr.
Dr. M. Ralph Kaufmann
Dr. Seymour Kaufmann
Dr. Hans Kaunitz
Dr. Herbert J. Kayden
Dr. Donald Kaye
Dr. D. Gordon I. Kaye
Dr. B. H. Kean
Dr. Aaron Kellner
Dr. Alan J. Kenyon
Dr. Muriel Kerr
Dr. Lee Kesner
Dr. Richard H. Kessler
Dr. Walter R. Kessler
Dr. Gerald T. Keusch
Dr. Andre C. Kibrick*
Dr. John G. Kidd*
Dr. Edwin D. Kilbourne
Dr. Margaret Kilcoyne
Dr. Thomas Killip
Dr. Charles W. Kim
Dr. Giho Kim
Dr. Yoon Berm Kim
Dr. Daniel Kimberg
Dr. Thomas J. Kindt
Dr. Barry G. King*
Dr. Donald West King
Dr. Glenn C. King*
Dr. Mary Elizabeth King
Dr. Lawrence C. Kingsland, Jr.
Dr. David W. Kinne
Dr. John M. Kinney
Dr. R. A. Kinsella*
Dr. Esben Kirk
Dr. D. M. Kirschenbaum
Dr. David Klapper
Dr. Bernard Klein
Dr. Herbert Klein
Dr. David L. Kleinberg
Dr. Abraham M. Kleinman
Dr. A. K. Kleinschmidt

*Life member.

310 ACTIVE MEMBERS

Dr. Percy Klingenstein
Dr. Margarete Knecht
Dr. Jerome L. Knittle
Dr. W. Eugene Knox
Dr. Joseph A. Kochen
Dr. Shaul Kochwa
Dr. Samuel Saburo Koide
Dr. Kiyomi Koizumi
Dr. M. J. Kopac*
Dr. Levy Kopelovich
Dr. Arthur Kornberg
Dr. Peter Kornfeld
Dr. Leonard Korngold
Dr. Irvin M. Korr*
Dr. Nechama S. Kossower
Dr. Charles E. Kossmann*
Dr. Arthur Kowalsky
Dr. O. Dhodanand Kowlessar
Dr. Philip Kozinn
Dr. Irwin H. Krakoff
Dr. Lawrence R. Krakoff
Dr. Alvan Krasna
Dr. Stephen J. Kraus
Dr. Richard M. Krause
Dr. Norman Kretchmer
Dr. Howard P. Krieger
Dr. Isidore Krimsky
Dr. Robert A. Kritzler
Dr. Robert Schild Krooth
Dr. Stephen Krop
Dr. Saul Krugman
Dr. Edward J. Kuchinskas
Dr. Friedrich Kueppers
Dr. I. Newton Kugelmass*
Dr. William J. Kuhns
Dr. Henry G. Kunkel
Dr. Sherman Kupfer
Dr. Herbert S. Kupperman
Dr. Marvin Kuschner
Dr. Henn Kutt
Dr. David M. Kydd
Dr. John S. LaDue
Dr. Chun-Yen Lai

Dr. Michael Lake*
Dr. Michael Lamm
Dr. R. C. Lancefield*
Dr. Robert Landesman
Dr. Frank R. Landsberger
Dr. M. Daniel Lane
Dr. William B. Langan
Dr. Gertrude Lange
Dr. Kurt Lange
Dr. Glen A. Langer
Dr. Louis Langman*
Dr. Philip Lanzkowsky
Dr. John H. Laragh
Dr. Daniel L. Larson
Dr. Etienne Y. Lasfargues
Dr. Sigmund E. Lasker
Dr. Richard P. Lasser
Dr. Leonard Laster
Dr. Raffaelle Lattes
Dr. John Lattimer
Dr. Henry D. Lauson
Dr. George I. Lavin*
Dr. Leroy S. Lavine
Dr. Christine Lawrence
Dr. H. S. Lawrence
Dr. Walter Lawrence, Jr.
Dr. Richard W. Lawton
Dr. Robert W. Leader
Dr. Stanley L. Lee
Dr. Sylvia Lee-Huang
Dr. Robert S. Lees
Dr. Albert M. Lefkovits
Dr. David Lehr
Dr. Gerard M. Lehrer
Miss Grace Leidy
Dr. Edgar Leifer
Dr. Louis Leiter*
Dr. Edwin H. Lennette*
Dr. Roger L. Lerner
Dr. E. Carwile LeRoy
Dr. Stephen H. Leslie
Dr. Gerson J. Lesnick
Dr. Harry Le Veen

*Life member.

Dr. Stanley M. Levenson
Dr. Arthur H. Levere
Dr. Richard D. Levere
Dr. Harold A. Levey
Dr. Robert Levi
Dr. Aaron R. Levin
Dr. Louis Levin*
Dr. Philip Levine*
Dr. Rachmiel Levine
Dr. Robert A. Levine
Dr. Cyrus Levinthal
Dr. Marvin F. Levitt
Dr. Barnet M. Levy
Dr. Harvey M. Levy
Dr. Lester Levy
Dr. Milton Levy*
Dr. Arthur Lewis
Dr. James L. Lewis
Dr. N. D. C. Lewis*
Dr. Marjorie Lewisohn
Dr. Allyn B. Ley
Dr. Koibong Li
Dr. Herbert C. Lichtman
Dr. Charles S. Lieber
Dr. Seymour Lieberman
Dr. Frederick M. Liebman
Dr. Martin R. Liebowitz
Dr. Fannie Liebson
Dr. Philip D. Lief
Dr. Edith M. Lincoln*
Dr. Geoffrey C. Linder*
Dr. Alfred S. C. Ling
Dr. George Lipkin
Dr. Martin Lipkin
Dr. Fritz Lipmann*
Dr. M. B. Lipsett
Dr. Iris F. Litt
Dr. Julius Littman
Dr. Stephen D. Litwin
Dr. George Liu
Dr. Teh-Yung Liu
Dr. Arthur Livermore
Dr. David P. C. Lloyd*

Dr. Joseph LoBue
Dr. Michael D. Lockshin
Dr. John N. Loeb
Dr. Robert F. Loeb*
Dr. Werner R. Loewenstein
Dr. Irving M. London
Dr. Morris London
Dr. L. G. Longsworth*
Dr. R. Lorente de Nó*
Dr. Donald B. Louria
Dr. Barbara W. Low
Dr. Jerome Lowenstein
Dr. Oliver H. Lowry
Dr. Bertram A. Lowy
Dr. Fred V. Lucas
Dr. Jean M. Lucas-Lenard
Dr. E. Hugh Luckey
Dr. A. Leonard Luhby
Dr. Daniel S. Lukas
Dr. Clara J. Lynch*
Dr. Harold Lyons
Dr. George I. Lythcott
Dr. Kenneth McAlpin*
Dr. Marsh McCall
Dr. W. S. McCann*
Dr. Kenneth S. McCarty
Dr. Maclyn McCarty
Dr. Robert McClusky
Dr. David J. McConnell
Dr. James E. McCormack
Dr. W. W. McCrory
Dr. Donovan J. McCune*
Dr. Walsh McDermott
Dr. Fletcher McDowell
Dr. Currier McEwen*
Dr. Paul R. McHhugh
Dr. Rawle McIntosh
Dr. Rustin McIntosh*
Dr. Cosmo G. MacKenzie*
Dr. John Macleod*
Dr. Robert G. McKittrick
Dr. James J. McSharry
Dr. Charles K. McSherry

*Life member.

DR. THOMAS MAACK
DR. NICHOLAS T. MACRIS
DR. MELVILLE G. MAGIDA
DR. T. P. MAGILL*
DR. JACOB V. MAIZEL, JR.
DR. OLE J. W. MALM
DR. BENJAMIN MANDEL
DR. WILLIAM M. MANGER
DR. MART MANNIK
DR. JAMES M. MANNING
DR. WLADYSLAW MANSKI
DR. KARL MARAMOROSCH
DR. CARLOS MARCHENA
DR. AARON J. MARCUS
DR. CYRIL CARLISLE MARCUS
DR. DONALD M. MARCUS
DR. PHILIP I. MARCUS
DR. STEWART L. MARCUS
DR. NORMAN MARINE
DR. MORTON MARKS
DR. PAUL A. MARKS
DR. DOUGLAS A. MARSLAND*
DR. DANIEL S. MARTIN
DR. RICHARD L. MASLAND
DR. BENTO MASCARENHAS
DR. RICHARD C. MASON
DR. ARTHUR M. MASTER*
DR. EDMUND B. MASUROVSKY
DR. ROBERT MATZ
DR. PAUL H. MAURER
DR. EVELYN A. MAUSS
DR. MORTON H. MAXWELL
DR. KLAUS MAYER
DR. AUBRE DE L. MAYNARD
DR. E. W. MAYNERT
DR. RAJARSHI MAZUMDER
DR. ABRAHAM MAZUR
DR. VALENTINO MAZZIA
DR. EDWARD MEILMAN
DR. GILBERT W. MELLIN
DR. ROBERT B. MELLINS
DR. ISMAEL MENA
DR. MILTON MENDLOWITZ

DR. WALTER L. MERSHEIMER
DR. WILLIAM METCALF
DR. KARL MEYER*
DR. LEO M. MEYER*
DR. ALEXANDER J. MICHIE
DR. CATHERINE MICHIE
DR. GARDNER MIDDLEBROOK
DR. G. BURROUGHS MIDER*
DR. PETER O. MILCH
DR. A. T. MILHORAT*
DR. DAVID K. MILLER*
DR. FREDERICK MILLER
DR. JOHN A. P. MILLETT*
DR. C. RICHARD MINICK
DR. GEORGE S. MIRICK*
DR. ORMOND G. MITCHELL
DR. WILLIAM F. MITTY, JR.
DR. WALTER MODELL*
DR. CARL MONDER
DR. WILLIAM L. MONEY
DR. DAN H. MOORE
DR. JOHN A. MOORE
DR. NORMAN S. MOORE*
DR. STANFORD MOORE
DR. ANATOL G. MORRELL
DR. AUGUSTO MORENO
DR. GILDA MORILLO-CUCCI
DR. AKIRO MORISHIMA
DR. ROBERT S. MORISON*
DR. THOMAS QUINLAN MORRIS
DR. KEVIN P. MORRISSEY
DR. ALAN N. MORRISON
DR. JOHN MORRISSON
DR. JANE H. MORSE
DR. STEPHEN I. MORSE
DR. NORMAN MOSCOWITZ
DR. MICHALE W. MOSESSON
DR. MELVIN L. MOSS
DR. HARRY MOST*
DR. ISABEL M. MOUNTAIN*
DR. WALTER E. MOUNTCASTLE
DR. ARDEN W. MOYER
DR. RICHARD W. MOYER

*Life member.

Dr. R. S. Muckenfuss*
Dr. Stuart Mudd*
Dr. G. H. Mudge
Dr. Meredith Mudgett
Dr. John V. Mueller
Dr. Hans J. Müller-Eberhard
Dr. Ursula Müller-Eberhard
Dr. M. G. Mulinos*
Dr. Otto H. Muller*
Dr. Robert S. Munford
Dr. George E. Murphy
Dr. James S. Murphy
Dr. M. Lois Murphy
Dr. Carl Muschenheim*
Dr. W. P. Laird Myers
Dr. Martin S. Nachbar
Dr. Ralph L. Nachman
Dr. David D. Nachmansohn*
Dr. Ronald L. Nagel
Dr. Gabriel G. Nahas
Dr. Tatsuji Namba
Dr. William Nastuk
Dr. Samuel Natelson
Dr. Gerald Nathenson
Dr. M. Nathenson
Dr. Stanley G. Nathenson
Dr. Clayton L. Natta
Dr. Enid A. Neidle
Dr. Norton Nelson
Dr. Harold C. Neu
Dr. Maria M. New
Dr. Walter Newman
Miss Eleanor B. Newton*
Dr. Shih-hsun Ngai
Dr. Warren W. Nichols
Dr. John F. Nicholson
Dr. John L. Nickerson*
Dr. Giorgio L. Nicolis
Dr. Julian Niemetz
Dr. Ross Nigrelli*
Dr. Jerome Nisselbaum
Dr. Charles Noback*
Dr. W. C. Noble*

Dr. M. R. Nocenti
Dr. Hymie L. Nossel
Dr. Richard Novick
Dr. Alex B. Novikoff
Dr. Ruth Nussenzweig
Dr. Victor Nussenzweig
Dr. Irwin Nydick
Dr. William B. Ober
Dr. Manuel Ochoa, Jr.
Dr. Severo Ochoa*
Dr. Herbert F. Oettgen
Dr. Michiko Okamoto
Dr. Arthur J. Okinaka
Dr. William M. O'Leary
Dr. Eng Bee Ong
Dr. Stanley Opler
Dr. Jack H. Oppenheimer
Dr. Peter Orahovats
Dr. Irwin Oreskes
Dr. Marian Orlowski
Dr. Ernest V. Orsi
Dr. Louis G. Ortega
Dr. Eduardo Orti
Dr. Elliott F. Osserman
Dr. Elena I. R. Ottolenghi
Dr. Zoltan Ovary
Dr. M. D. Overholzer*
Dr. Norbert I. A. Overweg
Dr. George H. Paff*
Dr. Irvine H. Page*
Dr. George Palade
Dr. Photini S. Papageorgiou
Dr. Paul S. Papavasiliou
Dr. George D. Pappas
Dr. A. M. Pappenheimer, Jr.
Dr. John R. Pappenheimer
Dr. E. M. Papper
Dr. Jean Papps
Dr. Frank S. Parker
Dr. Raymond C. Parker*
Dr. Gary Aiken Parks
Dr. Robert J. Parsons*
Dr. Pedro Pasik

*Life member.

DR. TAUBA PASIK
DR. MARK W. PASMANTIER
DR. PIERLUIGI PATRIARCA
DR. PHILIP Y. PATTERSON
DR. MARY ANN PAYNE
DR. O. H. PEARSON
DR. EDMUND D. PELLEGRINO
DR. ABRAHAM PENNER
DR. JAMES M. PEREL
DR. GEORGE A. PERERA
DR. ELI PERLMAN
DR. GERTRUDE PERLMANN
DR. JAMES H. PERT
DR. DEMETRIUS PERTSEMLIDIS
DR. MARY PETERMANN*
DR. MALCOLM L. PETERSON
DR. RUDOLPH PETERSON
DR. FREDERICK S. PHILIPS
DR. ROBERT A. PHILIPS*
DR. LENNART PHILIPSON
DR. EMANUEL T. PHILLIPS
DR. MILDRED PHILLIPS
DR. JULIA M. PHILLIPS-QUAGLIATA
DR. E. CONVERSE PIERCE, II
DR. JOHN G. PIERCE
DR. CYNTHIA H. PIERCE-CHASE
DR. LOU ANN PILKINGTON
DR. JOSEPH B. PINCUS
DR. JOHANNA PINDYCK
DR. KERMIT L. PINES
DR. MARGARET PITTMAN*
DR. ROBERT F. PITTS*
DR. CHARLES PLANK
DR. CALVIN F. PLIMPTON
DR. CHARLES M. PLOTZ
DR. FRED PLUM
DR. NORMAN H. PLUMMER*
DR. BEATRIZ G. T. POGO
DRi ALAN PAUL POLAND
DR. WILLIAM POLLACK
DR. MARCEL W. PONS
DR. EDWIN A. POPENOE
DR. J. W. POPPELL

DR. HANS POPPER
DR. KEITH R. PORTER
DR. JEROME G. PORUSH
DR. JEROME B. POSNER
DR. JOSEPH POST
DR. EDWARD L. PRATT
DR. RUDOLF PREISIG
DR. JOHN B. PRICE, JR.
DR. MARSHALL P. PRIMACK
DR. R. B. PRINGLE
DR. PHILIP H. PROSE
DR. JOHN F. PRUDDEN
DR. LAWRENCE PRUTKIN
DR. CHARLES B. PRYLES
DR. MAYNARD E. PULLMAN
DR. DOMINICK P. PURPURA
DR. FRANCO QUAGLIATA
DR. PAUL G. QUIE
DR. JAMES P. QUIGLEY
DR. MICHEL RABINOVITCH
DR. JULIAN RACHELE
DR. EFRAIM RACKER
DR. BERTHA RADAR
DR. C. A. RAGAN, JR.
DR. ILENE RAISFELD
DR. MORRIS L. RAKIETEN*
DR. HENRY T. RANDALL
DR. HELEN M. RANNEY
DR. FELIX T. RAPAPORT
DR. HOWARD G. RAPAPORT
DR. RICHARD H. RAPKIN
DR. FRED RAPP
DR. MAURICE M. RAPPORT
DR. SARAH RATNER*
DR. AARON R. RAUSEN
DR. RULON W. RAWSON
DR. BRONSON S. RAY*
DR. STANLEY E. READ
DR. GEORGE G. READER
DR. WALTER REDISCH
DR. COLVIN MANUEL REDMAN
DR. S. FRANK REDO
DR. GEORGE REED

*Life member.

Dr. George N. Reeke, Jr.
Dr. Gabrielle H. Reem
Dr. Carl Reich
Dr. Edward Reich
Dr. Franz Reichsman
Dr. Marcus M. Reidenberg
Dr. Christine Reilly
Dr. Joseph F. Reilly
Dr. Leopold Reiner
Dr. Donald J. Reis
Dr. Charlotte Ressler
Dr. Paul Reznikoff*
Dr. Goetz W. Richter
Dr. Maurice N. Richter*
Dr. Ronald F. Rieder
Dr. Harold Rifkin
Dr. Richard A. Rifkind
Dr. Robert R. Riggio
Dr. Walter F. Riker, Jr.
Dr. Conrad M. Riley
Dr. Vernon Riley
Dr. David Allen Ringle
Dr. Harris Ripps
Dr. Richard S. Rivlin
Dr. William C. Robbins
Dr. Carleton W. Roberts
Dr. Jay Roberts
Dr. Kathleen E. Roberts
Dr. Richard B. Roberts
Dr. Alan G. Robinson
Dr. William G. Robinson
Dr. Dudley F. Rochester
Dr. Olga M. Rochovansky
Dr. Morris Rockstein
Dr. Muriel Roger
Dr. William M. Rogers*
Dr. Bernard Rogoff
Dr. Ida Pauline Rolf*
Dr. Paul D. Rosahn*
Dr. Marie C. Rosati
Dr. Harry M. Rose*
Dr. Herbert G. Rose
Dr. Theodore Rosebury*

Dr. Gerald Rosen
Dr. John F. Rosen
Dr. Ora Rosen
Dr. Murray D. Rosenberg
Dr. Philip Rosenberg
Dr. Richard E. Rosenfeld
Dr. Isadore Rosenfeld
Dr. Herbert S. Rosenkranz
Dr. Arthur F. Rosenthal
Dr. William S. Rosenthal
Dr. William Rosner
Dr. Herbert Ross
Dr. Pedro Rosso
Dr. Eugene F. Roth
Dr. Alan B. Rothballer
Dr. Sidney Rothbard
Dr. Edmund O. Rothschild
Dr. M. A. Rothschild
Dr. Bruce Rowe
Dr. Lewis P. Rowland
Dr. Paul Royce
Dr. Albert L. Rubin
Dr. Benjamin A. Rubin
Dr. Ronald P. Rubin
Dr. Walter Rubin
Dr. Daniel Rudman
Dr. Maria A. Rudzinska
Dr. Paul Ruegeseggar
Dr. George D. Ruggieri
Dr. Mark G. Rush
Dr. Henry I. Russek
Dr. Urs. S. Rutishauser
Dr. David D. Rutstein*
Dr. David Sabatini
Dr. Ruth Sager
Dr. F. B. St. John*
Dr. Stanley Walter Sajdera
Dr. Lester B. Salans
Dr. Gerald Salen
Dr. Letty G. M. Salentijn
Dr. Lee Salk
Dr. Milton R. J. Salton
Dr. Paul Samuel

*Life member.

Dr. Herbert Samuels
Dr. Stanley Samuels
Dr. John Sandson
Dr. B. J. Sanger*
Dr. Shigeru Sassa
Dr. Jussi J. Saukkonen
Dr. Arthur Sawitsky
Dr. Philip N. Sawyer
Dr. Wilbur H. Sawyer
Dr. Brij Saxena
Dr. Robert G. Schacht
Dr. David Schachter
Dr. Russell W. Schaedler
Dr. Morris Schaeffer
Dr. Fenton Schaffner
Dr. Matthew D. Scharff
Dr. Joseph Schattner
Dr. Frederick G. Schechter
Dr. Andreas S. Scheid
Dr. I. Herbert Scheinberg
Dr. Isaac Schenkein
Dr. Barbara M. Scher
Dr. Lawrence Scherr
Dr. Gerald Schiffman
Dr. Fred J. Schilling
Dr. E. B. Schlesinger
Dr. R. W. Schlesinger
Dr. Jeffrey Schlom
Dr. Donald H. Schmidt
Dr. Willard C. Schmidt
Dr. Howard A. Schneider
Dr. J. B. Schorr
Dr. Paul Schreibman
Dr. Henry A. Schroeder*
Dr. Ernest Schwartz
Dr. Gabriel Schwartz
Dr. Irving L. Schwartz
Dr. James H. Schwartz
Dr. Morton K. Schwartz
Dr. David Schwimmer
Dr. John J. Sciarra
Dr. T. F. McNair Scott*
Dr. William Addison Scott

Dr. John C. Scott-Baker
Dr. John Scudder*
Dr. Beatrice C. Seegal*
Dr. Mildred S. Seelig
Dr. Barry M. Segal
Dr. Sheldon J. Segal
Dr. George Seiden
Dr. Samuel Seifter
Dr. Stephen J. Seligman
Dr. Ewald Selkurt
Dr. Fabio Sereni
Dr. Aura E. Severinghaus*
Dr. Robert E. Shank
Dr. James A. Shannon*
Dr. Harvey C. Shapiro
Dr. Herman S. Shapiro
Dr. L. L. Shapiro*
Dr. Lucille Shapiro
Dr. William R. Shapiro
Dr. Lewis Inman Sharp*
Dr. Aaron Shatkin
Dr. Joyce C. Shaver
Dr. Elliott Shaw
Dr. David Shemin
Dr. Paul Sherlock
Dr. Raymond Lionel Sherman
Dr. Sol Sherry
Dr. Maurice E. Shils
Dr. Bong-Sop Shim
Dr. W. C. Shoemaker
Dr. Charles D. Siegel
Dr. George Siegel
Dr. Morris Siegel*
Dr. Philip Siekevitz
Dr. Ernest B. Sigg
Dr. Selma Silagi
Dr. Robert Silber
Dr. Maximillian Silbermann*
Dr. Lous E. Siltzbach
Dr. Lawrence Silver
Dr. Richard T. Silver
Dr. Morris Silverman
Dr. Philip Silverman

*Life member.

Dr. William A. Silverman
Dr. Emanuel Silverstein
Dr. Martin E. Silverstein
Dr. Samuel C. Silverstein
Dr. Saul Silverstein
Dr. Michael Simberkoff
Dr. Eric J. Simon
Dr. Norman Simon
Dr. Joe L. Simpson
Dr. Melvin V. Simpson
Dr. Inder J. Singh
Dr. Gregory Siskind
Dr. William R. Sistrom
Dr. Anneliese L. Sitarz
Dr. Mark T. Skarstedt
Dr. Vladimir P. Skipski
Dr. Lawrence E. Skogerson
Dr. Robert J. Slater
Dr. Daniel N. Slatkin
Dr. George K. Smelser*
Dr. Frank Rees Smith
Dr. James P. Smith
Dr. M. De Forest Smith*
Dr. Elizabeth M. Smithwick
Dr. I. Snapper*
Dr. Edna Sobel
Dr. Louis Soffer*
Dr. Richard Luber Soffer
Dr. John A. Sogn
Dr. Arthur Sohval
Dr. Leon Sokoloff
Dr. Samuel Solomon
Dr. Alex C. Solowey
Dr. Martin Sonenberg
Dr. Chull Sung Song
Dr. Sun K. Song
Dr. Joseph A. Sonnabend
Dr. Carol F. Soroki
Dr. Hamilton Southworth
Dr. Paul Spear
Dr. Abraham Spector
Dr. Francis Speer*
Dr. Robert Sisson Spiers

Dr. Frank C. Spencer
Dr. Gabriel Spergel
Dr. Sol Spiegelman
Dr. Morton Spivack
Dr. David Sprinson
Dr. Norton Spritz
Dr. Katherine Sprunt
Dr. P. R. Srinivasan
Dr. Neal H. Steigbigel
Dr. Richard M. Stein
Dr. William Stein*
Dr. Philip R. Steinmetz
Dr. Herman Steinberg
Dr. Kurt H. Stenzel
Dr. Kenneth Sterling
Dr. Joseph R. Stern
Dr. Marvin Stern
Dr. Stephen Sternberg
Dr. Irmin Sternlieb
Dr. C. A. Stetson, Jr.
Dr. De Witt Stetten, Jr.
Dr. Fred W. Stewart*
Dr. John M. Stewart
Dr. W. B. Stewart
Dr. Walter A. Stewart*
Dr. C. Chester Stock*
Dr. Walter Stoeckenius
Dr. Herbert Carl Stoerk
Dr. Peter E. Stokes
Dr. Daniel J. Stone
Dr. Fritz Streuli
Dr. William T. Stubenbord
Dr. Jackson H. Stuckey
Dr. Horace W. Stunkard*
Dr. Osias Stutman
Dr. John Y. Sugg*
Dr. Barnet M. Sultzer
Dr. Martin I. Surks
Dr. Marcy Sussman
Dr. Joseph G. Sweeting
Dr. Roy C. Swingle
Dr. Margaret Prince Sykes
Dr. Wlodzimierz Szer

*Life member.

Dr. Milton Tabachnick
Dr. John Taggart
Dr. Igor Tamm
Dr. Donald F. Tapley
Dr. Suresh S. Tate
Dr. Edward Lawrie Tatum
Dr. Robert N. Taub
Dr. Harry Taube
Dr. Jurg Tauber
Dr. Sheldon B. Taubman
Dr. Howard Taylor, Jr.*
Dr. Constantin V. Teodoru
Dr. Robert D. Terry
Dr. Gail A. Theis
Dr. Henry M. Thomas
Dr. Lewis Thomas
Dr. David D. Thompson
Dr. Gerald E. Thomson
Dr. Neils A. Thorn
Dr. David A. Tice
Dr. Edward Tolstoi*
Dr. Helene W. Toolan
Dr. William A. Triebel
Dr. George L. Tritsch
Dr. Walter Troll
Dr. R. C. Truex*
Dr. Orestes Tsolas
Dr. Dan Tucker
Dr. Gerard M. Turino
Dr. Louis B. Turner
Dr. Gray H. Twombly*
Dr. Sidney Udenfriend
Dr. Johnathan W. Uhr
Dr. John E. Ultmann
Dr. Paul N. Unger
Dr. Harry E. Ungerleider*
Dr. Arthur Canfield Upton
Dr. Morton Urivetzky
Dr. Virginia Utermohlen
Dr. Carlo Valenti
Dr. Fred Valentine
Dr. Parker Vanamee
Dr. Ivo Van de Rijn

Dr. William G. Van der Kloot
Dr. Andre Varma
Dr. Mario Vassalle
Dr. Edward F. Vastola
Dr. Elliot S. Vesell
Dr. Carmine T. Vicale
Dr. F. Stephen Vogel
Dr. Henry J. Vogel
Dr. Mögens Volkert
Dr. Irving H. Wagman
Dr. Bernard M. Wagner
Dr. Lila A. Wallis
Dr. Roderich Walter
Dr. John L. Wang
Dr. S. C. Wang
Dr. Lewis W. Wannamaker
Dr. George E. Wantz
Dr. Bettina Warburg*
Dr. Robert C. Warner
Dr. Louis R. Wasserman
Dr. Alice M. Waterhouse*
Dr. Robert F. Watson*
Dr. Samuel Waxman
Dr. Annemarie Weber
Dr. Bruce Webster*
Dr. Jerome P. Webster*
Dr. Rene Wegria
Dr. Richard Weil, III
Dr. Virginia L. Weimar
Dr. Leo Weiner
Dr. Herbert Weinfeld
Dr. I. Bernard Weinstein
Dr. Leonard H. Weinstein
Dr. Stephen W. Weinstein
Dr. Irwin M. Weinstock
Dr. John M. Weir
Dr. Abner I. Weisman
Dr. Gerson Weiss
Dr. Harvey J. Weiss
Dr. Julius H. Weiss
Dr. Paul A. Weiss
Dr. Herbert Weissbach
Dr. Bernard Weissman

*Life member.

Dr. Norman Weissman
Dr. Gerald Weissmann
Dr. Daniel Wellner
Dr. Gerhardt Werner
Dr. Sidney C. Werner*
Dr. Arthur R. Wertheim
Dr. W. Clarke Wescoe
Dr. C. D. West
Prof. Otto Westphal
Dr. Joseph P. Whalen
Dr. Henry O. Wheeler
Dr. Frederick E. Wheelock
Dr. Abraham White
Dr. Abraham G. White
Dr. John C. Whitsell, II
Dr. Edkhart Wiedeman
Dr. Stanley Wiener
Dr. Norman Wikler
Dr. Herbert B. Wilcox, Jr.*
Dr. David L. Williams
Dr. M. Henry Williams
Dr. John Wilson
Dr. Victor J. Wilson
Dr. Sidney J. Winawer
Dr. Erich E. Windhager
Dr. Myron Winick
Dr. Asher Winkelstein
Dr. Robert M. Winters
Dr. Jonathan Wittenberg
Dr. Herbert Wohl
Dr. Abner Wolf*
Dr. George A. Wolf
Dr. Julius Wolf
Dr. Robert L. Wolf

Dr. Stewart G. Wolf, Jr.
Dr. James A. Wolff
Dr. Harvey Wolinsky
Dr. Sandra R. Wolman
Dr. Harrison F. Wood
Dr. Henry N. Wood
Dr. John A. Wood
Dr. John L. Wood*
Dr. James M. Woodruff
Dr. Kenneth R. Woods
Dr. Melvin H. Worth, Jr.
Dr. Walter D. Wosilait
Dr. Irving S. Wright
Dr. Melvin D. Yahr
Dr. Sehchi Yasumura
Dr. Chester L. Yntema*
Dr. Bruce Young
Dr. Fuli Yu
Dr. Tasai-Fan Yu
Dr. John B. Zabriskie
Dr. George A. Zak
Dr. Ralph Zalusky
Dr. Esmail D. Zanjani
Dr. Vratislav Zbuzek
Dr. James E. Ziegler, Jr.
Dr. Harry M. Zimmerman
Dr. Norton Zinder
Dr. Arthur Zitrin
Dr. Burton L. Zohman
Dr. Joseph Zubin*
Dr. Marjorie B. Zucker
Dr. Dorothea Zucker-Franklin
Dr. Benjamin W. Zweifach

*Life member.

DECEASED MEMBERS, FORMERLY ACTIVE AND ASSOCIATE

T. J. Abbott
Isidor Abrahamson
Mark H. Adams
Isaac Adler
David Adelersberg
Andrew J. Akelaitus
F. H. Albee
Harry L. Alexander
Samuel Alexander
F. M. Allen
Alf S. Alving
H. L. Amoss
Dorothy H. Anderson
W. B. Anderton
Wm. Dewitt Andrus
Herman Anfanger
W. Parker Anslow, Jr.
William Antopol
Virginia Apgar
R. T. Atkins
Hugh Auchincloss
John Auer
J. Harold Austin
O. T. Avery
Halsey Bagg
C. V. Bailey
Harold C. Bailey
Pearce Bailey
Eleanor DeF. Baldwin
Clarence G. Bandler
Bolton Bangs
W. Halsey Barker
Herbert J. Bartelstone
F. H. Bartlett
Louis Bauman
W. W. Beattie
Carl Beck
William H. Beckman
Edwin Beer
Sam M. Beiser

Rhoda W. Benham
A. A. Berg
Max Bergmann
Charles M. Berry
Solomon A. Berson
Hermann M. Biggs
Francis G. Blake
N. R. Blatherwick
Hubert Bloch
Sidney Blumenthal
Ernest P. Boas
Aaron Bodansky
Victor Bokisch
Charles F. Bolduan
Richard Walker Bolling
Ralph H. Boots
J. B. Borden
David Bovaird
Samuel Bradbury
Erwin Brand
A. Braslau
S. M. Brickner
Nathan E. Brill
J. J. Bronfenbrenner
Detlev Bronk
Harlow Brooks
F. Tilden Brown
Samuel A. Brown
Wade H. Brown
Maurice Bruger
Joseph D. Bryant
Sue Buckingham
Jacob Buckstein
Leo Buerger
Henry G. Bugbee
Frederick C. Bullock
Jesse H. M. Bullowa
Joseph L. Bunim
Claude A. Burrett
Glenworth R. Butler

George F. Cahill
W. E. Caldwell
Xenophon C. Callas
Wm. F. Campbell
Alexis Carrel
Herbert S. Carter
John R. Carty
L. Casamajor
Russell L. Cecil
William H. Chambers
Harry A. Charipper
John W. Churchman
W. LeGros Clark
Hans T. Clarke
F. Morris Class
A. F. Coca
Martin Cohen
Alfred E. Cohn
L. G. Cole
Rufus Cole
Charles F. Collins
Harvey S. Collins
Robert A. Cooke
Otis M. Cope
A. Curtis Corcoran
James A. Corscaden
Pol N. Coryllos
Frank Co-Tui
Walter P. Covell
E. V. Cowdry
Edwin B. Cragin
Lyman C. Craig
Floyd M. Crandall
G. W. Crary
Glenn E. Cullen
John G. Curtis
Edward Cussler
H. D. Dakin
C. Darlington
William Darrach
Leo W. Davidoff
Martin H. Dawson
Richard C. de Bodo
H. J. Devel, Jr.
Smith O. Dexter, Jr.

Henry D. Diamond
Joseph S. Diamond
L. S. Dietrich
Paul A. Dineen
Konrad Dobriner
Blake F. Donaldson
Edwin J. Doty
Henry Doubilet
W. K. Draper
Alexander Duane
E. F. DuBois
Theodore Dunham
C. B. Dunlap
L. C. Dunn
F. Duran-Reynals
Walter H. Eddy
Wilhelm E. Ehrich
Max Einhorn
Robert Elman
C. A. Elsberg
W. J. Elser
A. Elywyn
Haven Emerson
Earl T. Engle
Albert A. Epstein
Lowell Ashton Erf
Samuel M. Evans
James Ewing
Gioacchino Failla
K. G. Falk
L. W. Famulener
Morris S. Fine
Maurice Fishberg
Simon Flexner
Austin Flint
Rolfe Floyd
Joseph E. Flynn
Ellen B. Foot
N. Chandler Foot
Joseph Fraenkel
Edward Francis
Thomas Francis, Jr.
Robert T. Frank
Virginia K. Frantz
Rowland G. Freeman

Webb Freundenthal
Wolff Freundenthal
E. D. Friedman
Lewis F. Frissell
H. Dawson Furniss
Nicolas F. Gang
C. Z. Garside
Herbert S. Gasser
F. L. Gates
F. P. Gay
Samuel H. Geist
Bertram M. Gesner
H. R. Geyelin
William J. Gies
Herman Gladstone
J. H. Globus
Harry Gold
Ross Golden
S. Goldschmidt
S. S. Goldwater
Kenneth Goodner
Frederick Goodridge
Malcolm Goodridge
N. W. Green
Harry S. N. Greene
Isidor Greenwald
Magnus I. Gregersen
Louise Gregory
Menas S. Gregory
Louis Gross
Emil Gruening
Frederick Gudernatsch
H. V. Guile
Alexander B. Gutman
John H. Hall
John W. Hall
Robert H. Halsey
Franklin M. Hanger
Lawrence W. Hanlon
Meyer M. Harris
R. Stuart Hart
Frank Hartley
Robert A. Hatcher
Hans O. Haterius
H. A. Haubold

Louis Hausman
James A. Hawkins
Selig Hecht
George Heller
Carl M. Herget
W. W. Herrick
George J. Heuer
Howard H. Hines
Charles L. Hoagland
August Hoch
Eugene Hodenpyl
George M. Hogeboom
Arthur L. Holland
Franklin Hollander
A. W. Hollis
Emmett Holt, Jr.
J. G. Hopkins
Henry Horn
Herbert I. Horowitz
Frank Horsfall, Jr.
Hubert S. Howe
Paul S. Howe
Stephen Hudack
John H. Huddleston
F. B. Humphreys
H. M. Imboden
Moses L. Isaacs
Benjamin Jablons
Leopold Jaches
Holmes C. Jackson
Abraham Jacobi
Walter A. Jacobs
George W. Jacoby
A. G. Jacques
Joseph Jailer
Walter B. James
Edward G. Janeway
H. H. Janeway
Frode Jensen
James W. Jobling
Scott Johnson
William C. Johnson
Norman Jolliffe
Don R. Joseph
Louis Julianelle

FREDERICK KAMMERER
DAVID KARNOPSKY
HAIG H. KASABACH
LUDWIG KAST
JACOB KAUFMANN
F. L. KEAYS
EDWARD C. KENDALL
FOSTER KENNEDY
LEO KESSEL
BEN WITT KEY
E. L. KEYES
GEORGE KING
FRANCIS P. KINNICUTT
D. B. KIRBY
JOHN E. KIRK
STUART F. KITCHEN
HERBERT M. KLEIN
I. S. KLEINER
PAUL KLEMPERER
WALTER C. KLOTZ
ARNOLD KNAPP
HERMANN KNAPP
YALE KNEELAND, JR.
SEYMOUR KORKES
ARTHUR F. KRAETZER
BENJAMIN KRAMER
MILTON LURIE KRAMER
CHARLES KRUMWIEDE
L. O. KUNKEL
ANN G. KUTTNER
RAPHAEL KURZROK
WILLIAM S. LADD
ALBERT R. LAMB
ADRIAN V. S. LAMBERT
ALEXANDER LAMBERT
ROBERT A. LAMBERT
S. W. LAMBERT
ERNEST W. LAMPE
CARNEY LANDIS
GUSTAV LANGMANN
H. CLAIRE LAWLER
BURTON J. LEE
EGBERT LeFEVRA
E. S. L'ESPERANCE
P. A. LEVENE

MICHAEL LEVINE
SAM Z. LEVINE
ROBERT L. LEVY
CHARLES H. LEWIS
JACQUES M. LEWIS
EMANUEL LIBMAN
CHARLES C. LIEB
FRANK L. LIGENZOWSKI
ASA L. LINCOLN
WRAY LLOYD
JOHN S. LOCKWOOD
JACQUES LOEB
LEO LOEB
ROBERT O. LOEBEL
LEO LOEWE
ALFONSO A. LOMBARDI
C. N. LONG
PERRIN LONG
WARFIELD T. LONGCOPE
RAY R. LOSEY
ROSE LUBSCHEZ
SIGMUND LUSTGARTEN
JOHN D. LYTTLE
W. G. MacCALLUM
DUNCAN A. MacINNES
GEORGE M. MACKENZIE
THOMAS T. MACKIE
COLIN M. MacLEOD
WARD J. MacNEAL
F. B. MALLORY
A. R. MANDEL
JOHN A. MANDEL
F. S. MANDELBAUM
MORRIS MANGES
GEORGE MANNHEIMER
DAVID MARINE
W. B. MARPLE
KIRBY MARTIN
WALTON MARTIN
HOWARD MASON
JAMES A. L. MATHERS
HUNTER McALPIN
CHARLES McBURNEY
GERTRUDE S. McCANN
W. S. McCANN

W. Ross McCarty
Walter S. McClellan
J. F. McGrath
Earl B. McKinley
Franklin C. McLean
Philip D. McMaster
George McNaughton
Edward S. McSweeny
Frank S. Meara
W. J. Meek
Victor Meltzer
Adolf Meyer
Alfred Meyer
Michael Micailovsky
Henry Milch
Edgar G. Miller
George N. Miller
Samuel Charles Miller
Alfred E. Mirsky
H. C. Moloy
Carl Moore
Robert A. Moore
C. V. Morrill
A. V. Moschcowitz
Eli Moschcowitz
Abraham Moss
John H. Mulholland
John P. Munn
Equinn W. Munnell
Edward Muntwyler
J. R. Murlin
James B. Murphy
Clay Ray Murray
V. C. Myers
James F. Nagle
James Neill
Carl Neuberg
Selian Neuhof
Isaac Neuwirth
Walter L. Niles
Charles V. Noback
Jose F. Nonidez
Van Horne Norrie
Charles Norris
John H. Northrop

Nathaniel Read Norton
Francis W. O'Connor
Charles T. Olcott
Peter K. Olitsky
Eugene L. Opie
B. S. Oppenheimer
Hans Oppenheimer
Kermit E. Osserman
Sadao Otani
John Overman
Ralph S. Overman
Beryl H. Paige
Arthur Palmer
Walter W. Palmer
George W. Papanicolaou
A. M. Pappenheimer
William H. Park
Stewart Paton
John M. Pearce
Louise Pearce
Charles H. Peck
James Pedersen
E. J. Pellini
David Perla
E. Cooper Person
J. P. Peters
Frederick Peterson
Godfrey R. Pisek
Harry Plotz
Milton Plotz
G. R. Pogue
Albert Policard
William M. Polk
Abou D. Pollack
F. L. Pollack
Sigmund Pollitzer
Nathaniel B. Potter
Thomas D. Price
T. M. Prudden
Edward Quintard
Francis M. Rackemann
Geoffrey W. Rake
C. C. Ransom
Bret Ratner
George B. Ray

R. G. Reese
Jules Redish
Birdsey Renshaw
C. P. Rhoads
A. N. Richards
D. W. Richards
Henry B. Richardson
Oscar Riddle
Austen Fox Riggs
John L. Riker
Seymour Rinzler
David Rittenberg
Thomas M. Rivers
Kathleen Roberts
Andrew R. Robinson
Frank H. Robinson
William M. Rogers
W. Stanton Root
Martin Rosenthal
Nathan Rosenthal
M. A. Rothschild
F. J. W. Roughton
Peyton Rous
Wilfred F. Ruggiero
F. J. Ryan
George H. Ryder
Florence R. Sabin
Bernard Sachs
Wm. P. St. Lawrence
Stanley W. Sajdera
William A. Salant
T. W. Salmon
Benjamin Salzer
E. F. Sampson
Harold E. Santee
Wilbur A. Sawyer
Reginald H. Sayre
Herbert W. Schmitz
Rudolph Schoenheimer
Louis C. Schroeder
Herman Von W. Schulte
E. L. Scott
David Seegal
H. Shapiro
Harry H. Shapiro
George Y. Shinowara

Ephraim Shorr
Harold Shorr
William K. Simpson
M. J. Sittenfield
J. E. Smadel
A. Alexander Smith
Carl H. Smith
Homer W. Smith
R. Garfield Snyder
Harry Sobotka
F. P. Solley
H. J. Spencer
J. Bentley Squier, Jr.
W. C. Stadie
Norbert Stadtmüller
Henricus J. Stander
Daniel Stats
J. Murray Steele
Richard Stein
Antonio Stella
J. W. Stephenson
Kurt G. Stern
George D. Stewart
H. A. Stewart
Harold J. Stewart
E. G. Stillman
Ralph G. Stillman
L. A. Stimson
C. R. Stockard
George H. Stueck, Jr.
Arthur M. Sutherland
John E. Sutton
Paul C. Swenson
Homer F. Swift
W. W. Swingle
Sam Switzer
Jerome T. Syverton
L. James Talbot
E. L. Tatum
Sterling P. Taylor, Jr.
Oscar Teague
J. de Castro Teixeira
Edward E. Terrell
John S. Thacher
Allen M. Thomas
Giles W. Thomas

W. HANNA THOMPSON
KARL J. THOMPSON
WILLIAM S. TILLETT
EDGAR W. TODD
WISNER R. TOWNSEND
THEODORE T. TSALTAS
JAMES D. TRASK, JR.
H. F. TRAUT
NORMAN TREVES
FOLKE TUDVAD
JOSEPH C. TURNER
KENNETH B. TURNER
ROBERT A. TURNER
CORNELIUS J. TYSON
EDWARD UHLENHUTH
F. T. VAN BEUREN, JR.
PHILIP VAN INGEN
R. VAN SANTVOORD
DONALD D. VAN SLYKE
H. N. VERMILYE
WOLF VISHNIAC
KARL VOGEL
ALFRED VOGL
WILLIAM C. VON GLAHN
AUGUSTUS WADSWORTH
HEINRICH B. WAELSCH
H. F. WALKER
GEORGE B. WALLACE
WILBUR WARD
JAMES S. WATERMAN
JANET WATSON
HANS WEBER
LESLIE T. WEBSTER

R. W. WEBSTER
WEBB W. WEEKS
RICHARD WEIL
LOUIS WEISFUSE
JULIA T. WELD
SARA WELT
JOHN R. WEST
RANDOLPH WEST
GEORGE W. WHEELER
JOHN M. WHEELER
J. S. WHEELWRIGHT
DANIEL WIDELOCK
CARL J. WIGGERS
HERBERT B. WILCOX
H. B. WILLIAMS
ARMINE T. WILSON
MARGARET B. WILSON
PHILIP D. WILSON
JOSEPH E. WINTERS
DAN H. WITT
HAROLD G. WOLFF
I. OGDEN WOODRUFF
D. WAYNE WOOLLEY
HERMAN WORTIS
S. BERNARD WORTIS
ARTHUR M. WRIGHT
JONATHAN WRIGHT
WALTER H. WRIGHT
JOHN H. WYCKOFF
L. ZECHMEISTER
FREDERICK D. ZEMAN
H. F. L. ZIEGEL
HANS ZINSSER

8
9
0
1
2
3
4
5
6